Creative Problem Solving in Occupational Therapy

Creative Problem Solving in Occupational Therapy

With Stories About Children

Jeanne E. Lewin, MS, OTR/L

Founder and President
The Tramble Co.

OT Continuing Education, an Educational Division of The Tramble Co.
Frankfort, Illinois

Colleen A. Reed, MS, OTR/L

Associate Professor
Occupational Therapy Program
Chicago State University
Chicago, Illinois

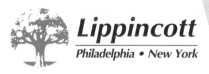

Lippincott
Philadelphia • New York

Acquisitions Editor: Margaret Biblis
Production Editor: Virginia Barishek
Production Manager: Helen Ewan
Production Service: P. M. Gordon Associates, Inc.
Compositor: Circle Graphics
Printer/Binder: Courier/Kendallville
Cover Designer: Deborah Lynam
Cover Printer: Lehigh Press

9 8 7 6 5 4 3 2 1

Library of Congress Cataloging-in-Publication Data
Lewin, Jeanne E.
    Creative problem solving in occupational therapy / Jeanne E.
Lewin, Colleen A. Reed.
        p.   cm.
    Includes bibliographical references and index.
    ISBN 0-397-55233-5 (pbk. : alk. paper)
    1. Occupational therapy.   2. Medical reasoning.   3. Problem
solving.   I. Reed, Colleen A.   II. Title.
RM735.L49   1998
615.8′515—DC21   97-48862
                                                                                                      CIP

Care has been taken to confirm the accuracy of the information presented and to describe generally accepted practices. However, the author, editors, and publisher are not responsible for errors or omissions or for any consequences from application of the information in this book and make no warranty, express or implied, with respect to the contents of the publication.

The authors, editors and publisher have exerted every effort to ensure that drug selection and dosage set forth in this text are in accordance with current recommendations and practice at the time of publication. However, in view of ongoing research, changes in government regulations, and the constant flow of information relating to drug therapy and drug reactions, the reader is urged to check the package insert for each drug for any change in indications and dosage and for added warnings and precautions. This is particularly important when the recommended agent is a new or infrequently employed drug.

Some drugs and medical devices presented in this publication have Food and Drug Administration (FDA) clearance for limited use in restricted research settings. It is the responsibility of the health care provider to ascertain the FDA status of each drug or device planned for use in their clinical practice.

We dedicate this book

to our families:
Fred Lewin
and Stephen, Kristen, and Katie Reed
for their love and support

and

to the creators and researchers of Creative Problem Solving (CPS):
Alex Osborn and Sidney Parnes for their pioneering work in CPS
and Scott Isaksen, Donald Treffinger, and K. Brian Dorval
for their current research and development of the CPS theory

and

to the creative spirit that resides in each of us.

Contents

12
Show and Tell: Test Your Knowledge of CPS   333

UNIT II
Practice Applying CPS to the Occupational Therapy Process   347

13
Practice Using CPS in the Context of Occupational Therapy Services   351

14
Design Your Own Therapy Expedition   443

About This Book

Here are a few **BITS** of background information about how this book is organized.

BIT #1: You Are About to Embark on a Very Special Journey

For instructional purposes, we have given this book a travel metaphor. The word *journey* suggests travel from one place to another. In this book you will travel from one section to another as you learn how to solve problems creatively within the occupational therapy process. Because you will be traveling, you will need an itinerary.

An itinerary is a travel plan that details where you will go and what you will do when you get there. Your itinerary is listed on a clipboard at the beginning of each section. There are 14 sections in the book. Sections 1–12 make up Unit I, and Sections 13 and 14 make up Unit II.

To help you begin a lifelong process of collaboration with clients, colleagues, and other allied health and medical professionals, many of the activities in this book suggest that you work in pairs or small groups. And some activities request that you share your thinking with your colleagues, who are your traveling companions. Sharing ideas with others is an important part of the problem solving process in therapy.

BIT #2: For Your Journey, You Will Need a Field Book

This text is a therapy field book. The term *field book* suggests a book meant to be used as a guide "in the field." This field book was written with the intent that you will consult it whenever you do not have a ready-made answer to a therapy-related problem or whenever you are faced with a dilemma that is beyond the scope of your textbooks or other publications. This field book's purpose is to give direction to your thinking as you travel through the therapy process and to help you learn to tap your creative abilities. Because it is often easier learning a new concept if the concept is first anchored to a familiar example, we use daily-life occurrences that may be unrelated to therapy when we introduce a new idea related to problem solving.

Throughout this field book you will read stories from the field of occupational therapy. Some are scenarios based on real cases and some are previously published articles. Each story was selected to illustrate some element of creative problem solving. You will use the stories as a point of departure for learning ways to enhance your own problem solving skills.

In Unit I, you will learn, step-by-step, how to use Creative Problem Solving (CPS). In Unit II you will apply the process with your own creative energies and imagination as your guide.

BIT #3: This Field Book Is Written to Be Reader Friendly

1. **References**. We put all reference notes at the end of each section rather than using in-text citations. The superscript numbers within the text relate to the notes, which list the references on which we base our assertions and sometimes include additional com-

ments. The Bibliography lists the references cited in the book as well as additional publications related to the subject of CPS.

2. **Pronoun usage.** We randomly use the pronouns *he* and *she* and *his* and *her* when referring to hypothetical individuals, such as therapy clients who are not specifically named.

3. **Client.** You will see references to "the client" throughout this field book. The dictionary defines client as one who engages the services of a professional. This book is illustrated with stories about children. And because every child has some close attachment to family, caregivers, and other significant individuals, we value everyone who contributes in some way to the child's well-being as an important participant in the therapy process. Thus there are three definitions for "the client," that depend on the usage context. The client may be (1) the child or (2) the child's family, caregivers, and significant others or (3) both the child and the family, caregivers, and significant others. Everyone who has some level of responsibility toward making the child's "dreams" ("dreams" are translated "therapy-related goals") become reality is part of the therapy process. We define the therapist-client relationship in all therapy-related interactions as the "therapeutic process."

BIT #4: To Develop Problem Solving Skills, You Will Need to Participate Actively with the Content

Learning is an active process. For real learning to occur, you must be engaged in experiences that connect your present knowledge to new information that you will need for future problem solving.[1] The goal of any learning exercise is to take in knowledge for the purpose of applying it later. In order for that transfer of knowledge to occur from one situation to another, certain strategies must be in place to help you analyze and "mindfully"[2] connect new information to the knowledge you bring to the situation. For this field book on problem solving, we have developed a system that supports learning for transfer.

To make the most of this field book and to ease the transfer of the information presented here to situations beyond this book, we encourage you to write in the book. Completing every activity in this field book is the best way to learn the problem solving process described here. We invite you to fill in the Reflective Journal entries and draw the Mind Maps that occur in every section, participate in the cooperative group experiences, and complete the Field Organizers and the stories, crossword puzzles, and word searches.

BIT #5: To Complete the Activities That Occur During the Journey, You Will Need to Pack a Supply Bag

You will need the following supplies:

◆ Orange, self-adhering dots, 1/4″
◆ Crayola™ crayons, 16-count box (Remember the anticipation you felt as a child when you were about to dive into a new box of crayons. We encourage you to use crayons to recapture that experience for drawing activities in this field book.)
◆ Three highlighter pens—yellow, blue, and green

Keep these supplies handy because you will be using them throughout your travels.

BIT #6: You Will Be Making Reflective Journal Entries to Record Personal Reflections on the Content as It Is Presented

Each Reflective Journal entry gives you an opportunity to record your thoughts about the territory through which you are traveling. The Reflective Journal entries have a statement and lead-in prompt.

The journal has three purposes. First, your journal entries will help to link your own experiences with the text material. Journaling is a way to identify patterns in your thoughts and feelings. We anticipate that through journaling you will recognize that your thinking strategies already include the ability to solve problems creatively.

Second, your journal entries will help you identify characteristics of your thoughts and perceptions at various points along your journey. Journaling provides you with an opportunity to listen to your judgment, the inner voice that is forever sizing up situations as they occur.

Third, and most important, your journal entries will allow you to examine your values and beliefs and how they influence the decisions that you make. Your decisions also reflect your personal thoughts and feelings. Through journaling you can examine the impact of your thoughts and feelings and your values and beliefs on the decision-making process. You can gain a lot by committing your reflections to paper and reviewing them later. We encourage you, throughout the journaling process, to share your reflections with your traveling companions in order to broaden your point of view.

BIT #7: You Will Learn to Use Thinking Keys to Unlock Your Thoughts

On your journey you will be introduced to thinking strategies, referred to as Thinking Keys.[3] A key is something that provides a means of access. Thinking Keys are mental strategies that open doors. Using each Thinking Key will allow you to examine a facet of creative problem solving and increase your understanding of how therapists solve therapy-related problems.

You will have many opportunities to practice using the Thinking Keys throughout this field book. As you practice using the Thinking Keys you may think that we are asking you to process your thoughts in slow motion, as though you were watching an 8-mm movie one frame at a time. We describe this process as freeze-frame thinking. Freeze-frame thinking will help you look at different aspects of a problem from a variety of viewpoints. The result is that you will develop a thorough understanding of your thinking processes that lead to solving complex problems. As you develop skill using the Thinking Keys your speed will increase.

Through practice using the Thinking Keys, you will develop skill in solving problems creatively. Each time you are introduced to a Thinking Key, you will see a key icon, like the one to the left. For later reference, all of the Thinking Keys introduced in this book are listed in Section 14. Each Thinking Key has a corresponding form for recording your ideas. The forms are called Field Organizers. Each Field Organizer is designed to help you develop a particular thinking strategy. For this reason, there is a key at the top of each organizer to remind you that as you use the form, you are using a key to open doors to your thinking. In Appendix B ("B" for "blank") you will find blank masters of all Field Organizers to photocopy as needed for on-the-job use or "field work."

BIT #8: You Will Be Creating Mind Maps

A Mind Map is a pictorial representation, a "map," of your thoughts. Mind mapping is a method of recording your ideas on paper as you generate them.[4] Through practice constructing Mind Maps, you will learn, as you conceptualize your thoughts, to respect the output from both sides of your brain. Unlike the linear outline format that is typically introduced in the primary grades, mind mapping promotes an unrestricted flow of ideas and provides a format for connecting your ideas into a network that is referred to as a map. The map is a free-form, live, dynamic vehicle by which to capture your ideas as they occur and commit them to paper.[5]

A Mind Map can include symbols along with words to express ideas. Write and draw with colored pens, markers, crayons, or pencils to add dimension to the ideas expressed in the map. Mind mapping is important to solving problems creatively because generating a Mind Map involves whole-brain thinking. Whole-brain thinking is an innate, not a learned, capacity.[6] When the brain conceptualizes a problem in an attempt to solve it, the brain goes through three steps. First, the right hemisphere identifies the "gestalt" or the big picture, which is the context. Next, once the context has been identified, the left hemisphere begins to review the details, or the content, filtering out what is needed in an attempt to identify possible solutions. Finally, the forebrain assimilates the information from both hemispheres and, with additional information from the senses and intuition, evaluates the data and makes a decision, which is the conclusion. There is strong evidence that all creative thinking involves these three steps: establishing context, content, and conclusion.[7]

Mind mapping is a note-taking strategy that allows you to generate thoughts all in one place and at the same time about the client, the situation in which the client's problem occurs, the diagnosis, and the occupational therapy process. You can then make associations between many different thoughts by connecting spokes to each thought that is committed to paper.

The saying "A picture is worth a thousand words" definitely applies to mind mapping. Images encourage creative thoughts and reinforce memory. Don't be bothered by such thoughts as "I can't draw" or "This isn't right." Take the advice of Jon Pearson, business consultant and graphic artist, who says that "when we try to do a picture all 'right' we are super-aware of WRONG. When we try to do it all 'wrong' we may be super-aware of PERMISSION and POSSIBILITY . . . . Trying to do things 'right' we sometimes stop seeing. Making things 'wrong' we see what we're not seeing."[8] Use symbols, words with embellished letters, and stick figures or just squiggles with body parts. If your Mind Map graphically expresses your thoughts and feelings, it has achieved its goal and it is "right."

Look at Figure I.1. It is a Mind Map of the information you have covered so far in this section.

The Mind Map begins with a journey at the center. The branch to the right connects the itineraries and the supplies needed for the trip to the field book that describes the journey. The branch below the journey associates Thinking Keys and Field Organizers to the thinking strategies you will learn as you proceed on the journey. To the left of the journey

Figure I.1. *Example of a Mind Map of the 9 Bits*

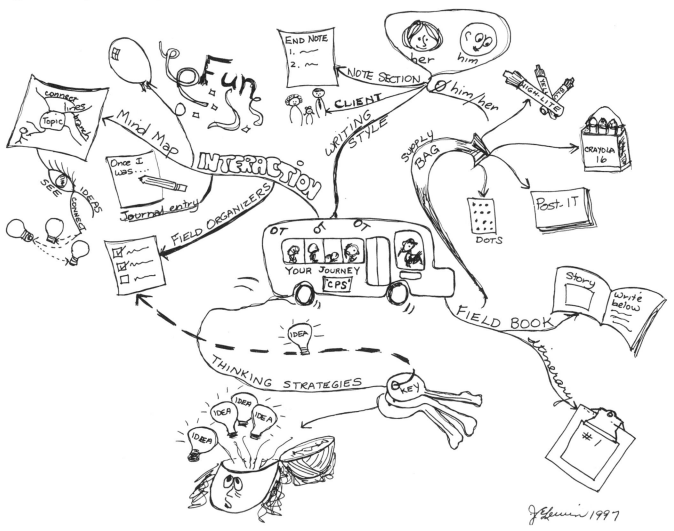

are branches for four kinds of interaction you can have with the content of the field book (completing Mind Maps and Field Organizers, journaling, and having fun). And the branch above depicts the writing style used in this field book.

Guidelines for Developing a Mind Map to Expand Your Ideas About a Problem

1. Clearly define the main problem—preferably in a colored graphic representation rather than in words—in the center of unlined paper.
2. Use images throughout the Mind Map. When using words, print them and put no more than one or two words on a line.
3. Show ideas radiating out from the central thought.
4. Begin to link the main concepts as you generate more details.
5. The more linkages that you generate between elements, the greater your ability to see how all of the elements are related.

Mind mapping is an open-ended process that allows you to add new information as it becomes available to you. Toward the end of every section in Unit I of this field book, you will be asked to create a Mind Map of the material you just read. Creating the Mind Maps will help you develop mind-mapping skills, and the Mind Maps will become study guides when you need to review the material.

In Unit II, you will create Mind Maps of each story. You will use the Mind Maps to organize your ideas about which elements of the story will be the focus of the problem-solving process.

BIT #9: You Will Be Doing Self-Assessments Along the Way

At the end of every section, just before the section reference notes, you will be asked to evaluate what you have just learned. The Self-Assessment is based on the itinerary items. You will use your colored dots (see Bit #4) in each Self-Assessment to identify the concepts you understand well and those that you need to review.

NOTES

1. R. N. Caine and G. Caine, *Making Connections: Teaching and the Human Brain* (New York: Addison-Wesley, 1994); L. B. Resnick, *Education and Learning to Think* (Washington, D.C.: National Academy Press, 1987).
2. E. Langer, *Mindfulness* (New York: Addison-Wesley, 1989).
3. The inventory of Thinking Keys included in this field book is not an all-inclusive list of Thinking Keys. Two excellent references on expanding your Thinking Key collection are M. Michalko, *Thinkertoys* (Berkeley, Calif.: Ten Speed Press, 1991), and R. Fobes, *The Creative Problem Solver's Toolbox* (Corvallis, Oreg.: Solutions through Innovation, 1993).
4. MindMap is a registered trademark of the Buzan organization. See T. Buzan, *Use Both Sides of Your Brain*, 3d ed. (New York: Penguin Books, 1989). For information about the mind-mapping seminars, contact the Buzan Center, 415 Federal Highway, Lake Park, FL 33403; telephone: 1-800-Y-MINDMAP. The Buzan Center offers a full range of books, courses, and videos on mind mapping. Other resources on mapping that demonstrate the process of generating cohesive thoughts through whole-brain processing are J. Wycoff, *Mindmapping* (New York: The Berkley Publishing Group, 1991); Nancy Margulies, *Mapping Inner Space* (Tucson, Ariz.: Zephyr Press, 1991); and G. Rico, *Writing the Natural Way* (Los Angeles: Jeremy P. Tracher, 1983).
5. Inspiration Software, Inc., PO Box 1629, Portland, OR 97207, provides an easy and fast mind-mapping tool on the computer. Nancy Margulies, author of *Mapping Inner Space*, presents mind mapping in an 90-minute video available from Zephyr Press, Tucson, Ariz.
6. J. Edward Clark, "The Search for a New Educational Paradigm," in A. Costa, J. Bellanca, and R. Fogarty, eds., *If Minds Matter: A Foreword to the Future* (Palatine, Ill.: Skylight, 1992), 1:25–40.
7. David Loye, *The Sphinx and the Rainbow* (Boulder, Colo.: Shambhala, 1983).
8. Jon Pearson, *Drawing on the Inventive Mind: Exercises in Thinking, Language, and Self-Esteem* (Los Angeles: Jon Pearson, 1992). Available from Jon Pearson, PO Box 25367, Los Angeles, CA 90025.

Acknowledgments

To begin our acknowledgments, we are grateful to Andrew Allen, the former Executive Editor of Allied Health Publications at Lippincott–Raven for supporting our idea of an interactive field book on thinking. Owing to Andrew's perceptive nature he understood the importance at this time of a publication that teaches creative and critical thinking skills. Margaret Biblis, who assumed the duties in 1997 of Executive Editor of Allied Health Nursing and Allied Health Publishing at Lippincott–Raven, shared Andrew's forward style of thinking and was also very receptive to the concept of our book and continued to offer full support to the project, for which we are very grateful. To Virginia Barishek, Production Editor at Lippincott–Raven, we extend heartfelt thanks for diligently working to see that this publication came together as we intended. We also wish to offer special thanks to our skillful copy editor, Debby Stuart, who was instrumental in shaping the original manuscript into a clear and cohesive textbook. We will forever be grateful for Debby's patience, enthusiasm, and good humor as she orchestrated the many hours of copyediting.

With deep gratitude we wish to acknowledge the organizers of the Creative Problem Solving Institute (CPSI), an internationally attended symposium that has been held annually in Buffalo, New York, since 1954. CPSI participants are educators, writers, business consultants, and product designers who have dedicated their lives to fostering an understanding of creative and critical thinking. In the summer of 1995 we "discovered" Creative Problem Solving and met many people who have contributed to the theory of creativity as it stands today. We wish to thank those at CPSI who helped us: Sidney Parnes, who directed us toward a rich literature on CPS, which we drew from to build the foundation for this field book; Brian Dorval, who introduced us to the importance of blending creative with critical thinking; Rolf Smith and Michael Donahue, whose discussion of their success with Thinking Expeditions inspired the therapy expedition metaphor used in this field book; Anthony LeStorti, who taught us about the concept of "mindtraps," which we adapted to situations in a therapy context; and Roger Firestein, who demonstrated the powerful link between creativity and positive thought (and led us to our visit with David Meier, at the Center for Accelerated Learning, who taught us the principles of accelerated learning). We also thank Alan Black for his vision and his willingness to share and Jon Pearson for being a model for thinking "out-of-the-box."

Before attending CPSI, we spent 18 months looking for what we found there: a thinking model that is a powerful system and flexible enough to apply across all contexts, yet simple to teach to others who wish to creatively expand their options while engaged in solving complex problems. In our training session at CPSI, we realized that the steps in Creative Problem Solving (CPS) are amazingly similar to those used by occupational therapists to solve therapy-related problems, and so CPS became the model by which we would teach problem-solving strategies within the occupational therapy process. For the insights gained during our CPSI training we extend many thanks to all the facilitators and group members.

K. Brian Dorval from the Creative Problem Solving Group and Donald J. Treffinger from the Center for Creative Learning, Inc., are creativity scholars and theorists to whom we owe an immense thanks. They kindly reviewed our manuscript and offered valuable feedback to our explanations of Creative Problem Solving. In addition, their book, *Creative Approaches to Problem Solving* (written along with Scott Isaksen), was a primary source for our organizational structure of CPS.

Writing a textbook is a dual challenge. The first task is to present the content clearly; the second is to present it in an engaging mode. And for helping us meet the latter challenge, we wish to acknowledge Geoffrey Caine, Renate Nummela Caine, and Sue Jones. We want to thank Geoffrey Caine and Renate Nummela Caine for their research and publications (*Making Connections* and *Mindshifts*) about brain-based learning. Their work was a driving force for us as we created the various activities in this field book. "How might Caine and Caine teach that concept?" we asked ourselves regularly. We are grateful to Sue Jones, educational consultant, who prompted us to re-examine certain activities in the book to keep the learning experiences consistent with the principles of brain-based learning.

To Peter Segne, business consultant, researcher, educator, and author, we owe many thanks. We were inspired to frame this textbook as a field book after studying *The Fifth Discipline Fieldbook: Strategies and Tools for Building a Learning Organization*.

We owe a debt of gratitude to Mihalyi Csikszentmihalyi, researcher, writer, and educator, for his ability to articulate so exquisitely the concept of the "just right challenge"— which he refers to as Flow. Like the work of Caine and Caine, Csikszentmihalyi's work kept us ever mindful of creating learning experiences that offered the just right challenge. Section 11 contains an application of the components of Flow within a therapy context.

To Helen L. Hopkins and Elizabeth Tiffany-Mather we offer many thanks for insights about occupational therapy as a problem-solving process, which they describe in *Willard and Spackman's Occupational Therapy*. From conversations with these two authors, as well as with Helen D. Smith and Elinor Anne Spencer, we deepened our understanding of the early traditions of occupational therapy, which relied heavily on creativity and imagination to solve problems faced in practice. We were privileged to have Helen Hopkins, Elinor Spencer, and Elizabeth Tiffany-Mather review the book and provide us with helpful editorial comments. For editorial comments made on selected portions of the book, we wish to thank Abby Brown, Debra Fountain-Ellis, Leslie Roundtree, and Jim Searle.

To E. Louise Betteridge, the author of the story around which we teach CPS, we offer thanks for sharing her personal vision of creative problem solving in such an interesting and engaging manner. Thanks also to Victor Espinoza and Diana Bal for discussing their creative problem-solving experiences in occupational therapy. We have included their stories in Section 14. Thanks to Bruce E. Tapper, author of Victor Spinoza's story, "Putting Cosmetic Prostheses to Work," for having the insight to draw out Victor's unique capacity for problem solving. We thank Sam and his parents, Anne and Barry Miller, for allowing us to use his story in Section 13. In one sense, this project is dedicated to all of the children and their families we have worked with over the years who present with one complex problem after another.

Special thanks are due to Terry Street, an exceptional artist and special friend who created the scenes in Section 4. Terry's drawings make learning Uniform Technology fun. She developed what educators Caine and Caine refer to as "felt" meaning for each of the terms before she generated their visual representations.

Thanks also go out to the many occupational therapy students from Chicago State University who demonstrated time and time again the power of CPS to tap the wellspring of a person's imagination. Thanks also to the many faculty at Chicago State University and William H. Ray, Phillip Murray, and Charles S. Brownell Elementary Schools, whose comments in faculty development workshops during the course of this project advanced our understanding of issues surrounding the role of creativity in learning and teaching thinking to students.

Writing a book in this high-tech electronic age goes beyond having a dictionary, sharpened pencils, and a good eraser. Section 4 is full of fun and interactive activities because of the tech support of several people. For this reason, we owe thanks to Marc Albert, at Visions Technology in Education, who graciously guided us through the crossword and word search software and regularly sent software upgrades. Also, the tech staff at Inspiration Software, Inc., patiently answered our many questions about the formation of the concept maps of the uniform terminology sections.

With a deep sense of gratitude and heartfelt thanks we recognize the special people in our personal lives whose abundance of love and support throughout this four-and-a-half-year project made this publication possible.

Jeanne thanks her husband, Fred Lewin, for being a constant source of inspiration and warm hugs during the many challenges that were ever present through this project. He was always there to listen and provide editorial advice, especially when a new word or advice on clarity of thought was needed.

Colleen offers much love to Katherine and Kristen, her high-maintenance angels, for sharing a significant portion of their childhood with this book and for avoiding the temptation to blow up the computer when the book seemed to take over their lives. She offers admiration and much love to Stephen Reed, her husband, for being a "master of many trades," and love to her mother and father, Frances and Theodore, for teaching her to love and be open minded, and to her sister, Mary, and her brother, Tony, for dedicating their lives to the pursuit of creativity. And to God to whom she owes all her blessings.

Learning About CPS

*O*nce upon a time, occupational therapists provided their services in hospitals and community outpatient clinics, most of which were part of a medical model. Life was different in those early days of practice. Therapy customers were called patients. Now the term *patient* is fading, except in hospital settings. And the people many occupational therapists work with are called clients or students, depending on the setting in which therapy services are delivered. With the introduction of managed care systems and the growth in the number of therapists serving children in school systems and in the community, the challenges related to the delivery of services have greatly increased. With those increased challenges has come an urgent need to solve problems creatively.

Fundamental to solving problems creatively in therapy is the ability of a therapist to learn a client's life story. A life story is a complex network of scenarios, involving many different people, each holding a unique set of values and perspectives. The effective practitioner considers the composite of a client's life story and recognizes where he or she interfaces with the client's story. Skillful therapists evaluate the context of the client's situation, gather data, generate ideas, and ultimately create and implement a treatment plan in much the same way as a sculptor creates a masterpiece.

So how does a student gain the skills of the skillful therapist? And how does the experienced therapist who switches from working in one area of practice to another "hit the road running" in the new area of practice? One strategy for students and experienced therapists alike is to learn thinking strategies that provide a structure for examining the context of any challenging situation. Hence, the need for a *field book about thinking*.

This is a book about *how* to think about ill-structured problems (problems for which there are no "ready-made" solutions) and arrive at a "better" solution within the context of the challenging situation. Because there are few situations in therapy where there is the "best" solution, we strive to select the "better" one from among the choices available at the time of our decision.

In Unit I, you will be introduced to a mental model for examining many choices in order to determine the "better" solution. The model is called Creative Problem Solving, or simply CPS. You will be guided step by step through the use of Thinking Keys and their respective Field Organizers, designed to expand your thinking about challenges that have more than one "correct" answer.

As occupational therapists and educators, we recognize that for our brain to enjoy learning new information, we must interact and "play" with the information. We also recognize that basing learning on memorization does little to facilitate the transfer of that learning to real-life situations. But that transfer can occur easily when the learner can anchor new learning to his or her own life experiences. Thus, out of a desire to create an interactive learning environment that is fun and meaningful for you, we have incorporated learning strategies into the design of Unit I. These include Reflective Journal entries, Thinking Keys and Field Organizers, Mind Mapping, crossword puzzles and word searches, and metaphors (such as the overall metaphor of going on a journey) and everyday examples.

U N I T

I

Each section of your journey through this field book begins with an itinerary of the "stops" you will make in that section. Your journey begins in Section 1 with a brief discussion about clinical reasoning, then moves into the realm of creativity and imagination. In this section you will learn about the important role of creativity in today's health care environment wrought with constant change.

Section 2 presents the history and basic components of CPS. Section 3 returns you to the realm of occupational therapy to show how the process of therapy is like an expedition and to present an overview of the mindset of a therapy guide. In Section 3, you will be introduced to the first set of Thinking Keys and Field Organizers.

In Section 4, you will make another important stop to learn about the paradigm of occupational therapy through the system of Uniform Terminology. The crossword puzzles, word searches, and creative writing activities will allow you to literally play with the vocabulary as you learn it.

The next major stop on your journey will last from Section 5 through Section 11, where you will learn about CPS through Louise and her "Nose-Blowing Expedition." Louise is an occupational therapist who taught a group of children in an early childhood education program how to blow their noses. Because we feel that Louise was an extremely creative problem solver, her story forms the foundation on which we teach CPS. Her story appears in Section 5. In Sections 6–11, you will learn how to think "off of the page" as you generate novel, creative solutions to the nose-blowing problem, much like those explicitly expressed by Louise. As you learn about CPS, you will pick up the Thinking Keys.

In Section 12, you will have an opportunity to play with the concepts learned in Sections 1–11. Section 12 is a game that challenges you to recall details related to the paradigm of occupational therapy and CPS. We want you to have fun playing with the new information introduced in Unit I as you compete with classmates or against yourself before you enter the last leg of the journey in Unit II.

Have a good journey. And keep in mind that while we may not always be able to execute the "best" possible decision in therapy, we can strive to make the "better" decision under a particular set of circumstances that frame the situation. CPS is one creative and systematic way to arrive at the "better" decision.

Clinical Reasoning, Creative Problem Solving, and Occupational Therapy

Itinerary #1

At the end of the first part of your journey, you will be able to explain:

✓ the difference between clinical reasoning and CPS

✓ the role of creativity in problem solving

✓ the role of imagination in problem solving

✓ the difference between thinking in-the-box and thinking out-of-the-box

✓ why CPS skills are important where change is a constant

Clinical Reasoning and Creative Problem Solving—What's the Difference?

What is meant by creative problem solving? How does creative problem solving fit into the occupational therapy process? What is the difference between clinical reasoning and creative problem solving? Answers to these questions are the subject of this field book. Let's begin with a discussion of clinical reasoning, since it is a term that is currently used to describe how therapists solve problems.

The literature frequently uses the terms *clinical reasoning, clinical decision making*, and *clinical problem solving* interchangeably when defining the thinking processes of practitioners in clinical practice. Clinical reasoning refers to a model that describes a combination of general thought processes a therapist uses when making decisions about a client.

The American Occupational Therapy Foundation, in 1984, under the leadership of Nedra Gillette and Stephanie Hoover, supported a major research project to advance the profession's understanding of clinical reasoning. The principle investigators of this study, Maureen Hayes Fleming, an occupational therapist, and Cheryl Mattingly, an anthropologist, describe their work in *Clinical Reasoning: Forms of Inquiry in a Therapeutic Practice.*[1] Their ground-breaking research identified various kinds of complex thinking that therapists use during the therapeutic process. Throughout this field book we use the term *therapeutic process* to refer to the therapist-client relationship in all therapist interactions.

The thinking patterns Fleming and Mattingly describe reveal that therapists process information at many different levels simultaneously. For instance, while engaged in a therapy activity with a client, therapists think about a client's program goals, psychological status, emotional well-being, and medical condition all at the same time. Because therapists are able to process information this way, they can continually switch the focus of the treatment throughout a session and thus stay in tune with the client's needs.

Skilled therapists can switch the focus within a single therapy session in much the same way a skilled juggler keeps many plates spinning on the top of vertical rods, while continuously adding more plates. Both the therapist and the juggler deal with one part of an action while remaining mindful of the coherency of each action within the whole scene. Once the juggler has one plate spinning atop the supporting rod, another plate needs attending to. During a treatment session, the therapist, like the juggler, manages several issues at one time. Just as one problem gets solved, another one may pop up. Or the solution to one problem creates a new problem in another area of performance.

How can a therapist simultaneously work on one problem area of a client's treatment while being mindful of other problem areas? A therapist does this by adjusting her focus, by moving between looking at a small part of the picture and looking at the picture as a whole. This technique allows the therapist to sort through a huge amount of information to determine the most appropriate course of action to take.

Fleming and Mattingly also found that therapists make multiple decisions by relying on technical knowledge combined with the personal knowledge they bring to the situation. Thus, the decisions therapists make are based not only on what options seem logical but on what options feel right.

Fleming and Mattingly's research revealed unique patterns of clinical reasoning used by skilled therapists and has led occupational therapists to a better understanding of specific ways clinicians think when they successfully solve problems. One kind of clinical reasoning is called the Three Track Mind. In this model of thinking, the therapist goes back and forth between three mental tracks when working with a client. Fleming and Mattingly refer to the three thinking tracks as (1) procedural, (2) interactive, and (3) conditional reasoning.

When the therapist is thinking in the procedural reasoning track, he is thinking about the client's functional limitations, such as why she cannot bend over to tie her shoes. When thinking in the interactive reasoning track, the therapist is thinking about how to collaborate with the client so that they work together to develop treatment goals. When thinking in the conditional reasoning track, the therapist is thinking about activities in which the client will participate. Thoughts along the conditional reasoning track might lead the therapist to decide whether the client's session will involve activities such as gardening, cooking, or jewelry making.

Understanding *what* skilled therapists do in therapy is like being able to see daylight at the end of a long, dark tunnel. But seeing the light does not mean you know how to get to it. Likewise, when you observe a skilled practitioner at work, you can only imagine the path the therapist took to reach the decisions that led to the actions you observed.

The question then becomes *how* does a student or a new therapist develop the skills to think like a skilled practitioner? How do therapists who are changing from one practice area to another learn the steps of solving problems in a new practice area? How does a skilled practitioner continuously refine her own problem solving skills?

One way to look at the developmental progression of a therapist's clinical reasoning is to follow it along the five-stage continuum described by D. A. Schöen: novice, advanced beginner, competent, proficient, and expert.[2] The therapist at the novice level of practice rigidly applies the rules and principles of clinical practice learned in school and picked up by observing more experienced therapists; the novice abides by certain rules and principles regardless of the context in which the problem occurs. Advanced beginners learn that the rules and principles must be modified to fit the needs of a particular situation. The competent therapist has the confidence to adjust the rules and procedures to fit the situation; her judgment is not blindly directed by what she has read or seen others do. The proficient therapist feels secure enough to flexibly alter treatment procedures because she has a clear idea about the way the treatment program fits into the client's "life space" at discharge. Therapists who are at the expert level of proficiency organize their treatment programs around the clues they pick up from their own investigative "sleuthing" of the way the client presents himself at the time of the initial evaluation. In contrast to the novice, expert practitioners recognize the client's problems and potentials for change quickly because they cluster the clues into patterns. Expert practitioners have an inventory of patterns on which to reflect because of their years of experience in the particular area of practice.

The novice-to-expert model describes the qualities of the therapist's thinking patterns. It does *not*, however, explain the steps the new graduate or the therapist who changes his area of practice might take to develop good decision making skills. Today's health care market is hallmarked by constant change; to meet the challenges presented by an environment of change, therapists need to develop skills in creative and critical thinking. Practitioners who will be working in the twenty-first century need to have an inventory of creative and critical thinking strategies at their disposal, ready to apply wherever necessary so they can "hit the road running." Future health care environments will not be as supportive of novice-to-expert mentoring relationships as they have been in the past. Practitioners must learn to trust their own intuition and understand that ultimately their best mentor is themselves. (In Section 3, you will learn more about the influence of intuition on decision making.)

Clinical Reasoning

Before moving on, let's discuss clinical reasoning. We believe that the term *clinical reasoning* does not accurately describe the global nature of a therapist's thinking processes. "Reasoning" in "clinical reasoning" captures only a portion of the identified ways in which therapists think. "Reasoning" applies to the intellectual, rational side of thinking. It refers to logical and sequential thinking, the ability to analyze and to judge. When we analyze something, we determine *what is* and then make a decision based on that determination. Effective therapists need to think beyond what is. They need to help the client create a vision of an improved future state.

Reasoning is the thinking we associate with our head. But skilled therapists do not think solely with their heads. They also use their hearts to solve problems. When they "think" with their hearts they are using their emotional intelligence. Daniel Goleman defines emotional intelligence as "self-awareness and self-control, persistence, zeal and self-motivation, empathy and social deftness."[3] These qualities that Goleman associates with emotional intelligence form the basis of a person's character. Skilled therapists demonstrate the ability to balance their emotional intelligence with their rational mind.

Just as the word *reasoning* does not fully capture the wide range of thinking used by therapists, the word *clinical* does not capture the scope of today's practice settings. Clinics are only one place among many where therapists see clients. Therapists also work in homes, schools, residential facilities, work sites, and therapy departments as administrative managers, to mention only a few locations. We need to broaden our perspective about the way we think about where therapists practice.

Therapists are moving out of the clinic and into the communities where people live. In response to this change says Linda Learnard, a community-based occupational therapist from Maine, "We really need to focus on teaching people skills in their environment. The most appropriate rehabilitation method is to work on skills with people where they need them." When therapists work only in the clinic, she adds, "we teach people things out of context from the way they occur." A therapist might plan, for example, to do a cooking activity with a client, but the scheduled therapy session is not coordinated with the client's regular mealtime. Learnard would prefer to teach clients "at regular mealtimes in their own kitchens on their cranky gas stoves that sometimes refuse to light."[4] The movement in health care and education is to do just this, to teach clients skills that will allow them to function at their highest level within their "home" communities.

Creative Problem Solving

Whether a therapist is working with an adult in her own kitchen or with a toddler at home in his parents' living room or with an adolescent with autism in supported employment at a restaurant, unique therapy-related problems are continually arising. Sometimes the problem may be hard to define, and sometimes the problem may seem insurmountable. What is important for the therapist is to choose the best way to frame the problem. The perspective one uses to frame the problem plays an important role in providing one with the mindset needed to go forth and solve the problem. By learning intentional thinking strategies directed at solving problems creatively, occupational therapy practitioners equip themselves with a systematic and disciplined way of thinking about daily challenges.

A challenge is a stimulating undertaking. The idea that something is a challenge stimulates feelings of energy and entices one to move ahead with effort to meet the challenge. The word *challenge* is generally associated with the perception of positive thinking and internal drive to succeed. In contrast, the word *problem* is often associated with negative emotions such as doubt, uncertainty, and difficulty. When a therapist views a seemingly insurmountable problem as a challenge, a special mindset begins to evolve. When you view a problem as a challenge you are motivated to solve it. And if you are motivated to solve the problem, you begin to think creatively.

REFLECTIVE JOURNAL ENTRY 1.1

Complete the following thoughts:

1. The most challenging problem I ever solved creatively was . . .

2. After I met the challenge I felt . . .

Learning how to sharpen your creative skills at solving problems creatively involves learning a set of thinking strategies. Thinking strategies help organize your thoughts. Helen Hopkins, an occupational therapist, author, and educator, says that problem solving in occupational therapy requires creativity and imagination, along with knowledge, skills, and good professional judgment to find the best solution for each client.[5] This field book provides a set of thinking strategies to help you develop your creativity and imagination in order to enhance your problem solving ability within the therapy process.

This is a "how to" book that teaches thinking strategies. You will learn HOW to think about problems from different perspectives; HOW to generate a variety of options to solve problems; HOW to broaden the scope of a problem before focusing on one part of it.

Therapists at all levels of experience can benefit from learning new thinking strategies and sharpening those they already know. The strategies are instrumental in helping them to meet the challenges of daily practice. This field book offers the reader a problem solving model that is organized into three components and six stages. Each stage contains the thinking strategies we call Thinking Keys to help guide your thinking within a particular phase of the problem solving process.

The problem solving model that you are about to learn is Creative Problem Solving, or simply CPS, as it is called by the educators and researchers who created the model. We selected this problem solving model because it is compatible with the occupational therapy process. We are presenting an adaptation of the CPS model described by Donald Treffinger, Scott Isaksen, and K. B. Dorval.[6] CPS will broaden and deepen your thinking as you work through each stage of the occupational therapy process, beginning with the referral, and moving through assessment, goal setting, treatment planning, and intervention.

CPS is a widely researched problem solving model.[7] It has been used for decades in the business world and is one of the longest standing frameworks for the practical application of decision making. In this field book you will learn how to use CPS to systematically solve treatment-related problems that do not have ready-made solutions. The CPS model can be applied to all therapy frames of reference. It provides a solid foundation for making sound judgments related to decision making. (CPS is described in greater detail in Section 2.)

While it might be interesting to read about the different forms of clinical reasoning used by therapists, learning about the way other practitioners solve problems will not necessarily provide you with the "right" information to solve problems under any circumstance, nor will learning step-by-step directions to a predetermined answer.[8] Effective problem solving relies on the individual's ability to organize information in such a way that he can access that information and apply it to the problem that begs a solution.

Creativity in Problem Solving

In therapy, creativity is an essential ingredient to solving problems. When you apply creativity to problem solving, your thoughts about the problem are embedded in the context of the situation in which the problem occurs, and you generate solutions derived from personal perceptions and thinking.

There are two kinds of solutions to a problem: creative and ready made. Creative solutions are solutions that are tailored to the specific situation in which the problem occurs. Creative solutions are in direct contrast to "ready-mades." A ready-made is a solution that was used to solve a previous problem under a different set of circumstances at a different time. Just as you might choose a ready-made suit off a shop rack, you might select a ready-made solution because it best "fits" the situation. Ready-mades are convenient and should be considered first when making a decision because they can save both time and expense. But because ready-mades are "pieces of thinking" that are taken from someone else, such as a teacher, a publication, or television, use them with discretion. Don't lose sight of the fact that a ready-made is a substitute for your own thinking (see Section 5, under "Ill-Structured and Well-Structured Problems").

In most therapy situations, the uniqueness of the situation calls for a novel solution. There are infinite applications of creativity within the therapy process. The following are three examples.

1. **Fabricating an assistive device.** An occupational therapy practitioner, employed by a home health agency, is working with an adolescent who has diabetes and an above-the-elbow amputation. The client needs to be able to administer his own insulin. The therapist's challenge is two-fold. First, he must recognize the client's need for a wall-mounted insulin injection device. And then he must design and fabricate the device. The driving force behind the therapist's equipment design is his vision of the client's special need to operate the device independently using one arm, and his creativity to design and fabricate the device.

2. **Selecting treatment media.** A therapist working with a child in the child's home is having difficulty finding toys that will entice her young client to move about. She uses creativity when she thinks about what toys might motivate the child. Suddenly the family pet, a slow-moving basset hound, saunters past. Challenged by the need to teach her client new movement patterns and stimulated by the sight of the dog, the therapist decides to replace toys with the dog. The child will learn new ways to move while petting and brushing the family dog.

3. **Selecting treatment strategies.** A therapist working with a child with asthma uses creativity when she selects an atypical strategy to help the child manage his asthma. She teaches him behavior modification techniques and shows him how to use visualization.

These examples illustrate that creativity is not limited to people in the world of the performing and visual arts. Creativity belongs to everyone.

Imagination in Problem Solving

Skillful therapists are creative problem solvers. Creativity is an important element within the therapy process. The skilled therapist applies creativity as he helps clients and their families achieve optimal performance at home, at school, or at the workplace, playing, working, or relaxing. Creativity comes naturally when the therapist looks at a situation from a new perspective or with a fresh insight. Creative energy charges the imagination.

> *REFLECTIVE JOURNAL ENTRY 1.2*
>
> *Relax for a moment and allow yourself to give way to your sense of imagination. Close your eyes for two minutes and imagine yourself in a favorite place. Then open your eyes and complete the following statement:*
>
> *The first thing that came to mind was . . .*

Most likely your response demonstrated that you can become totally absorbed in another level of thought without much effort. Just as your imagination took you to another place, your imagination has the power to open your mind to new and different, "out-of-the-box" ideas. Out-of-the-box thinking refers to thoughts that are outside the usual or expected way of looking at a thing, an event, or a situation. Out-of-the-box thinkers frame their thinking with statements that begin, "What if . . ." or "How about . . ."

When you are comfortable using your imagination as you work, you enjoy what you are doing, just as you did when you were a child. The reason children seem to have such vivid imaginations is that they don't know all the rules for why something won't work. You can observe imagination at work when you watch a young child engrossed in a favorite toy. As the child plays, he uses the toy in many different ways, new and old.

Enhancing your imagination as an adult involves recapturing the unfettered imagination of your childhood. You were good at using your imagination when you were a child because you practiced and practiced imagining how things could be. All your "What if" and "How about" questions that drove your family to distraction revealed your imagination at work; you were wondering how things might be seen from a variety of perspectives. As you grew older, you learned the "should be" and "should not be" rules of life. You may even have stopped asking the "What if" and "How about" questions.

"Unless you use it, you lose it," is a familiar saying. Individuals whose thinking becomes grounded in the "should be" and "should not be" rules of life lose their ability to generate creative thoughts. In time, they forget how to use their imagination. By age 40 a person is only 2 percent as creative as at age 5. Studies show that creativity scores can drop about 90 percent between the ages of 5 and 7 years.[9] The tale you will read on pp. 10–11 illustrates what happens to our creativity when we try to do everything "just right."

Thinking In-the-Box and Out-of-the-Box

As you read the tale of the twin lines, imagination helps you to think out-of-the-box as well as differently in-the-box. In the following pages, you will explore the concept of thinking in-the-box and out-of-the-box.

> ### REFLECTIVE JOURNAL ENTRY 1.3
>
> *Think of a problem you solved creatively. (It can be the same problem you used in Reflective Journal Entry 1.1 or a different one.) Then complete the following statements:*
>
> 1. *The problem I solved creatively was . . .*
>
> 2. *My creative solution was . . .*

Recall your mindset when you solved the problem described in Reflective Journal Entry 1.3. With a yellow highlighter, shade 10 words in the Mindset Word List on p. 12 that best characterize your mindset at the time that you solved the problem.

> ### REFLECTIVE JOURNAL ENTRY 1.4
>
> *Now think of another problem solving situation, but this time, choose a problem that you failed to solve. Briefly describe the problem and why you failed to solve it.*
>
> 1. *A problem that I failed to solve was . . .*
>
> 2. *In retrospect, I failed to solve the problem because . . .*

A Tale of the Twin Lines

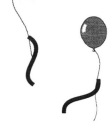

Once upon a time, in a far away land, twin lines were born.

The twins had a very happy early linehood. As little lines, they used their imagination to explore the world around them.

As little lines, the twins did not know what lines could and could not do, so they experimented endlessly and joyfully.

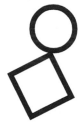
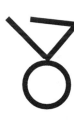

They curled up into balls, turned into triangles, squares and circles. Days passed ever so quickly as the twins explored the world which they were so curious about.

Eventually they had to leave their world of freedom and go to school to learn how to be a BIG line.

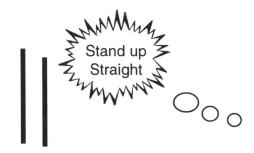
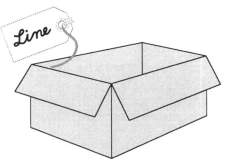

Being obedient little lines, the twins did what they were told, when they were told. The twins were eager to share with their Line teachers the many different ways they could become unline-like. However, the teachers were so busy teaching the little lines how to be BIG lines, they were not interested in any unline ideas.

Eventually the twins stopped trying to tell the BIG lines about their ideas. In time, they even forgot about having all their creative ideas. The twins learned to act the way every other line did, in the box, labeled LINE. They learned all the right rules and regulations of living in the LINE box.

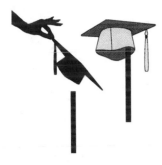

Eventually the twins graduated from LINE school with a diploma; they took jobs with the Proper LINE Corporation.

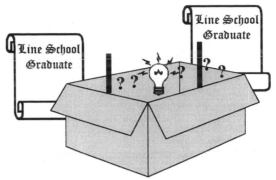

The twins were quick to learn how to do well in the LINE box at their new jobs. Their main responsibility was to solve problems. They went to work every day and were neither happy nor sad. They had learned to do what they were told to do and, after awhile, stopped feeling much of anything.

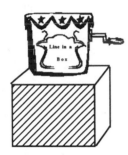

One day when neither twin line could come up with a solution to a problem they were working on, they took a break and went to the cafeteria. At the table where they sat there was a box with a crank handle. At first, the twins thought it was a toy a little line had left behind.

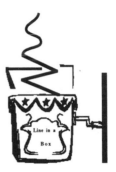

One of the twins turned the handle around and around until, much to his surprise, a little line popped out of the box. It was a "Line in the Box." This box was just like the one the twins had when they were little lines. The lines laughed and laughed as they thought about how they had forgotten about their funny little toy.

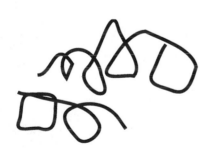

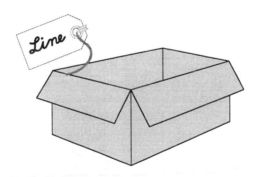

The Line in the Box triggered the twins to reminisce about the days when they thought about line ideas out of the "box." They felt the joy of their early linehood come rushing back. They were so excited about remembering the creative ways they used to do things, they decided to go back to work and think about the world outside of their box. Their creative spirit felt alive again. The twins were so energized by remembering how they had used their imagination during their early linehood, they promised themselves never again to lose sight of their creative spirit by thinking *only* in the box.

THE END

C. Reed; J. Lewin 1997

Inspired by Frank Prince, *C and the Box: A Paradigm Parable* (San Diego, Calif.: Pfeiffer & Co., 1993).

Recall your mindset when you failed to solve the problem described in Reflective Journal Entry 1.4. With a pencil, circle 10 words in the Mindset Word List that best characterize your mindset at the time that you were trying to solve the problem.

Mindset Word List

fearful	aggressive	challenged	free	passive
daring	brave	adventuresome	analytical	gentle
inventive	empathetic	independent	procedural	original
innovative	energized	harmonious	motivated	wavering
ordinary	enterprising	sluggish	stagnant	fair-minded
dreamy	friendly	tense	guarded	hostile
kind-hearted	good-natured	authoritative	self-righteous	linear
flexible	happy	secure	critical	judgmental
discordant	harmonizing	amiable	expansive	disagreeable
unconventional	humble	adaptable	theoretical/abstract	easily influenced
judgmental	indifferent	humorous	cautious	open-minded
imaginative	intuitive	passionate	explorative	rigid
tolerant	inviting	dogmatic	centered	fearful
weak	lacking	mindful	neglectful	expressive
practical	logical	controlling	reserved	courteous
relaxed	loyal	sincere	considerate	encouraging
respectful of other points of view	nonconforming	inquisitive	alert to endless possibilities	able to make connections
caring	observant	neglectful	stubborn	synthesizing
insightful	perceptive	sensitive	curious	contrary
realistic	practical	pragmatic	holistic	colorful
deliberate	resourceful	cooperative	ingenious	courageous
yielding	risk-taking	resistive	uncertain	welcoming
expressive of wonder	self-confident	self-actualized	impartial	positive
dependent	sensitive	supportive	accepting	biased
hesitant	spontaneous	structured	unique	empathetic
alive	sympathetic	hasty	generous	self-reliant
uncertain	vulnerable	scared	transformed	imagine big thoughts

Referring only to the words that you circled and highlighted, select those words that you feel characterize thinking out-of-the-box. Write the words somewhere outside the box in Figure 1.1. Next, select the words that characterize your thinking in-the-box. Write those words in the box in Figure 1.1.

Figure 1.1. *Thinking In-the-Box and Out-of-the-Box*

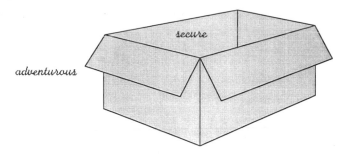

REFLECTIVE JOURNAL ENTRY 1.5

Count the number of out-of-the-box words and the number of in-the-box words you came up with and complete the following thoughts:

1. *The number of out-of-the-box words I came up with is _____.*

2. *The number of in-the-box words I came up with is _____.*

3. *When I compare my thinking in these two situations, I would classify my thinking as _____ (fill in choice) because . . .*
   out-of-the-box or in-the-box

You can hone your skill in thinking out-of-the-box and being creative by nurturing your imagination. Practice expanding your mind beyond the rules of "should be" and "should not be." Begin to think outside of the box again by asking questions that start with "What if" and "How about." Therapy practitioners need an expansive, creative mindset to solve the problems they face daily in practice. And feeling comfortable asking the "What if" and "How about" questions is one way to begin thinking creatively.

The Importance of CPS Skills Where Change Is a Constant

Rapid changes in health care systems, Cyberspace, telecommunications, and computer and other technologies has inundated us with more information and options than most of us can deal with at one time. To thrive in a world of constant change, one must be able to process a multitude of facts quickly. Old ways of doing things no longer suffice.

In the decade between 1990 and 2000, there will be a 100 percent increase in raw knowledge, and there will be another 100 percent increase by 2010. American society is changing. One of the major changes is that American families are continually on the move because of job relocation. And because of these moves the extended family support systems have been seriously affected. It is also commonplace today to have both parents working outside of the home and to have the child's main adult contact be a babysitter at home or in a day care center. Single-parent homes are on the rise. The average amount of individual contact between parent and child is now approximately 15 minutes a day.[10] To involve the family in a child's therapy program, for example, you can no longer rely on the methods of the past to work with family members. Developing creative thinking skills is vitally important to your ability to respond to the challenges in today's culture where change is a constant.

Therapists need to act quickly and in a thoughtful manner. They need to be able to shift gears at a moment's notice. And shifting gears quickly requires a high degree of flexibility. Developing the skills to think creativity and critically on demand will help you become a flexible thinker, open to considering another perspective, another point of view, another way.

When therapists help people manage their problems, they are not dealing with absolutes. Every situation is unique because every interaction you have with a person is unique. Whether you are dealing with a client, the client's family, or the client's significant other, you are managing a new situation, and each new situation offers a new challenge. Therapists need to consider many different options, because in therapy there are few totally right or totally wrong answers. Consequently you need a high tolerance for ambiguity.

Consider the following scenario: You are working with two children who have the same diagnosis. When you view each child's problem as a "medical diagnosis," the problems sound alike. If you were using only the medical diagnosis to guide your thinking toward the intervention, more than likely you would embark on a decision making path that looked very similar for both children. But, when you approach each of the two children with the same diagnosis from a creative problem solver's viewpoint, you learn to place a high value on each child's individual differences. You value the differences in each child's family support system, individual resources of the family, and how each family member views the child's disability. Because family or caregiver support systems vary and because socioeconomic factors can influence the quality of the therapy services, the medical diagnosis alone is insufficient in guiding your thinking about the child and the family.

Knowing what the medical diagnosis is and having basic information about the usual ways that the disease or injury affects one's abilities does not tell you about the unique coping abilities of the individual client. Differences in age, personal outlook, family support system, and socioeconomic resources demand that each individual be treated in a unique manner. Because no two people are alike, your therapy-related decisions cannot be based on the medical diagnosis alone.

REFLECTIVE JOURNAL ENTRY 1.6

Read the following sentence and complete the statements that follow.

I recall one time when I had two problems that were similar, yet I dealt with them very differently.

1. *The first problem was . . .*

2. *The second problem was . . .*

3. *The similarities were . . .*

4. The differences were . . .

5. I handled the problems differently because . . .

For the two problems described above you were able to use different solutions because you were sensitive to the unique elements within each problem. You changed your perspective according to the unique elements of each problem. Learning to appreciate the unique elements of a situation is a basic part of developing skill in CPS.

So come journey with us through this field book to learn CPS, a model that relies on creative and critical thinking. CPS is a systematic process for organizing your thoughts about clients and the challenges that face them. You will hone your problem solving skills by using the thinking strategies referred to as Thinking Keys. You will use the Thinking Keys to develop problem solving skills within the occupational therapy process. Like the keys you depend on to open your front door or start your car, each Thinking Key will open a different "door" to your thinking.

You have just completed Section 1 of your journey. Now it is time for a review. At the end of every section you will review your reading by creating a Mind Map and evaluate what you have learned by completing a Self-Assessment.

When you create a Mind Map, include as many details as you feel are necessary to capture the content of the section. You can use your Mind Map as a study guide for later review of the material. To help you get started, in Sections 1 and 2, we began your map with a few main concepts. Each time you come to the end of a section, the Mind Map Guidelines box will be your cue to create a Mind Map. You may find it easier to draw your map with the page turned sideways.

A small clipboard (reminding you of the itinerary for the section) will signal the Self-Assessment. To complete the Self-Assessment, you will need to do the following:

1. Remove the green and red crayons from your supply bag.
2. Read the list of itinerary items and evaluate your level of understanding of the material summarized by each item.
3. For each item, ask yourself: Do I understand this concept well enough that I can explain it to a traveling companion? or Is this concept a little "fuzzy"?
4. If you understand the concept well enough that you can explain it to a traveling companion, use the green crayon to fill in the circle to the left of the item. If, however, the concept is still "fuzzy" or unclear to you, color the circle red.
5. Go back through the section and review the "red dot" concepts before continuing to the next section of your journey.

Create a Mind Map of Section

1

Mind Map Guidelines

1. Radiate ideas from the section's main concept.
   - Use images (be sure to use color).
   - Headline text—one or two words per line.
   - Print text (for easy reading).
2. Link the main concepts and generate more ideas from the linkages.
3. Have fun!

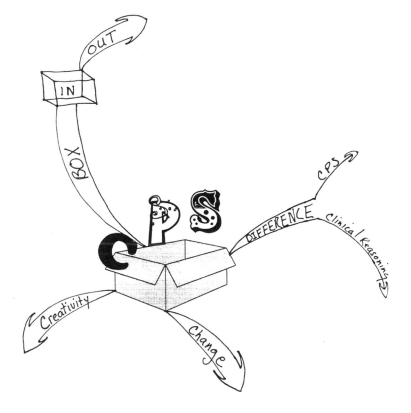

Section 1
SELF-ASSESSMENT

Now that I have completed the first part of my journey, I can explain:

○ the difference between clinical reasoning and CPS.

○ the role of creativity in problem solving.

○ the role of imagination in problem solving.

○ the difference between thinking in-the-box and thinking out-of-the-box.

○ why CPS skills are important where change is a constant.

NOTES

1. Mattingly and Fleming, *Clinical Reasoning: Forms of Inquiry in a Therapeutic Practice* (Philadelphia: F. A. Davis, 1993). This publication describes the authors' research, which consisted of videotaped therapy sessions and interviews with the occupational therapist who implemented the sessions. The authors conclude that the thinking in occupational therapy often centers on "story making." Occupational therapists view each therapy session as a piece of a broader life story of that client rather than an employment of technical skills (such as UE-ROM, meaning "evaluate upper extremity range of motion") as an end in itself. Hence, Mattingly and Fleming conclude that thinking in occupational therapy differs from that of traditional medicine. Occupational therapists do not limit their clinical thinking to the medical diagnosis and do not base treatment on the expected dysfunction, which is linked to specific treatment activities and procedures.

2. P. Brenner, *From Novice to Expert: Excellence and Power in Clinical Nursing Practice* (Reading, Mass.: Addison-Wesley, 1984); H. L. Dreyfus, and S. E. Dreyfus, *Mind over Machine: The Power of Human Intuition and Expertise in the War of the Computer* (New York: Free Press, 1986); R. Dutton, *Clinical Reasoning in the Physical Disabilities* (Baltimore, Md.: Williams & Wilkins, 1995); D. A. Schöen, *The Reflective Practitioner: How Professionals Think in Action* (New York: Basic Books, 1983); D. Y. Slater, and E. S. Cohn, "Staff Development Through Analysis of Practice," *American Journal of Occupational Therapy* 45 (1991): 1038–44.

3. D. Goleman, *Emotional Intelligence* (New York: Bantam Books, 1995).

4. B. Ruben, "For Maine OT, Community-Based Care Is Key to Recovery," *OT Week*, March 8, 1990.

5. H. L. Hopkins, "Problem Solving," in H. L. Hopkins and H. D. Smith, eds., *Willard and Spackman's Occupational Therapy*, 8th ed. (Philadelphia: J. B. Lippincott, 1993).

6. D. Treffinger, S. Isaksen, and K. B. Dorval, *Creative Problem Solving, Introduction*, rev. ed. (Sarasota, Fla.: Center for Creative Learning, 1994). This is a well-referenced and comprehensive explanation of the creative problem solving (CPS) theory that has 50 years of research and development behind it. The book also provides exercises, worksheets, and discussions of issues related to the foundations for using creativity in problem solving.

7. A. Osburn, *Applied Imagination*, 3d ed. (New York: Charles Schribner's Sons, 1963).

8. B. May and J. Newman, "Developing Competence in Problem-Solving: A Behavioral Model," *Physical Therapy* 60, no. 9 (September 1980): 1140–45. The authors present a recommended model for problem solving in physical therapy. Their model centers on the cognitive, affective, and psychomotor domains originally described in B. Bloom, *Taxonomy of Educational Objectives Handbook I: Cognitive Domain* (New York: David McKay, 1956); and D. Karthwohn, B. Blook, and B. B. Masia, *Taxonomy of Educational Objectives Handbook II: Affective Domain* (New York: David McKay, 1964).

9. M. Ferguson, *The Aquarian Conspiracy* (Los Angeles: Jeremy P. Tarcher, 1980).

10. M. Cetron and O. Davies, *The American Renaissance* (New York: St. Martin's Press, 1989).

Introduction to Creative Problem Solving

SECTION

2

Itinerary #2

At the end of the second part of your journey, you will be able to:

✓ explain the origin of Creative Problem Solving

✓ identify the three components and six stages of CPS

✓ explain how CPS and the occupational therapy process work together

✓ compare the Generating Phase with the Focusing Phase in CPS

✓ compare Deferred Judgment with Affirmative Judgment

✓ list two guidelines associated with Deferred Judgment

✓ list three guidelines associated with Affirmative Judgment

Origin of Creative Problem Solving

The process presented in this field book, Creative Problem Solving (CPS), is based on the research of Scott G. Isaksen, K. B. Dorval, and Donald Treffinger. Their work grew out of the Osborn-Parnes CPS model.[1] Alex Osborn, an advertising executive, created the first CPS model in the late 1930s, and Sidney Parnes, a psychologist, developed it further.[2]

Osborn is recognized as the father of brainstorming and is credited in *Webster's International Dictionary* as the originator of the term *brainstorming*. Osborn developed the strategy that became known as brainstorming when the company for which he was working asked him to organize an ideation session. The people who participated in the session dubbed their experience "brainstorming" to describe their act of spontaneity in generating quantities of ideas at the same time.[3] Osborn recognized that for a session to be brainstorming, certain principles must be strictly followed.

Osborn believed that to solve problems creatively, you need to generate many possible solutions before selecting one. He also believed that brainstorming occurs most easily when ideas are allowed to flow in the absence of any type of judgment—positive or negative. The principal of "deferred judgment" is central to brainstorming (see Section 9 for more about brainstorming). Based on research and his experience, Osborn found that when people judge ideas prematurely, they dismiss the value of many ideas that potentially could be useful.

Osborn's concept of brainstorming has its roots in India. Close to five hundred years ago, the Hindu teachers who worked with religious groups practiced Prai-Barshana. Prai means "outside yourself" and Barshana means "question." During Prai-Barshana, no discussion or criticism was allowed. All ideas were evaluated at a later time by the same group who generated them.

All ideas need to be nurtured, according to Osborn, since you never know from which idea a solution will emerge. His original CPS model provided a way of thinking about an issue. The first step was to generate many ideas. The second step was to evaluate the ideas. No idea was to be evaluated until after all of the possible ideas, including wild ones in need of "taming," were identified. The skill of generating ideas first and evaluating their merit later is important in therapy.

In addition to brainstorming, Osborn placed a high value on incubation, or what he called purposeful "relaxation." The dictionary has several definitions of incubation. The first two relate to the familiar uses of the word: (1) to sit on eggs for the purpose of hatching and (2) to keep premature babies in favorable conditions for growth. However, the third definition, to develop or produce (ideas) as if by hatching, fits Osborn's use of the word. Incubation applied to CPS refers to "the phenomenon by which ideas spontaneously well up into our consciousness."[4] Osborn said that incubation is what invites illumination, or sudden flashes of brilliance, on a situation begging a solution.

Incubation can result in "ah-ha" experiences. Those moments after you have stopped consciously thinking about a problem, ideas seem to jump into your head. There really is some validity to the concept of putting a problem away and "sleeping" on it. After a period of relative inactivity, a time-out to *not* think about a problem, a great idea can suddenly emerge.

REFLECTIVE JOURNAL ENTRY 2.1

Complete the following thought:

I recall having an ah-ha experience when . . .

Incubation is part of our "thinking environment." It is a constructive kind of procrastination. The ideas are set aside with the intent that we will revisit them at a later date. We need to allow time for the idea to incubate or germinate. And we need to recognize and respect the outcome when the "ah-ha" occurs. Incubation, like brainstorming, is an essential activity in CPS.

Three Components and Six Stages of CPS

CPS has three components and six stages. The three components are referred to as Get Ready, Get Set, and Go Forward. Get Ready to understand the problem, Get Set to find a solution, and Go Forward with an action plan. In "Get Ready to understand the problem," you focus on identifying the problem. In "Get Set to find a solution," you generate options that have never been tried. And in "Go Forward with an action plan," you turn the options into useful ideas that will effectively and efficiently solve the problem.[5]

Stages and Components of CPS

Get Ready to understand the problem

1. Opportunity Finding
2. Data Finding
3. Problem Finding

Get Set to find a solution

4. Idea Finding

Go Forward with an action plan

5. Solution Finding
6. Acceptance Finding

Within each component of CPS there are one or more stages. Each stage of the process helps you "find" information that will move you toward solving the problem. Hence the names Opportunity Finding, Data Finding, and so forth.[6] Each stage is made up of thinking strategies (which we refer to as Thinking Keys) that help guide your thinking within that particular stage of CPS.

CPS is an organizing framework that encompasses a variety of thinking strategies. Individuals and groups may choose to use one or more of these strategies in order to deal effectively with a particular task or challenge. While the CPS model is a deliberate approach to decision making, it is also meant to be flexible and dynamic. **As you learn about CPS, keep in mind that you may use any of the components (and the stages within them) in any order, depending on the nature of the problem.** This is an important point to remember as you learn the process because we present the model in a linear, step-by-step manner.[7] (Our detailed discussion of the process begins in Section 6.) The model can also be presented graphically. Treffinger, Isaksen, and Dorval show the six stages (each represented by a diamond) within the three components of CPS (see Figure 2.1).

In our graphic representation of CPS, the six stages form a circle to remind you of the interconnectedness of the stages (see Figure 2.2). The star shape in the middle of the six interconnected diamonds symbolizes the light generated by a bright star. CPS is like a shining beacon that sheds light on the problems you need to solve in therapy; it provides the thinking strategies that help you systematically develop creative solutions to problems you encounter in practice.

As you progress through this field book, you will work on the stages of CPS one by one. Each time you begin work on a new stage, you will see that stage highlighted with a dark background on the star diagram. The small reproduction of the model on the right side of

Figure 2.1. *Independent Components of CPS. (Reprinted with permission from Donald Treffinger, Scott Isaksen, and K. B. Dorval,* Creative Problem Solving, Introduction, *rev. ed. [Sarasota, Fla.: Center for Creative Learning, 1994].)*

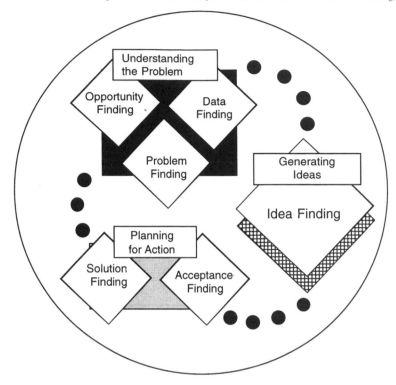

Figure 2.2 shows what the star will look like, for example, when you are working on Opportunity Finding.

Throughout this field book, you will read stories about therapists, their clients, and their experiences with decision making. When you analyze the stages through which these therapists traveled to solve each problem, you will be able to identify most, if not all, six stages of CPS.

Figure 2.2. *Six Stages of CPS*

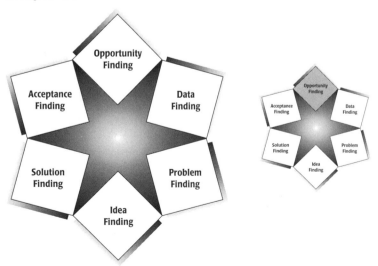

How CPS and the Occupational Therapy Process Work Together

You may be wondering, "At what point in the occupational therapy process do I use CPS?" or "Can CPS replace the occupational therapy process?" CPS is not a substitute for the occupational therapy, or OT, process. CPS is a thinking model to superimpose on the stages in the OT process. CPS augments your thinking during the various components of the OT process.

The introductory comments about CPS in Section 1 explain how this model broadens and deepens your thinking as you work through the OT process. Occupational therapists work in many different structures and systems to promote optimal health and functioning in others. In addition to providing treatment, occupational therapists engage in tasks such as program development, scheduling, budgeting, staff supervision, and instruction of colleagues (i.e., other therapy practitioners and interdisciplinary team members). Within the scope of treatment, the therapist also provides family education to the client's caregivers. In this field book, however, we limit the discussion of CPS to the therapist in a direct service role.

The occupational therapist Helen L. Hopkins has stated, "A generic approach to problem solving may prove useful to the therapist at all levels [of practice]: administrative, supervisory, and clinical.[8] CPS does provide the reader with a "generic approach to problem solving." After you learn CPS and become comfortable using it to solve therapy-related problems, we hope that you will expand your usage of CPS to other problems that require creative solutions.

We arbitrarily divided the OT process into seven stages that define the primary aspects of practice. The stages are as follows: the referral for therapy services, assessment, goal setting, treatment planning, treatment implementation, discharge planning and implementation, and follow-up.

When CPS is superimposed on the OT process (see the chart below), each part of the OT process corresponds to a CPS component. Occupational therapy referral, assessment, and goal setting correspond to understanding the problem. Treatment planning corresponds to finding a solution. Implementation of the treatment plan, discharge planning and implementation, and follow-up correspond to going forward with the action plan. Both the OT process and CPS value and encourage a mutual understanding with open communication between all individuals involved.

Occupational Therapy Process	Creative Problem Solving Process
	Get Ready to understand the problem
Referral	1. Opportunity Finding
Assessment	2. Data Finding
Goal Setting	3. Problem Finding
	Get Set to find a solution
Treatment Planning	4. Idea Finding
	Go Forward with an action plan
Treatment Implementation	5. Solution Finding
Discharge Planning	6. Acceptance Finding
Follow-up	

Like CPS, the OT process is flexible. If, for example, your new client's therapy-related problem has already been identified by a previous therapist, you would skip the referral, assessment, and goal setting stages and move on to the treatment planning component of the OT process. The same strategy holds true for CPS. You would skip over Opportunity Finding and move onto the stage that will best clarify your thinking about making a decision about the client's needs when the problem has been clearly identified.

To repeat, although you will be learning CPS in an apparent sequence—you will be introduced to Opportunity Finding first and Acceptance Finding last—we want you to understand that the sequence in which the stages are taught is not the only route to take. As you learn the stages and start to apply CPS "in the field," you will use those stages that are most appropriate to the situation.

In the first part of the OT process, you must determine whether the client's problem falls within the realm of occupational therapy services. The thinking strategies in "Get Ready to understand the problem" augment your ability to systematically consider all the factors related to the client's problem in order to determine whether occupational therapy is an appropriate service. If, after reviewing all of the data surrounding the **referral**, you determine that therapy services are appropriate, you move on to **assessment** and **goal setting**. You must (1) decide the best course of action and (2) set goals that reflect that course of action.

The thinking strategies used in the first component of CPS, "Get Ready to understand the problem," will help you explore comprehensively all therapy options available to the client. **Goal setting** then includes combining your interpretation of what you see (i.e., your perception of the client's problems) with what you hear (i.e., the client's perception of the problem) into measurable, functional, achievable goals. Goal setting is a collaborative effort between you and the client (or if the client is a young child, the client's caretakers).

The second component, "Get Set to find a solution," supports the second part of the OT process, **treatment planning**. Treatment planning takes into consideration all the information gathered during the assessment phase. The more you are able to consider all the relevant factors related to a client's problem, the better you will be at developing activities that will help the client meet his goals. The thinking strategies in "Get Set to find a solution" enhance your ability to generate a huge number of treatment ideas, some that are commonplace and others that are out of the ordinary. The thinking strategies in this component also help to make your activities more interesting and meaningful for the client.

The thinking strategies in the third component of CPS, "Go Forward with an action plan," supports the third part of the OT process. The third part of the OT process addresses the methodology of the therapy process—the ideas behind all of the planning are transformed into action. **Treatment implementation, discharge planning**, and **follow-up** address the change agents, the "who, what, where, when, and why" change will occur. They are similar in that they involve helping the client move from his current reality to a desired future state of well-being. The thinking strategies in this third component help you systematically determine which treatment activities are the better options to help the client achieve that desired future state.

CPS enhances a therapist's ability to use the OT process. Like the specialized tools and strategies artisans use to help them perform their jobs more efficiently, CPS is a process that will help you to help clients solve their problems. By learning the thinking strategies associated with CPS, you will improve your skill in solving problems related to practice.

The Generating and Focusing Phases in CPS

Each stage in CPS has two phases, the Generating Phase and the Focusing Phase.[9] The Generating Phase is the first part of each stage and the Focusing Phase is the second part.

The Generating Phase allows you to consider all options related to the issue under consideration. Think of it as the expansion phase, because it begs you to open your mind and broaden your perspective of each element of the problem. In the Generating Phase, the focus is on discovering through the use of imagination more than one right answer. Remember, there are few absolutes in CPS. Your goal is to recognize the "better" answer within the context of the specific situation. There may not always be one "best" option. Settling for the first or "obvious" answer will limit the probability that you will make the "better" decision.

The more ideas that you identify in each Generating Phase, the more options you will have to select from when you enter the Focusing Phase. When the two phases of CPS are

Figure 2.3. *The Two Phases of Each Stage of CPS*

Generating Phase
The top half of the diamond represents the Generating Phase. You open up and stretch your mind here.

Focusing Phase
The bottom half of the diamond represents the Focusing Phase. You narrow your list of options here.

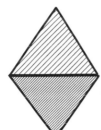

The diamond is represented here as one unit, without the split shown above to indicate that in each stage of CPS, you flow from the Generating Phase to the Focusing Phase. Then, to the next stage, which begins again with the Generating Phase, and so on.

represented by a diamond shape (see Figure 2.3), the Generating Phase is represented by the broadening or expansion of the triangle from its apex and the Focusing Phase is represented by the broad base narrowing or contracting toward the apex.

You may be asking yourself, "How do I know when to move on to the Focusing Phase?" When you can no longer identify any more ideas or when you begin to repeat ideas, you are ready to proceed to the Focusing Phase. The Focusing Phase gives you an opportunity to evaluate the information you gathered in the Generating Phase. In the Focusing Phase, as you evaluate your options you are also recognizing priorities about the data. You are sorting out what information is directly relevant to solving the problem and what information is interesting but does not move you directly toward a positive outcome. This process of consolidation is what eventually leads you to making conclusions or better decisions about how to solve the problem.

Remember that in each stage of CPS, you first expand your thinking to identify as many ideas as possible. That is the Generating Phase. Then you immediately follow with your evaluation of those ideas, by contracting your thoughts in the Focusing Phase.

Deferred Judgment and Affirmative Judgment

As you travel through the Generating and Focusing Phases, you must follow two important rules. The rules are referred to as Deferred Judgment and Affirmative Judgment. Deferred Judgment and Affirmative Judgment are like the rules of the road, the CPS road. They help regulate the flow of ideas just as traffic rules help to keep motor vehicles flowing.

Whenever you are in the Generating Phase you will use the rule of Deferred Judgment. And whenever you are in the Focusing Phase you will use the rule of Affirmative Judgment.

Generating Phase ⟶ Deferred Judgment
Focusing Phase ⟶ Affirmative Judgment

Deferred Judgment means that you refrain from reviewing your ideas until after you have stopped generating the list of options. Judging new options while you are still generating them results in your rejecting ideas without giving them a fair chance. When you judge your ideas prematurely, you risk narrowing your options. And narrowing your options is something you want to avoid in the Generating Phase. Think of the Generating Phase as the "idea inspiration" phase.

To exercise your ability to generate ideas without judging them, perform the Nine Dot exercise in Figure 2.4. As you try to find solutions to the Nine Dot exercise, reflect on what boundaries you place on yourself. Note that six sets of the nine-dot pattern are provided so that you will have five opportunities to make a fresh start.

DIRECTIONS

1. Choose one nine-dot pattern to begin on. Then, without lifting your pencil from the paper, draw exactly four straight, connected lines that will go through all nine dots, drawing through each dot only once.[10]
2. If you are familiar with this exercise, consider in what ways you can connect all of the dots using only one line. Expand the limits of your thinking and generate some wacky ideas.
3. See Appendix A for one solution.

Figure 2.4. *Nine Dot Exercise*

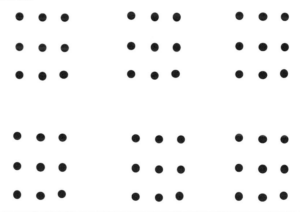

REFLECTIVE JOURNAL ENTRY 2.2

Complete the following thoughts:

1. As I attempted to solve the Nine Dot exercise I found myself thinking . . .

2. One of the boundaries that I had to work through was . . .

The Nine Dot exercise is a brain teaser designed to trigger thoughts about what kinds of boundaries you impose on yourself when you solve problems. A typical boundary people impose on themselves when doing this exercise is that the lines they draw must begin and end on a dot. If you impose a similar boundary, the possibility of working outside of the dots does not exist. To solve the Nine Dot exercise it is necessary to see that the dots do not define the entire territory within which you work. The lesson of this exercise is: **When you are aware of the kinds of boundaries you place on your thinking, you can more easily expand the limits of those boundaries according to the demands of the situation.**

The more readily you can stretch the limits of your boundaries and think outside-of-your-box, the easier it will be for you to put off judging your ideas in the Generating Phase. So don't give in to your inner censor that says, "That's a dumb idea. . . . How could you do that? . . . That idea will never work." Keep an open mind. When you consider all of the options—the good, the bad, and the weird—with an open mind, you will increase the potential of your arriving at a truly creative solution. To be an effective problem solver, you need to express *every* idea that you can think of related to the situation. In the Generating Phase, every idea is a great idea and therefore worthy of consideration at a later time. That later time, as you now know, is the next phase, the Focusing Phase.

As you generate ideas, write them down. Choosing not to record your ideas violates the rule to defer judgment. Not recording an idea suggests a critical rejection of the idea. In the Generating Phase, there are no bad ideas, only undeveloped ones. Consider them all diamonds in the rough.

In the Focusing Phase, you will use Affirmative Judgment. When you use Affirmative Judgment, your thinking shifts into a "critical thinking" evaluative mode. Now is the time to judge your ideas. Affirmative Judgment in the Focusing Phase allows you to consider the positives and the negatives. It is a balance to your thinking in the Generating Phase, where you used your imagination to come up with many different ideas without evaluating any of them.[11]

Direct your efforts at choosing the *better* ideas or options from your list. There may not always be a *best* option. Affirmative Judgment allows you to direct your attention selecting those ideas that seem the most useful and promising to help the client solve his problem.

How often have you thought about what was "right" about a problem situation? Critical thinking is often only about finding fault and excluding that which is irrelevant. When you use Affirmative Judgment, you form your opinions about the merit of your ideas as they relate to solving the problem. You seek to identify the positives and negatives as well as the interesting ideas, or the ideas that may take on greater meaning at a later time but that for now are not clearly either positive or negative.

When you affirmatively judge ideas, you learn to look at both sides of the issue. The following three questions can help you select an idea from a multitude of possible ideas.

◆ What are the benefits of this idea?
◆ What are the drawbacks of this idea?
◆ What more information can I gather about each idea's interesting points that will help me to arrive at a solution?

When using Affirmative Judgment recognize that *every option* on your list holds the *potential* of bringing you closer to your solution. To fully consider each idea generated you must keep an open mind. Ask yourself, "How might this idea work?" Avoid thinking, "This idea will not work because . . ."

REFLECTIVE JOURNAL ENTRY 2.3

Complete the following thought:

The last time I can remember asking myself, "How will this idea work?" was when . . .

Never rule out an idea before thoroughly considering its value. You don't want to risk discarding you diamonds in the rough!

Direct your attention toward constructing possibilities rather than eliminating them. Sometimes exploring the ideas that at first appear to be the least likely path can lead to a constructive and useful solution. Remember, your goal is to find effective solutions to the problem. Sometimes a whole idea isn't "great." But *parts* of the idea may be useful. When you remain open to ideas, solutions can be found in some very unlikely places. Consider constructing a new idea from the pieces of two different "not so great" ideas.

Project your thoughts into the future by asking yourself, "How might this idea work out?" The word *might* focuses your attention on the possibilities that the idea brings to CPS. Next, think about the consequences of your actions further into the future. Ask "What's next?" The more thoroughly you can think through the consequences of a tentative decision, the greater the likelihood your ultimate decision will be a sound one.

Guidelines for Deferred Judgment in the Generating Phase

There are two guidelines in the Generating Phase that are related to Deferred Judgment.[12] (You will practice applying these guidelines to CPS later.) The guidelines target ways to come up with many, many options, the primary goal of the Generating Phase.

Guidelines for Deferred Judgment
1. Strive for quantity.
2. S t r e t c h your mind.

Strive for Quantity

Strive to generate a large number of ideas because quantity yields quality. Alex Osborn says, "The more ideas you think up, the more likely you are to arrive at the potentially best leads to a solution."[13] Osborn goes on to explain that while there are no hard and fast techniques of coming up with the right solution, certain principles in the form of procedural guides will enhance the probability of your coming up with high quality options from which to choose later. Therefore, in the Generating Phase, strive for many ideas, including wild ideas, in anticipation of polishing them later.

Build one idea onto another. You are encouraged to "hitchhike," to combine or hitch one idea on top of another. By strengthening your ability to recognize ways you can interrelate ideas, you will create better and better ideas. The more ideas you generate, the better your opportunities to find a useful, creative solution. Be mindful that the evaluation of ideas comes *after* the ideas are generated. So in the Generating Phase just let 'em rip.

Generating ideas is sort of like collecting sea shells on the beach. When you collect shells, at first you harvest every one that you pick up, even the not-so-beautiful ones. You defer judgment to sort the extraordinary "keepers" with the ordinary "toss back into the ocean" shells because you never know whether the one shell you toss back might be the only one of its kind for the day. Similarly, when you generate ideas, deferring judgment allows you to harvest a large number of thoughts.

Maintain a mindset that the best way to generate premium thoughts is to strive for a quantity of ideas. Like the shells on the beach, the first idea that comes to mind is not likely to be the extraordinary "keeper." You are more likely to find a "keeper" when you have a quantity of ideas from which to choose.

Stretch Your Mind

The first guideline, Strive for quantity supports the second guideline, Stretch your mind. When you strive to generate as many ideas as possible, you stretch your mind to accept all ideas that pop into your head. Accepting all ideas that pop into your head is a novel approach in a culture where one is rewarded for giving the "right" answer and admonished for giving the "wrong" one. When you defer judgment, freewheeling is encouraged. The definition of freewheeling is "unrestrained behavior." When you are freewheeling you allow the ideas—all ideas, even outrageous and silly ones—to flow. You'll have an opportunity to tame the "wild" ideas into practical ones later in the process. When you defer judgment you are encouraged to do "unrestrained" thinking.

As you practice freewheeling, you will become more and more comfortable with stretching your mind and you will begin to see an increase in the numbers of ideas generated. Be flexible. Consider all options, no matter how original, wild, off-the-wall, out-of-the-box, or elaborate they are. After you produce a quantity of ideas, you can pick and choose among the options that best match your situation.

REFLECTIVE JOURNAL ENTRY 2.4

Complete the following thought:

1. My mind flows with ideas when I . . .

2. I find it hard to think of lots of ideas when I . . .

If you have a habit of critiquing your thoughts as you generate them, you may have difficulty thinking up large volumes of ideas. If you have a habit of analyzing your thoughts as they are created, try freewheeling when you are by yourself. It may take you some practice to express your thoughts without feeling self-conscious about being judged by others. Take the advice of Alex Osborn, the originator of brainstorming, who once said that it is easier to tame down a wild idea than to invigorate a weak one. So respect whatever comes to mind during the Generating Phase.

Guidelines for Affirmative Judgment in the Focusing Phase

So often the word *judgment* brings to mind negative thoughts. Affirmative Judgment is more than considering the negatives. Affirmative Judgment directs your attention to the possible and the impossible aspects of the options. There are three guidelines in the Focusing Phase that are related to Affirmative Judgment.[14] The guidelines apply at all times and are deeply rooted values within CPS.

Guidelines for Affirmative Judgment

1. Consider all ideas.
2. Be deliberate and explicit.
3. Consider novelty.

Consider All Ideas

Consider, or contemplate, the possibles, the probables, and the impossible ideas. This first guideline reminds you to value all ideas at first. Sometimes it helps to rate the ideas on a "do-ability" scale that ranks them as possible (those having some potential), probable (under certain conditions, there's a chance that the idea might work), and impossible (no chance for the idea working because of limited resources, inadequate time, or inappropriate place). The "do-ability" of each idea depends on the available supports that allow it to become a reality. Consider what you like and what you think will result in a productive solution within the context of the situation.

REFLECTIVE JOURNAL ENTRY 2.5

Complete the following thought:

A wild idea that I thought would never work, but did, was the time I . . .

In addition to the possibles and the impossibles, consider the probable ideas. The "probables" are those ideas that might work under some, but not all, conditions. The "probable" ideas are too valuable to discard because you sense that you may use them in the future. Keep them for now if they have any chance of working; you can always discard them later if they turn out to be useless. The "probable" category gives you a place to store ideas. Listen to your intuitive self. It should always be a part of your decision making process.

Be Deliberate and Explicit

Carefully and clearly evaluate your ideas. Think through each idea and be able to explain the reasons you chose the idea. Hidden agendas and unspoken assumptions can force you to take dangerous detours. It's best to avoid "side trips." They will prevent you from reaching a solution farther down the road. Be honest with yourself. Ask yourself whether there are any hidden agendas, ulterior motives, or unspoken assumptions that are driving your thoughts toward the decision.

In each stage of CPS, Affirmative Judgment leads you to make effective decisions. Throughout CPS, you are striving to close the gap between what you know about the situation and where you plan to end up. Keep focused on your vision—your ultimate destination. Purposefully and clearly identify what is most important to you in making the decision. Prioritize your ideas. Think "first things first." When you apply Affirmative Judgment, what you value most becomes the criteria against which you begin to judge your ideas.

When you use Affirmative Judgment, explicitly define the criteria that you are using to choose your options. The criteria should be a balance between logical thought and your personal feelings and values. Use your head to ask yourself practical questions ("Do I need to do this to reach my goal?" "Is this a wish more than a need? Can I live without it and still reach my goal?"). Consult your heart to explore how you feel about the decision you are about to make ("Does this choice feel right?"). Be mindful. You may have a great idea, but that "great idea" may not be the better option for solving your problem under your particular set of circumstances.[15]

Consider Novelty

Value the originality and the appropriateness of each idea. Capitalize on the opportunity to select a new, never-done-before idea. Ask yourself whether the idea is appropriate within the context of the situation. Evaluate whether the idea fits the situation. Does the option have the power to move you closer to your solution? Appropriate ideas, like a compass on a ship, help you to stay on course and navigate toward a solution.

30   Unit I ◆ Learning About CPS

Novelty and appropriateness play active roles in CPS. Therefore, novelty and appropriateness are necessary criteria when using Affirmative Judgment in each stage of the process. Note how the guidelines are related in the two phases.

Rules of the Road and Guidelines in the Generating and Focusing Phases

Generating Phase ⟶
    Deferred Judgment

Guidelines:

1. Strive for quantity.
   + Hitchhike.
2. Stretch your mind.
   + Freewheel.

Focusing Phase ⟶
    Affirmative Judgment

Guidelines:

1. Consider all ideas.
2. Be deliberate and explicit.
3. Consider the novelty.

Create a Mind Map of Section

2

Mind Map Guidelines
1. Radiate ideas from the section's main concept.
   + Use images (be sure to use color).
   + Headline text—one or two words per line.
   + Print text (for easy reading).
2. Link the main concepts and generate more ideas from the linkages.
3. Have fun!

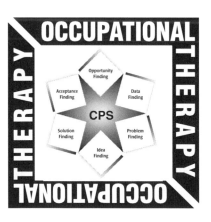

Section 2
SELF-ASSESSMENT

Now that I have completed the second part of my journey, I can:

○ explain the origin of Creative Problem Solving.

○ identify the three components and six stages of CPS.

○ explain how CPS and the occupational therapy process work together.

○ compare the Generating Phase with the Focusing Phase in CPS.

○ compare Deferred Judgment with Affirmative Judgment.

○ list two guidelines associated with Deferred Judgment.

○ list three guidelines associated with Affirmative Judgment.

NOTES

1. Scott Isaksen, K. B. Dorval, and Donald Treffinger, *Creative Approaches to Problem Solving* (Dubuque, Iowa: Kendall/Hunt, 1994).
2. Parnes noted that each stage of CPS should begin with an expansion of ideas—a diverging of one's thinking without evaluation—and conclude with a contraction phase, during which the most important data is organized into categories. Isaksen, Dorval, and Treffinger further refined the Osborn-Parnes CPS model. Their book *Creative Approaches to Problem Solving* provides an extensive history of CPS and the CPS model. Isaksen and Treffinger later added "Mess Finding," the component of CPS that targets the primary concern, challenge, or opportunity.
3. Alex Osborn, *Applied Imagination*, 3d ed. rev. (New York: Charles Scribner's Sons, 1963). Osborn is responsible for the inclusion of the word *brainstorming* in *Webster's International Dictionary*, with the definition: "To practice a conference technique by which a group attempts to find a solution for a specific problem by amassing all the ideas spontaneously contributed by its members" (151).
4. Ibid., 312.
5. Isaksen, Dorval, and Treffinger, *Creative Approaches to Problem Solving*. Get Ready to understand the problem, Get Set to find a solution, and Go Forward with an action plan are our conceptualization of CPS; we borrowed the phrase "understand the problem" from the Creative Problem Solving Group in Buffalo.
6. We changed the stage labeled Mess Finding by Isaksen and Treffinger to "Opportunity Finding" but retained its position in CPS.
7. Donald Treffinger, *Creative Problem Solving and School Improvement*, Idea Capsules (Sarasota, Fla.: Center for Creative Learning, 1996).
8. H. L. Hopkins, "Problem Solving," in H. L. Hopkins and H. D. Smith, eds., *Willard and Spackman's Occupational Therapy*, 8th ed. (Philadelphia, Pa.: Lippincott, 1993).
9. The names of the phases of CPS are referred to as Divergent and Convergent Phases. To clarify the actions taken in each phase, we changed the names of the phases to Generating and Focusing. The guidelines for thinking within each phase remain the same as those described by Isaksen, Dorval, and Treffinger.
10. Sidney Parnes, *Visionizing* (Buffalo, N.Y.: Creative Education Foundation Press, 1992).
11. R. Firestein and Donald Treffinger, "Ownership and Converging: Essential Ingredients of Creative Problem Solving," *Journal of Creative Behavior* 17, no. 1 (1983): 32–38.
12. These guidelines are an adaptation and consolidation of the guidelines originally described by Alex Osborn and most recently by Isaksen, Dorval, and Treffinger in *Creative Approaches to Problem Solving*.
13. Osborn, *Applied Imagination*, 124.
14. These guidelines are an adaptation and consolidation of the guidelines originally described by Osborn (in ibid.) and most recently by Isaksen, Dorval, and Treffinger, in *Creative Approaches to Problem Solving*.
15. S. Johnson, *"Yes" or "No": The Guide to Better Decisions* (New York: HarperCollins, 1992).

The Therapy Process Is Like Being on an Expedition

Itinerary #3

At the end of the third part of your journey, you will be able to:

✓ compare the therapy process to an expedition

✓ use the "What's Next? Question Series" Thinking Key to project a therapy idea into the future

✓ use the "If–Then" Thinking Key to create a hypothesis statement

✓ identify the mindset of a therapy guide

✓ use the "What If . . . ? Question Series" Thinking Key to anticipate possible outcomes

✓ explain how questions support a therapy guide's quest for knowledge

✓ use the "Stop, Drop, and Listen" Thinking Key to enhance your empathy

✓ use the "Watch for Cues and Look for Patterns" Thinking Key to analyze a story for relevant information

✓ explain why a therapy guide needs to understand paradigms

✓ use the "Consider Other Viewpoints" Thinking Key to reframe a problem

✓ use the "Think Positive" Thinking Key to frame a problem

✓ use the "What Paradigm Is Operating?" Thinking Key

✓ describe how intuition helps a therapy guide make decisions

The Therapy Process as an Expedition

As you travel through this field book learning thinking strategies to enhance your problem solving skills, you will find the route clear and predictable. On this kind of journey you know what to do and what to expect because of your previous experiences learning from a textbook.

There is a second kind of journey, however, in addition to the kind described above. This journey occurs each time you move through the therapy process with a client and his family. Unlike the first kind of journey, the outcome of the second kind is often difficult to predict because the journey takes place largely in unfamiliar territory—the territory of another person's life. The nature of this second kind of journey prompted our making an analogy to an expedition.

An expedition is a journey undertaken by a group of explorers into territory that is unknown or little known. The explorers are seeking knowledge about the natural features or the inhabitants of the territory. When you begin a therapy relationship with a client, you must also travel into territory that is full of unknowns. Your purpose for traveling, like that of the explorer on an expedition, is to learn about the lives of the people you encounter and the territory in which they live.

The more thoroughly you understand the unique aspects of a client's "life circumstance," the more effective you will be in helping her deal with the problem that initiated the referral to therapy. In this field book the therapy process is presented in the context of an expedition. We call this journey a therapy expedition. As you make your way through the therapy expeditions in this field book, you will use the occupational therapy (OT) process along with Creative Problem Solving (CPS) to direct your mental actions.

On a therapy expedition the therapist is a guide. Therefore, from this point forward, imagine yourself as a guide on a therapy expedition. As the expedition guide, you will prepare a map of the route you and the client will take. The goals and their related treatment plan are the map of the therapy process. You will use the "therapy map" to navigate the trip. This map will help you monitor where the client and the client's family are at any point along the expedition route.

To determine the best route to take, you must learn to consider all of the information about the client's problem and the context in which the problem occurs. The more proficient you become in seeing the therapy situation from the client's perspective the greater your potential of selecting a therapy route that will lead to an efficient and effective solution.

You will need to examine your thoughts and feelings to determine possible routes that you will travel. You need to delve into your intellectual consciousness to retrieve textbook and other fact-based information that pertains to the client's situation. You must also respect the feelings you have that reflect your personal beliefs and intuition about the client's life environment. Together, you and the client will decide on the destination of the therapy expedition. You will create a mental picture of the expedition route in as much detail as possible. As you consider whether the envisioned path is the most direct route, ask yourself the following questions:

1. In what ways will this expedition route meet the client's and his family's real need?
2. Am I keeping an open mind that will allow me to consider all of the options?
3. What patterns do I see in this current problem that match previous problems that required a creative solution?
4. In what ways can reflecting on previous problems give me confidence to pursue the route that I am about to take in the present expedition?

As you envision the expedition on which you and the client will embark, you can develop further insights about the effectiveness of your proposed solution. To do this, use the **"What's Next? Question Series" Thinking Key** to map a tentative direction. The "What's Next? Question Series" will help to gradually project your thoughts into the future state in which a therapy expedition "lives."[1]

Meet Jason, a nine-year-old child who receives therapy support services as part of his public school program. If Jason's therapy guide decides, for example, to carve a therapy expedition route that involves modifying the classroom's physical structure or educational program, she will ask What's Next? questions to extend her thinking to consider future possibilities for Jason.

Look at the "What's Next? Question Series" Field Organizer. Column A is a list of the therapy guide's thoughts as she considers different strategies or routes she might take on the expedition. In column B the question "What's next?" is asked for each of the strategies. Column C is a list of answers. Practice using the "What's Next? Question Series" Thinking Key.

DIRECTIONS

1. Read the proposed actions listed in column A, rows 1–4.
2. Ask the question "What's next?" (column B) for each of the actions.
3. In column C, rows 3–4, record an action that might follow from the question "What's next?" Note: Use rows 1–2 to model your responses.

FIELD ORGANIZER

"What's Next? Question Series"

A Describe one part of the therapy plan	B Ask "What's next?"	C Respond to the question "What's next?"
1. Move Jason's seat in his language arts class up to the front of the room where he is less likely to get distracted.	"What's next?"	Monitor whether Jason is less distracted and better able to pay attention when he sits in the front row.
2. Ask Jason to record his daily assignments in a simple school organizer and take it home for his parents to review and sign.	"What's next?"	Determine whether having Jason record his own daily class assignments results in his completing more assignments on time.
3. For one grading period ask Jason to use an electronic speller to decrease the number of spelling errors he makes on his writing assignments.	"What's next?"	
4. Seek permission for Jason to use a water bottle during class to help satisfy his need to suck on something more socially acceptable than his clothing.	"What's next?"	

Have you ever met someone whose thinking is so directed toward the details of an issue that he or she has difficulty seeing the whole picture? You may even have described this person as being unable "to see the forest for the trees." The "What's Next? Question Series" helps you see the forest, or the bigger picture. This Thinking Key helps you broaden your perspective on possible solutions to a problem. The broader your perspective on the problem, the better able you are to generate possible solutions, and the more likely you are to discover the most direct route from the starting point to the end point on your therapy map.

Using the data derived from the "What's Next? Question Series" Thinking Key, the therapist develops a hypothesis. A hypothesis is a forward projection based on some information known about a situation. To generate a hypothesis you will use the **"If–Then" Thinking Key**. The therapy guide working with Jason proposed that "If" Jason were seated in the front of the room, "Then" his on-task attending behaviors might improve. Practice using the "If–Then" Thinking Key with reference to Jason by completing the "If–Then" Field Organizer.

DIRECTIONS

1. Read the "If" portion of the hypotheses in column A, rows 1–4.
2. Complete the "Then" portion of the hypotheses in column B, rows 3–4. Note: Use rows 1–2 to model your responses.

FIELD ORGANIZER
"If–Then"

A IF . . .	B THEN . . .
1. **IF** Jason's desk were moved to the front of the room	**THEN** he might be more attentive to classroom lessons.
2. **IF** Jason used a simple school organizer to record his daily assignments	**THEN** he might be able to complete his assignments on time.
3. **IF** Jason used an electronic speller	**THEN**
4. **IF** Jason had permission to use a water bottle during class	**THEN**

The hypothesis (identified in the "If–Then" Field Organizer) guides the therapist's thinking as she develops her goals and designs the treatment program that supports the therapy process. When you form a hypothesis, you are projecting your thoughts into the future. Just as you learned to seek out background information about the client's past, you must learn to envision and project thoughts about the client's future. Background information provides you with a starting point from which to begin the therapy process. The hypothesis provides you with a "frame" to structure the forward thinking needed in generating the client's treatment goals and strategies.

The hypothesis helps you develop expectations about the client's performance. An expectation allows you to imagine a future outcome.[2] Your projection of the future is based on a combination of what you know of the situation and what you hope will be the outcome of the situation.[3] To make the expectation come true, therapists must structure the therapy process on an expedition as an unfolding narrative.[4] Thus a therapy expedition is a continuous process of developing one hypothesis after another. Through this continuous flow of hypothesis formation, you are developing one act after another. In a way, a therapy guide is like a playwright creating a script. The client is the "lead character" on the therapy expedition.

Mindset of a Therapy Guide

A therapy guide possesses certain qualities that allow him to structure an expedition as an unfolding narrative. These qualities create a mindset that helps her make a successful therapy expedition. Among these many qualities are five we highlight here: (1) tolerance for ambiguity, (2) willingness to take risks, (3) flexibility, (4) open-mindedness, and (5) empathy. The discussion will begin with the concept of a therapy guide's tolerance for ambiguity.

A Therapy Guide Is Tolerant of Ambiguity

On a therapy expedition there are frequently several solutions to a problem rather than one "best" solution. Consequently, a therapy guide must be able to tolerate ambiguity. Tolerating ambiguity means two things. First, the therapy guide accepts that there are several possible ways to view a problem. Second, she welcomes the opportunity to think through each aspect of the problem before deciding on a solution.

More than likely, at one time or another, you have had to make a decision that involved choosing from among several courses of action because there was not one clear choice. Before you made the decision in that situation, you had to deal with the ambiguity of having several choices that all looked good. Take a moment now to close your eyes and recall a time when you had to make one "best" choice from many "good" ones.

REFLECTIVE JOURNAL ENTRY 3.1

Complete the following thoughts:

1. The last time I can remember having to tolerate ambiguity was when . . .

2. I realized, after I made the decision (described in #1), that it was in my best interest to wait and think through every aspect of the situation before I made the decision because . . .

3. When I take the time to think a problem through I usually . . .

Use the **"What If . . . ? Question Series" Thinking Key** to help you think through some of the possible outcomes (to sort out the worst and best case scenarios) of a decision. Turn to the "What If . . . ? Question Series" Field Organizer. The series of questions and answers are related to Matt, an eight-year-old who attends Ms. Suthers' special education class every afternoon.

Matt is an active student who seems able to focus on his school work only when he is in motion. He's always jumping up to go to the pencil sharpener to sharpen his already sharp pencils. He makes so many trips to the wastepaper basket during the day that his teacher wonders whether he has any materials left in his desk to work on.

Practice using the "What If . . . ? Question Series" Thinking Key.

DIRECTIONS

1. Read column A, rows 1–4, to review the possible strategies the therapy guide plans to think through before speaking to Ms. Suthers.
2. Identify one possible outcome (worst or best case scenario) of the "What if . . . ?" statements in column A, rows 3–4, and record your responses in column B, rows 3–4. Note: Use rows 1–2 to model your responses.

A **What if . . .**	**B** **Describe a possible outcome**
1. Matt was permitted to have a work station in his classroom that permitted him to stand up to do some of his work?	Other children in the classroom might also want to stand; but if they really did not need to stand to complete their work, they might tire easy and want to sit down.
2. Matt sat on an air cushion on which he could move around while still being seated?	Other children might want to sit on the air cushion; but if they did not feel a need to move constantly, they might tire of the unstable surface.
3. a corner of the room was designated as the Energy Corner, where Matt and all his classmates could go throughout the day to do squats to either rev up or tone down their energy level?	
4. when Matt starts to get restless in the classroom, he could take a walk and simultaneously participate in a task that would engage his large muscles (e.g., transporting heavy bags of dictionaries to specified locations in the school)?	

The "What If . . . ? Question Series" Thinking Key can be used to think through all the ramifications and the possible consequences of an action during therapy. Asking the "What If . . . ? Question Series" helps the therapy guide envision future events. When you avoid looking for quick answers and instead stop and ask, "What if?" in an effort to expand your thoughts about the consequences of an action, you are developing your ability to tolerate ambiguity.

A Therapy Guide Is a Risk Taker

When a therapy-related problem lacks a definitive, clear-cut solution, the therapy guide must feel comfortable not having the one "right answer." The moment a therapy guide recognizes that there is no one right answer to the problem, he becomes a risk taker. A therapy guide must learn to be comfortable with risk taking. Thinking like an explorer can prepare you mentally to take risks. A therapy guide, like an explorer, thrives on discovery. Every therapy-related interaction challenges the guide to discover a way to solve the client's problem.

> ### REFLECTIVE JOURNAL ENTRY 3.2
>
> *Complete the following thoughts:*
>
> *1. The time I had to make a risky decision was when . . .*
>
> *2. At first, I doubted whether I was making the right choice because . . .*

3. I decided to take the risk because I had to . . .

4. The emotions I felt afterward were . . .

You may be thinking, "What if I take a risk on a therapy expedition and the decision I make is the wrong one?" The answer: You will never know unless you try it. Your results are your best teachers. Keep an inventory of your decisions. Journaling is one way to do this. Your journal will be your personal resource to guide your future decisions.

REFLECTIVE JOURNAL ENTRY 3.3

Complete the following thoughts:

1. The time I learned from a mistake was when . . .

2. Two things I learned from making the mistake described above were:

   a.

   b.

When you are about to take a risk and engage in a new, unfamiliar activity, you are moving close to the borders of your comfort zone. Your comfort zone is that intangible psychological area that represents the realm of the familiar. It is where you feel safe.[5] As you start to move out of your comfort zone, you may find internal warning signals "flashing" in an effort to stop your thoughts or actions. When you approach the edge of your comfort zone, the following thoughts may begin to fill your head: "You've gone too far. . . . It's time to back up. . . . You're making a fool of yourself. . . . Stop before you get yourself in trouble."

Therapy guides take necessary risks with confidence because they trust their intellect and their intuition. They have a sense of the limits when they are on a therapy expedition. They know how far to go, when to push the edges and when to pull back. Therapy guides, as risk takers, are motivated and equipped to master challenges as a part of their daily routine.

A Therapy Guide Is Flexible

To travel in unfamiliar territory, a therapist on a therapy expedition must be prepared to "shift gears" at any time. Shifting gears means that she is able to change her course of action whenever necessary to meet the demands of the situation.

For an example of a therapist with a flexible mindset, imagine the following scenario:

Ericka is a therapist who works in an early childhood school program. She is about to begin a gross motor group with the class. The children are seated on the floor around Ericka, and the record is positioned on the turntable, ready to play.

Just as Ericka reaches to turn on the record player, Sara jumps up and grabs the record off of the turntable. When Ericka asks Sara to hand her the record, the child defiantly smashes it on the floor, splintering it into multiple pieces. With the record unplayable, Ericka cannot continue her plan.

After dealing with disciplinary actions related to the breaking of the record, Erika shifts gears and quickly creates a new plan. Rather than provide music for a music movement group, she distributes the rhythm band instruments to half of the group, instructing them to play and instructing the remaining half of the group to move to the rhythm sounds created by their classmates.

Shifting gears requires a high degree of flexibility. Ericka's flexibility allows her to remain open to whatever events come along. In a therapist, flexibility is essential at all times because no matter how well you plan, when you travel on a therapy expedition, you will have to deal with the unexpected. The outcome of the trip is never guaranteed. Detours are inevitable. On a therapy expedition, the unexpected will occur. Furthermore, when dealing with people and their life issues, change is a constant.

Children, especially, need new equipment as they grow. In fact, children face new challenges with each stage of development. Solutions that worked one week may not work the next. In general, the younger the child, the quicker the change from week to week. Being flexible is at the core of a therapy guide's ability to manage creatively the challenge that change brings about. When you prepare yourself to expect change, you learn to value change as an opportunity rather than an obstacle. Therapy guides value change. They view it as a move forward.

REFLECTIVE JOURNAL ENTRY 3.4

Complete the following thoughts:

1. *The time I really looked forward to a situation changing was when . . .*

2. *The time I dreaded that a situation would change was when . . .*

3. *I rate my overall ability to deal with change as follows* (make a vertical mark across the line on the scale below to indicate how you rate your ability to deal with change):

   Low _____ *High*

4. *I am satisfied/dissatisfied* (circle one) *with my overall level of flexibility in most situations because . . .*

5. *Some things that I might do to increase my level of flexibility are . . .*

As a therapy guide you learn to recognize the "gaps" that change creates in a client's performance. A child, for instance, moves from one classroom to another, and the increased height of a toilet changes his level of independence. In his previous classroom he could perform his own toileting needs, but now the toilet is higher and interferes with his ability to be independent. Change in the child's classroom created a change in the child's level of independence. This change created a gap in the child's performance.

As a therapist, you are continuously recognizing gaps and creating strategies for closing the gaps between "what is" and "what should be" in the lives of the clients you serve. Flexibility allows you to develop strategies to close the gaps between the now in a client's life and a more productive future. Remaining flexible helps you view therapeutic problems as *challenges*. Viewing problems as challenges helps you, in turn, to generate solutions to those challenges.

A Therapy Guide Is Open-Minded

To therapy guides, problems are seen as challenges rather than roadblocks to understanding a situation. Thinking about problems as a challenge gives you the freedom to further explore in what ways you might understand a situation. Therapy guides learn to view problems as challenges by fostering a positive mindset. Thinking positively about a problem sparks the creative energy needed to meet the demands of the challenge by opening up your mind to value all kinds of options.

When you let go of the expectation that there is one right way to do things, you can learn to be open to solving problems many different ways. A therapy guide assumes a mindset of openness because there are few absolutes in therapy. No one treatment strategy works for everyone.

Roger von Oech, a business consultant who specializes in stimulating creativity in others, recommends looking beyond the "first right answer."[6] von Oech advises that when you focus your efforts on looking for more than one right answer you turn on your imagination. Imagination moves you.

Try your skill at being open to ideas beyond the obvious. Look at Figure 3.1 and ask yourself, "What is this a picture of?" Record your ideas in your Reflective Journal Entry 3.5.

Figure 3.1. *What Is This a Picture Of?*

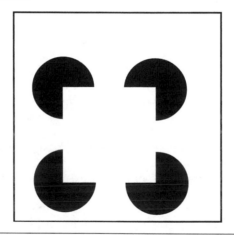

REFLECTIVE JOURNAL ENTRY 3.5

Complete the following thought:

I think Figure 3.1 is a picture of . . .

Perhaps you saw a square formed by the four black shapes. When you look again, can you see anything different? For example, can you see any of the following:

- Pac-man tag team
- two-legged animals with split hooves standing face to face
- chocolate sandwich cookies, each with a piece cut out
- four hungry circles

Keep an open mind and see how many other ways you can view Figure 3.1. Add your ideas to the list below. There are no wrong answers. Be wild; let yourself go.

What Is This a Picture Of?

1.
2.
3.
4.
5.

Beware of the Herculean influence your ego exerts on your thinking. Therapy guides need to remain open to new possibilities when helping a client solve problems. The ego protects your comfort zone and therefore has the power of setting up mental "roadblocks" to accepting new ideas. Be mindful that your ego can reject ideas even before they have a chance to be fully developed! So when you are on a therapy expedition be prepared to "set your ego aside for a moment [and] ask others what they [see]."[7] After listening to what they say, you can reflect on whether their insights might help you deepen your understanding of the situation to which you are seeking a solution.

Edward de Bono, a British educator who has written extensively on decision making, recommends that when one is involved in decision making, one should send the ego on a holiday. To ensure that the ego does not enter into the problem solving process, he created a system called "Six Thinking Hats."[8]

A Therapy Guide Is Empathetic

Empathy is the fifth and last quality of a therapy guide we highlight. We discuss empathy last because empathy weaves humanity through the other four special qualities of the therapy guide. When empathy becomes entwined with tolerance for ambiguity, willingness to take risks, flexibility, and open-mindedness, it adds richness, texture, and sensibility to the other qualities. Drawing on empathy allows a therapy guide to transform daily interactions with clients into a lifescape colored by the union of heart and mind.

Empathy is the foundation for developing caring, compassion, and altruism. Empathy allows you to see a situation from another person's perspective; it supports your ability to respect that person's feelings about the situation despite the differences in your perspectives. With empathy you are able to "hear" the feelings behind what another person says and to be attuned to how that person feels.

Empathy is rooted in self-awareness. Before you can be attuned to the needs of others, you must first be in touch with how you feel. The more you can identify feelings within yourself, the more you are able to sense the feelings of another person. And self-awareness is rooted in self-control, or the ability to manage your emotions. Thus, self-control leads to self-awareness and ultimately the ability to develop empathy.[9]

It is not enough only to read about empathy; you need to explore your own empathetic responses. To do so, you will enter the life story of people involved with the care of a child with special needs. You will imagine yourself "in the shoes" of the people you meet in a story entitled "The Other Side of the Mirror," and you will record your responses in a series of journal entries. The story, which appears below, was written by Mary Ann Gidewell, an occupational therapist and a parent of two children with special needs. Gidewell wrote the story because, in her words, "Perhaps my unique perspective of therapist and parent will assist other occupational therapists to better understand and help parents on the other side of the mirror."[10]

DIRECTIONS

1. Read the entire story, "The Other Side of the Mirror."
2. Continue on. You will find the story reprinted in sections. Each section is followed by a journal entry. For these journal entries, in contrast to those you have made so far, you will be asked to respond to the story from the perspective of one of the people in the story. For your convenience, the story is printed twice. The second copy of the story is interrupted by the journal entries.
3. Before making each journal entry, take a moment to prepare the mindset needed to "cross over" into the feelings of the person about whom you will be journaling. Each entry will cue you to do this.

The Other Side of the Mirror

Mary Ann Gidewell, OTR/L

Six-year-old Erik fell as he approached the school bus steps. He doubled over in pain and screamed as I gathered him into my arms.

"Do you want me to drive you to school?" I asked.

"No, mom," he insisted, "I *have* to catch my bus!"

I carried him over to his seat where his seven-year-old sister Elizabeth patted him and said, "I'll take care of him, Mom."

After stepping off the bus, I watched it rumble down the hill in the predawn light. My heart sank at the pain in Erik's knee and young life. He has cerebral palsy. He had stumbled over a tiny rock that a normal child could have ignored. His life, like the fall, has been a roller coaster of ups and downs.

Before starting a family, I worked as an occupational therapist and screened children for developmental delays. I prepared home programs, and treated or referred the patients to other professionals. Sometimes we used observation mirrors that allowed parents to watch sessions. At the time I wondered why parents reacted so differently to their child's problems. One mother told me, "Until it happens to you, you will never understand." She was right. It *did* happen to me. Now I *do* understand.

Two of my children have mild handicaps—mild when we seek services—significant when they compete with normal children. Our experiences are similar to other parents we've met with this problem. Perhaps my unique perspective of therapist and parent will assist other occupational therapists to better understand and help parents on the other side of the mirror.

When an occupational therapist encounters a new patient, he/she draws on previous textbook or clinical experience to prepare evaluations and treatments for that diagnosis. It may be her twentieth patient with such a problem. The therapist has the luxury of professional detachment: deal with the patient half an hour or less, observe, evaluate, record, plan, treat or refer but leave the other 10,050 minutes of weekly care to someone else. There's another patient waiting to be seen, and the therapist cannot emotionally handle the full-time, life-long burden of every patient.

The parents approached an initial conference quite differently. This is the *first* time for them. This is a crisis. Their reactions vary according to insight, background, onset and severity of the problem, prognosis, and information they already have. This is their little darling. They dreamed of him/her in their little hearts long before he

actually entered their lives. Although they realized he might not be a star athlete, they never expected real problems. Just having to go for developmental testing makes them ache with fear that something is terribly wrong.

Initially parents or professionals may deny that there is a problem. Unless the handicap is severe, developmental delays are discounted with an attitude, "The child will grow out of it." However, time becomes a cruel enemy as the baby cannot simply keep up with others its age. Fear of the unknown drives the parents into further denial, or to an endless quest to find help.

Once she suspects a problem, the mother focuses so on the child she begins to ignore her own health, appearances, housework, other children and spouse. When the father begins to realize the child is slow, he considers the long-term impact on the child, the family, and the budget. Depression, even blame, surround the family. Sleep patterns becomes erratic, and love-life becomes impaired or non-existent. The fear of the unknown becomes a chronic physical ache in the "gut."

When proper evaluations begin, the parents' reactions may seem inappropriate to the therapist. While she explains important facts, they listen between the lines and watch her non-verbal communications. They may prefer to hear results only from the physician. They even doubt the wisdom of selecting this doctor/clinic/therapist. If test reports are poor, they assume there's an error. In some cases, however the initial findings, whatever they are, bring great relief. At least the parents know they are not crazy—there really *is* a problem.

Parents of handicap children experience a chronic grief process. At first there is a tremendous shock and pain. They just want to hold the little guy and cry. Numbly they wonder what the future holds for their little one and for themselves. There is grieving for the normal child that "might have been." Guilt haunts the parents in many ways: Why did this happen to us? Are we being punished? Why didn't we see this problem earlier? Could we have helped him more? Could this have been prevented? Will it happen again?

Mom becomes over-protective: No one else understands my child; No one knows what this is doing to our family; There is no other person to trust for his care; The therapist just doesn't realize how smart he is. The parents, like two empty wells, reach for each other for comfort and emotional support. Dad may be overwhelmed, feeling emotionally inadequate and financially threatened.

(continued)

He may escape the pain by working longer hours. Some fathers, shaken that they may have produced something genetically defective leave the child and marriage altogether. The mother may face long hours of grief at home alone, or she may complicate her fatigue by placing the child with a baby-sitter and going to work.

Mom's personality changes in subtle ways that she doesn't even realize. The natural, protective drive to love and nurture her child becomes an all-consuming passion of a Mama Tiger fighting for her cub's life. If only she can find the right doctor, medicine, or therapy, then the baby will be normal. The search for answers begins as she gathers information from friends, professionals, articles, or books. Depending on findings and finances, the parents take the child from specialist to specialist. Determined to do all they can to help their child, they reason that his future depends on their effort alone. Mom feels, "If I don't fight, my child won't make it!" Health professionals dread to see Mom coming.

In a short while the parents become angry: Why didn't the doctor tell us sooner? Did the baby's delivery cause this? Who is to blame? Why can't my child get the help he needs? This anger may be directed against each other, towards medical personnel, school officials, family, neighbors, God, or even the child himself. It may be turned inward into a major depression.

By the time regular therapy sessions begins, the family has a small idea of the commitment ahead of them. Dad has to produce cash to cover costs, or must arrange for insurance or medical assistance. There are permission forms to complete, release of information data to compile. Mom must find baby-sitters for siblings (and cash to cover that cost), arrange for transportation, and bring reluctant little junior to a strange place during regular nap time. If mom is allowed to watch, she realizes how little the baby will actually do this for a stranger named a therapist. Sometimes she understands what the therapist is doing, but other times she is baffled. Finally Mom takes the home program for twenty goals, and drags the diaper, special equipment, stroller, screaming baby, and her broken heart home. There she looks over the list of technical jargon and tries to remember important instructions. Then she wonders if she will ever catch up on the housework and laundry.

The first time Mom tries the home program, her patient hates everything. His jealous siblings want equal time for each activity. By the time the multiple sessions are over it's time for dad's return home from work. He expected a reasonable meal, a peaceful home, and some appreciation for his hard day. Instead he finds piles of "therapeutic equipment," unfinished housework, grouchy kids, tired wife, and sandwiches. Mom feels the pressure,

"If I don't do the home program, the baby won't get better." Yet sometimes, after months of faithful working, there has been no improvement to encourage her daily efforts.

Another day, after struggling with exercise and dressing for over an hour, Mom takes the little ones shopping. Everyone stares at the baby's special equipment, reminding the parents, "this kid is different!" Perhaps the mother misunderstood instructions, or perhaps the splints actually don't work but cause blisters, and soon the equipment is forgotten. The child fought every time they were put on, and the parents couldn't see results anyway.

Eventually the child grows big enough to baffle even the experts on discipline. If his bites on neighborhood children have won him the name "Jaws," can he be held accountable? How much of this sweet child is medical, neurological, behavioral, emotional, developmental, normal child or just plain spoiled brat? His public tantrums or socially inappropriate behaviors humiliate and frighten his parents, who withdraw from society and stay home. Society is not as sympathetic if the handicap is invisible. The guilt for not doing enough, or doing too much, is continual.

Over time, the family encounters a new therapist every six months, several different physicians, painful medical tests, medications, hospitalizations (maybe surgery), and eventually school. The parents must communicate the child's medical history and needs to different professionals who, with varying points of view, might offer conflicting advice. Mom does not see official reports, and probably could not interpret the technical terminology. Yet she must stay alert for details like medical doses and legal rights at an IEP (Individualized Education Plan) Meeting.

School testing and placement can take up to a year to complete. Each school district within the county, state, or nation independently determines eligibility for services. If the family moves, they must begin the qualification process all over again. Middle-class children with mild handicaps may not be eligible for: special education programs; school therapies; government funding for private therapy; or third-party insurance reimbursement. Yet these children must compete with normal peers on state basic skills tests. The family must finance services on one income, since Mom is needed for the child's home therapy and educational programs. It may take Mom and Junior two or more hours to complete nightly homework, and then they face that occupational therapy home program with twenty goals.

Eventually the family must make a choice: to focus on the grief and suffering, or to accept their child's handicap as *part* of their lives. Acceptance does not mean that they like the handicap—deep inside they pray it will go away. This is not denial but hope. Parents have no road map with guarantees ahead. They simply want to do their best to help their little one reach his maximum potential. They begin to see him with all his wonderful possibilities, and even know joy as he accomplishes the impossible. Some days they almost believe life will be fine, and then a sudden medical crisis drags them down. Just when they feel utter despair, the child meets a goal and gives them thrilling new hope. The roller coaster of ups and downs will continue for the rest of their lives.

If they survive the stress, they try to see that other children with handicaps have a chance to make it, too.

Mary Ann Gidewell, "The Other Side of the Mirror," *Occupational Therapy Forum* 11, no. 11 (March 18, 1987): 1–6. Reprinted with permission.

The Other Side of the Mirror (with Journaling)

Six-year-old Erik fell as he approached the school bus steps. He doubled over in pain and screamed as I gathered him into my arms.

"Do you want me to drive you to school?" I asked.

"No, mom," he insisted, "I *have* to catch my bus!"

I carried him over to his seat where his seven-year-old sister Elizabeth patted him and said, "I'll take care of him, Mom."

REFLECTIVE JOURNAL ENTRY 3.6

Take a moment to cross over into Elizabeth's world. Imagine yourself as Elizabeth and complete the following thought:

As I sit here next to my brother, I feel . . .

Take a moment to cross over into Erik's world. Imagine yourself as Erik and complete the following thought:

As I sit here next to my sister, I feel . . .

After stepping off the bus, I watched it rumble down the hill in the predawn light. My heart sank at the pain in Erik's knee and young life. He has cerebral palsy. He had stumbled over a tiny rock that a normal child could have ignored. His life, like the fall, has been a roller coaster of ups and downs.

REFLECTIVE JOURNAL ENTRY 3.7

Take a moment to cross over into Mary Ann Gidewell's world. Imagine yourself as Mary Ann Gidewell and complete the following thought:

As I stand watching Erik and Elizabeth ride off to school, I feel . . .

Before starting a family, I worked as an occupational therapist and screened children for developmental delays. I prepared home programs, and treated or referred the patients to other professionals. Sometimes we used observation mirrors that allowed parents to watch sessions. At the time I wondered why parents reacted so differently to their child's problems. One mother told me, "Until it happens to you, you will never understand." She was right. It *did* happen to me. Now I *do* understand.

Two of my children have mild handicaps—mild when we seek services—significant when they compete with normal children. Our experiences are similar to other parents we've met with this problem. Perhaps my unique perspective of therapist and parent will assist other occupational therapists to better understand and help parents on the other side of the mirror.

When an occupational therapist encounters a new patient, he/she draws on previous textbook or clinical experience to prepare evaluations and treatments for that diagnosis. It may be her twentieth patient with such a problem. The therapist has the luxury of professional detachment: deal with the patient half an hour or less, observe, evaluate, record, plan, treat or refer but leave the other 10,050 minutes of weekly care to someone else. There's another patient waiting to be seen, and the therapist cannot emotionally handle the full-time, life-long burden of every patient.

REFLECTIVE JOURNAL ENTRY 3.8

Take a moment to cross over into the world of a therapist who is getting ready to see a new client while another one is also waiting to be seen for therapy. Imagine yourself as that therapist and complete the following thought:

As I prepare to see this new client for the first time, knowing that another client is waiting to be seen, I feel . . .

The parents approached an initial conference quite differently. This is the *first* time for them. This is a crisis. Their reactions vary according to insight, background, onset and severity of the problem, prognosis, and information they already have. This is their little darling. They dreamed of him/her in their little hearts long before he actually entered their lives. Although they realized he might not be a star athlete, they never expected real problems. Just having to go for developmental testing makes them ache with fear that something is terribly wrong.

REFLECTIVE JOURNAL ENTRY 3.9

Take a moment to cross over into the world of the parents of a child with special needs awaiting the initial evaluation of their child. Imagine yourself as one of those parents and complete the following thought:

As we prepare to see the therapist about our child for the first time, I feel . . .

Initially, parents or professionals may deny that there is a problem. Unless the handicap is severe, developmental delays are discounted with an attitude, "The child will grow out of it." However, time becomes a cruel enemy as the baby cannot simply keep up with others its age. Fear of the unknown drives the parents into further denial, or to an endless quest to find help.

Once she suspects a problem, the mother focuses so on the child she begins to ignore her own health, appearances, housework, other children and spouse. When the father begins to realize the child is slow, he considers the long-term impact on the child, the family, and the budget. Depression, even blame, surround the family. Sleep patterns becomes erratic, and love-life becomes impaired or non-existent. The fear of the unknown becomes a chronic physical ache in the "gut."

When proper evaluations begin, the parents' reactions may seem inappropriate to the therapist. While she explains important facts, they listen between the lines and watch her non-verbal communications. They may prefer to hear results only from the physician. They even doubt the wisdom of selecting this doctor/clinic/therapist. If test reports are poor, they assume there's an error. In some cases, however the initial findings, whatever they are, bring great relief. At least the parents know they are not crazy— there really *is* a problem.

Parents of handicap children experience a chronic grief process. At first there is a tremendous shock and pain. They just want to hold the little guy and cry. Numbly they wonder what the future holds for their little one and for themselves. There is grieving for the normal child that "might have been." Guilt haunts the parents in many ways: Why did this happen to us? Are we being punished? Why didn't we see this problem earlier? Could we have helped him more? Could this have been prevented? Will it happen again?

REFLECTIVE JOURNAL ENTRY 3.10

Take a moment to cross over into the world of the parents of a child with special needs feeling the grief of the normal child "that might have been." Imagine yourself as one of those parents and complete the following thought:

As I think about the normal child "that might have been," I feel . . .

Mom becomes over-protective: No one else understands my child; No one knows what this is doing to our family; There is no other person to trust for his care; The therapist just doesn't realize how smart he is. The parents, like two empty wells, reach for each other for comfort and emotional support. Dad may be overwhelmed, feeling emotionally inadequate and financially threatened. He may escape the pain by working longer hours. Some fathers, shaken that they may have produced something genetically defective leave the child and marriage altogether. The mother may face long hours of grief at home alone, or she may complicate her fatigue by placing the child with a baby-sitter and going to work.

Mom's personality changes in subtle ways that she doesn't even realize. The natural, protective drive to love and nurture her child becomes an all-consuming passion of a Mama Tiger fighting for her cub's life. If only she can find the right doctor, medicine, or therapy, then the baby will be normal. The search for answers begins as she gathers information from friends, professionals, articles, or books. Depending on findings and finances, the parents take the child from specialist to specialist. Determined to do all they can to help their child, they reason that his future depends on their effort alone. Mom feels, "If I don't fight, my child won't make it!" Health professionals dread to see Mom coming.

In a short while the parents become angry: Why didn't the doctor tell us sooner? Did the baby's delivery cause this? Who is to blame? Why can't my child get the help he needs? This anger may be directed against each other, towards medical personnel, school officials, family, neighbors, God, or even the child himself. It may be turned inward into a major depression.

By the time regular therapy sessions begins, the family has a small idea of the commitment ahead of them. Dad has to produce cash to cover costs, or must arrange for insurance or medical assistance. There are permission forms to complete, release of information data to compile. Mom must find baby-sitters for siblings (and cash to cover that cost), arrange for transportation, and bring reluctant little junior to a strange place during regular nap time. If mom is allowed to watch, she realizes how little the baby will actually do this for a stranger named a therapist. Sometimes she understands what the therapist is doing, but other times she is baffled. Finally Mom takes the home program for twenty goals, and drags the diaper, special equipment, stroller, screaming baby, and her broken heart home. There she looks over the list of technical jargon and tries to remember important instructions. Then she wonders if she will ever catch up on the housework and laundry.

REFLECTIVE JOURNAL ENTRY 3.11

Take a moment to cross over into the world of a mother of a child with special needs who is torn between trying to be cooperative with a therapist and feeling angry because she is not seeing "results" from the therapy program. Imagine yourself as that mother and complete the following thought:

After so many months, I wonder whether therapy is making a difference. I feel . . .

The first time Mom tries the home program, her patient hates everything. His jealous siblings want equal time for each activity. By the time the multiple sessions are over it's time for dad's return home from work. He expected a reasonable meal, a peaceful home, and some appreciation for his hard day. Instead he finds piles of "therapeutic equipment," unfinished housework, grouchy kids, tired wife, and sandwiches. Mom feels the pressure, "If I don't do the home program, the baby won't get better." Yet sometimes, after months of faithful working, there has been no improvement to encourage her daily efforts.

Another day, after struggling with exercise and dressing for over an hour, Mom takes the little ones shopping. Everyone stares at the baby's special equipment, reminding the parents, "this kid is different!" Perhaps the mother misunderstood instructions, or perhaps the splints actually don't work but cause blisters, and soon the equipment is forgotten. The child fought every time they were put on, and the parents couldn't see results anyway.

REFLECTIVE JOURNAL ENTRY 3.12

Take a moment to cross over into the world of a mother or father of a child with special needs who feels the stares of people whenever they are out in public. Imagine yourself as that parent and complete the following thought:

When my child and I are out in public, all the stares make me feel . . .

Eventually the child grows big enough to baffle even the experts on discipline. If his bites on neighborhood children have won him the name "Jaws," can he be held accountable? How much of this sweet child is medical, neurological, behavioral, emotional, developmental, normal child or just plain spoiled brat? His public tantrums or socially inappropriate behaviors humiliate and frighten his parents, who withdraw from society and stay home. Society is not as sympathetic if the handicap is invisible. The guilt for not doing enough, or doing too much, is continual.

Over time, the family encounters a new therapist every six months, several different physicians, painful medical tests, medications, hospitalizations (maybe surgery), and eventually school. The parents must communicate the child's medical history and needs to different professionals who, with varying points of view, might offer conflicting advice. Mom does not see official reports, and probably could not interpret the technical terminology. Yet she must stay alert for details like medical doses and legal rights at an IEP (Individualized Education Plan) Meeting.

School testing and placement can take up to a year to complete. Each school district within the county, state, or nation independently determines eligibility for services. If the family moves, they must begin the qualification process all over again. Middle-class children with mild handicaps may not be eligible for: special education programs; school therapies; government funding for private therapy; or third-party insurance reimbursement. Yet these children must compete with normal peers on state basic skills tests. The family must finance services on one income, since Mom is needed for the child's home therapy and educational programs. It may take Mom and Junior two or more hours to complete nightly homework, and then they face that occupational therapy home program with twenty goals.

Eventually the family must make a choice: to focus on the grief and suffering, or to accept their child's handicap as *part* of their lives. Acceptance dose not mean that they like the handicap—deep inside they pray it will go away. This is not denial but hope. Parents have no road map with guarantees ahead. They simply want to do their best to help their little one reach his maximum potential. They begin to see him with all his wonderful possibilities, and even know joy as he accomplishes the impossible. Some days they almost believe life will be fine, and then a sudden medical crisis drags them down. Just when they feel utter despair, the child meets a goal and gives them thrilling new hope. The roller coaster of ups and downs will continue for the rest of their lives.

If they survive the stress, they try to see that other children with handicaps have a chance to make it, too. The End.

A therapist who is able to cross over to the other side of the mirror—to use Gidewell's metaphor—has developed an ability to empathize with another human being. To review:

Special Qualities of a Therapy Guide

Tolerance for ambiguity

Willingness to take risks

Flexibility

Open-mindedness

Empathy

How Questions Support a Therapy Guide's Quest for Knowledge

As a therapy guide you will be traveling in the Land of Other Peoples' Life Stories. Because the territory is unfamiliar to you, you need to ask the children and families and caregivers with whom you work what they expect from the therapy process. The clearer you are about what a client wants, the more effective you will be in delivering therapy services. Asking questions is an integral part of a therapy guide's job. The word *question* comes from the Latin *quaerere*, meaning "to seek." This is the same root as for the word for *quest*. The therapy guide is on one continuous quest for information.

A therapy guide recognizes that people have their own travel plans. Like a trustworthy guide who is there for the sole benefit of the traveler, you know that you are providing services that help people get to where they want to go. In your quest for information, you need to ask them *what* the problem is, *how* the problem affects them, *when* do they experience the problem, *where* do they have the problem, and *why* are they concerned about the problem. You also need to ask in *what ways* might their problem be solved and in *what ways* would they like you to help them.

Therapists help people solve their problems. To help a client solve her problem you must be curious and ask many questions. Questions will help you gather the information you need to define the problem. The more explicitly you can define the problem, the closer you will be to finding a solution.

An effective way to gather information about a client's problem is to ask open-ended questions. Open-ended questions are structured so that one cannot answer them with a simple yes or no. In contrast, closed questions are so structured that one can answer only yes or no. Open-ended questions result in answers that are richer than yes or no. Open-ended questions, such as those that begin, "In what ways might you . . ." set the stage for a whole range of possible responses. The answers you receive from asking open-ended questions will bring you closer to helping a client solve his problem. Follow inventor Buckminster Fuller's advice to "dare to be naive," and you will be asking a good question.

Use the Open-Ended Questions Worksheet to practice formulating open-ended questions by rephrasing closed questions.

DIRECTIONS

1. Read the closed questions in column A.
2. For every closed question, create one or more open-ended questions and write them in column B. Note: Use rows 1–2 to model your responses. See whether you can generate additional open-ended questions for rows 1–2.
3. After you complete the worksheet, compare your open-ended questions with those created by a traveling companion. You will see that there are many ways to restate each of the closed questions.

Open-Ended Questions Worksheet

A Closed Questions	B Open-Ended Questions
1. Does Keiko play with toys?	*How would you describe Keiko's play behavior?*
2. Will Nathan feed himself?	*How much help does Nathan need when eating?*
3. Does Shondra dress herself?	
4. Can you bring Tasha to therapy on Tuesdays?	
5. Does Kendall like to play with blocks?	

Open-Ended Questions Worksheet (Continued)

A Closed Questions	B Open-Ended Questions
6. Does Latifah participate in after-school extra-curricular activities?	
7. Has Alexis been introduced to computers yet?	
8. Does Majid complete all of his homework assignments?	
9. Do you assign Marcus household chores?	
10. Does Jacques freely express his emotions?	

The way you ask questions, as well as the sensitivity with which you listen as the client responds, can either help you build a relationship or put distance between you and those with whom you interact. You develop skill at asking questions when you learn to balance your knowledge about a person with your *respect* for that person. The person comes to you with his "life territory." By asking questions that reflect your admiration and esteem for the person's life territory, you can discover important information.

Listening to a person's story with respect and an open mind allows you to learn about the person's values, interests, and aspirations. You gain insights about the person beyond what you could ever read in a medical chart or school record. Respectfully asking questions allows you to enter the person's life story. When you enter someone else's life story, you begin to understand what is important to that person and through this understanding you, the therapist, begin to build a relationship with the client. The relationship or bond that you form with the client has a powerful influence throughout the therapy expedition.

Whatever the age and the level of understanding of the client, the client side of therapist-client relationship should include both the client and the family or primary caregiver.

REFLECTIVE JOURNAL ENTRY 3.15

Reflect on the bond you have with a close friend or relative. Consider how you demonstrate mutual respect and complete the following thought:

1. We demonstrate mutual respect by . . .

Reflect on those times when your viewpoints are incompatible with those of the person referred to above. Reflect on whether, when you talk through your differences with this person you think about how you will discuss your differences and how you will phrase questions. Then complete the following thought:

2. When I am discussing differences with _____ (name), I . . .

Reflect on how effective your questions are in helping you deal with or resolve your differences with the person referred to above. Then complete the following thought:

3. Generally the way I phrase questions . . .

Occupational therapy has been called a "reflective practice."[11] As an occupational therapist you learn to reflect on the life stories of the clients with whom you work. When you reflect on a person's life story, you ponder it, you turn the story around in your mind, you contemplate each element deeply and thoroughly. As you reflect, you compare the elements of the client's life with your personal inventory of values, beliefs, and knowledge. You look at the client's life from many different perspectives. Reflecting helps you stay on course throughout a therapy expedition by strengthening your respect for the context of a client's life.

The questions that you ask on a therapy expedition can be a gift to the person to whom the question is being asked. When you ask questions with thoughtfulness and empathy, you can show the client that you care about her and are genuinely interested in what she has to say. Supportive and artfully worded questions can dynamically build relationships.

To ask questions that expand rather than distance a relationship, a therapy guide draws on his ability to empathize. The **"Stop, Drop, and Listen" Thinking Key** can help you develop your ability to empathize. Before practicing the "Stop, Drop, and Listen" Thinking Key, let's explore the use of each term in this key, beginning with Stop.

The Stop in "Stop, Drop, and Listen" means that when you are inquiring about a client's problem, you must stop and be fully present. The quality of the therapy expedition depends on your ability to stop and give your complete attention to the situation. But coming to a full stop does not necessarily mean physically stopping. It means stopping your thoughts to clear your mind so that you can take in new information. "The power of a clear mind is beyond description."[12]

REFLECTIVE JOURNAL ENTRY 3.16

Complete the following thoughts:

1. *When I am talking to someone and I know that the person is not paying complete attention to me, I feel . . .*

2. *When I fail to give my complete attention to another person, I imagine the other person feels . . .*

When you are working with one client and your mind is filled with thoughts about a different client or a personal situation such as your plans to get your tire changed after work or whether you remembered to take the chicken out of the freezer to defrost, it is difficult to absorb new information. If your attention is not focused on the outcome of the situation with the client, you will compromise the natural flow of the therapeutic process. But if you come to the therapeutic relationship with a clear mind, you will enhance the therapeutic process.

The Drop in "Stop, Drop, and Listen" has a figurative meaning. To develop your ability to empathize, you have to be willing to drop (or suspend) your point of view and begin to see the problem from the client's point of view. The importance of dropping your opinions in order to gain new insights is illustrated in the following story about a Japanese Zen master who received a college professor wishing to learn about Zen practices.

> It was obvious to the master from the start of the conversation that the professor was not so much interested in learning about Zen as he was in impressing the master with his own opinions and knowledge. The master listened patiently and finally suggested they have tea. The master poured his visitor's cup full and then kept pouring.
>
> The professor watched the cup overflowing until he could no longer restrain himself [and said,] "The cup is overfull, no more will go in."
>
> "Like this cup," the master said, "you are full of your own opinions and speculations. How can I show you Zen unless you first empty your cup?"[13]

This story illustrates the paradox that you must empty your "cup" of preconceived notions in order to see things anew. So is the case in any therapeutic interaction. Until you empty your cup of the past, or at least pour a little out to receive new information, you will be unable to receive any new perspectives. Information that clients give you will simply overflow the cup because it will have nowhere else to go.

REFLECTIVE JOURNAL ENTRY 3.17

Complete the following thoughts:

1. *The time I was in a conversation with someone who did not seem open to what I was saying, I felt . . .*

2. *If I don't hear what other people are saying, it is usually because I . . .*

The listen in "Stop, Drop, and Listen" means that you must do more than hear. When you are busy thinking, seeing, or saying something from your perspective, you are not listening to what another person is saying to you. A therapy guide knows that the success of an expedition is greatly influenced by her ability to listen, not just hear.

If you have ever read a familiar story to a child and tried to either take a short cut or simply miss a part, you may have found the child quick to correct the "mistake." The child is listening so closely to the story that the omission is obvious. In order to foster an optimal relationship with a client, a therapy guide needs to listen to the client's story with the intensity of a child listening to a favorite story.

When you are really listening to what the client is saying, you can hear the words as well as what is being said between the words. Read "Bradley's Story" and practice listening. Listen to what Bradley, his mother, and his teacher, Ms. Cook, are saying. Listen also for what messages are embedded deep in each person's reaction to the situation.

Bradley's Story

Bradley, a four-year-old child, was leaving home for school at his community Early Childhood Program. He was wearing his hat and coat, his book bag was slung over his shoulder, and his favorite Power Ranger miniature doll was tightly clenched in the palm of one hand. Bradley always felt more confident leaving home when he could hold something from home, usually a small, plastic object, in his hand.

Bradley's mother knew, from previous discussions with Bradley's teacher, Ms. Cook, that Ms. Cook did not like having students bring toys from home to school. But because she wanted to send Bradley to school feeling secure, she told him he could carry the small object.

When Bradley arrived at school, Ms. Cook said to him, "You must keep your toy in your book bag. You may take it home with you. At school, we have a lot of other fun toys for you to play with."

Bradley refused to give up the small object. He continued to clutch the toy as tightly as he was able to in his left hand. When his teacher approached, Bradley started to scream, "No . . . no . . . no!" then flung himself face down on the floor in front of the teacher, kicking and continuing to scream, "No . . . no . . . no!"

Who is correct? Bradley's mother, who chose to send him to school with the toy to help him feel secure? Or Ms. Cook, who wanted Bradley to play with the toys at school? Use the

"Stop, Drop, and Listen" Field Organizer to reflect on Bradley's situation. You will need to "read between the lines" to complete column C.

DIRECTIONS

1. Read column A to recall who said what in "Bradley's Story."
2. In column B, record any preconceived assumptions that you may have about the comments in column A, rows 2–3. Note: Use row 1 to model your responses.
3. In column C, rows 2–3, describe your *perception* of what Ms. Cook and Bradley were really saying in column A. Note: Use row 1 to model your responses.

FIELD ORGANIZER

"Stop, Drop, and Listen"

A WHO said WHAT?	B Assumption to Be Dropped	C Behind these words or actions the person is saying . . .
1. Bradley's <u>mother</u> told him he could take his toy from home to school.	Bradley's mother is uncooperative and does not respect the rules of the school.	I know from working closely with an occupational therapist that Bradley feels more secure and better able to make the transition from home to the bus and then into school when he is allowed to hold a favorite toy from home. I know that if Bradley is not permitted to carry his toy, he will get very upset and everyone will suffer.
2. <u>Ms. Cook</u> said she does not like having students bring toys from home to school.		
3. <u>Bradley</u>, kicking, screamed, "No . . . no . . . no!"		

As a therapy guide heeds the call to "Stop, Drop, and Listen," she has prepared her mind to watch for cues. On a therapy expedition the therapy guide uncovers relevant information. Each piece of relevant information is a cue.[14] Cues help the guide understand the client and the client's life situation that initiated the referral to occupational therapy. You will use the **"Watch for Cues and Look for Patterns" Thinking Key** along with the "Stop, Drop, and Listen" Thinking Key.

A cue is like one piece of a jigsaw puzzle. Just as each puzzle piece is a small part of the total picture of the completed puzzle, a cue is a small part of the client's life circumstances. With a puzzle, the number of pieces is finite, and you have an opportunity to see the completed picture. In a therapist-client relationship, however, you can never view the client's complete life circumstances. The client's life, unlike the static design of a puzzle, continues to evolve and develop. And therefore, your search for cues continues throughout the therapist-client relationship.

Even though you continually search for cues, recognizing cues is not enough. You still will not have the total picture. To come closer to identifying the whole picture, you need to look for relationships between the cues. As you begin to see how cues relate to one another, patterns will emerge. Because the human mind is programmed to recognize patterns you will begin to visualize the whole picture from just a few parts.[15] And just as when you assemble a puzzle, finding adjacent pieces expands or broadens your ability to understand the whole picture. So, too, the more cues you can assemble into patterns, the more accurately you can use patterns to develop goals and treatment during a therapy expedition.

To understand the relationship between cues and the recognition of patterns, consider the following comment by a therapist whose client is a child named Sandra: "From my observations of Sandra on the playground, I conclude that she has high muscle tone on the right side of her body."

Why did the therapist feel that Sandra had high muscle tone even before he had examined her? As the therapist observed Sandra run on the playground, something about the way Sandra moved triggered the therapist to think that "something didn't look right." Out of the quick, initial observation of Sandra emerged Cue #1—Sandra displays abnormal movement patterns. The therapist's thought that followed Cue #1 was, "What looks different?" The answer to the question became Cue #2—Sandra's right arm and leg are held in a fixed position.

By connecting Cue #1 and Cue #2 with what he knew about movement disorders, the therapist started to form an opinion about Sandra's muscle tone. His opinion about muscle tone was a compilation of previous knowledge about diagnostic categories combined with kinesiology, anatomy, and physiology. Although the diagnosis and the client's history are not a central focus of occupational therapy, knowledge of the medical condition can direct your thinking toward recognizing patterns from identified cues.[16]

Use the "Watch for Cues and Look for Patterns" Field Organizer to help you understand the client's problem in the story about a boy named Gregory. The directions are in two parts.

DIRECTIONS

1. Read the story "One Morning in the Life of Gregory."
2. Next, reread the story with a highlighter pen and mark all the cues that are relevant to understanding Gregory's behavior.
3. Turn to the "Watch for Cues and Look for Patterns" Field Organizer. Begin with "Part I: Cues." Compare the cues you highlighted in the story with those listed in column A.
4. In column B, row 5, describe your perception of the cue in terms of its relevance to you as a therapy guide. Note: Use rows 1–4 to model your responses.
5. Turn to "Part II: Patterns" and read the pattern in row 1. Look for patterns among the cues you highlighted in the story and record the patterns in rows 2–5. Note: Use the pattern in row 1 to model your responses.

One Morning in the Life of Gregory

Gregory is a quiet, polite four-year-old who attends an Early Childhood Program in a suburb of a large city. He seems to enjoy school. Although he usually rushes to be the first one in line, Gregory waits for the teacher to lead the group of children from the bus into the school. On most days, he eagerly participates in all activities with his classmates.

One day in late April, Gregory hurriedly climbs down the steps of the school bus. He runs into the school, breaking away from the group of his classmates and his teacher. Upon entering the classroom, Gregory rushes over to the play area.

"Gregory, hang up your jacket, and your book bag. Then you may play," Ms. Black, the classroom aide said, using a firm, directive voice.

"No!" Gregory shouts defiantly, as he stomps toward the sandbox in the far corner of the classroom.

FIELD ORGANIZER

"Watch for Cues and Look for Patterns"

A Cue	B What might this cue mean?
Part I: Cues	
1. Gregory is a quiet child.	Gregory might be a quiet, calm child, or perhaps he is less active because he processes information more slowly than his classmates. I wonder how much initiative he demonstrates when involved in a new activity and how quickly he interacts with the rest of the class. Does he need prodding? Does he ask questions when he doesn't understand something? Or does he watch what his classmates do before performing?
2. He waits for the teacher to lead the group into school.	Gregory is an obedient child who follows directions. I wonder whether he has been disciplined for breaking away from the group and running into the building.
3. He eagerly participates in all classroom activities.	He seems to enjoy school. I wonder whether he is always so compliant.
4. One day, instead of waiting for his class to enter the school, he breaks away from the group.	I wonder what happened at home today. Or was he running away from one of the children on the bus? Or was he so excited that he couldn't wait to tell the classroom staff something? Whatever the cause, this was a dramatic change in his behavior from the quiet demeanor he displays on most days.
5. Gregory shouts "No!" at the classroom aide after she directs him to hang up his jacket and his book bag.	

Part II: Patterns

1. Gregory is quiet, likes school, waits for teacher to lead children into school after arriving on the bus and eagerly participates in activities.

2.

Through the recognition of patterns, you begin to identify similarities in and differences between situations. You also begin to develop insights about what is possible within a particular situation.[17] Therapy guides who work with children with special needs deal with possibilities related to two challenges: They need to (1) recognize cues to help them make decisions that will enhance the child's ability to function "today" and (2) understand how the cues of today will influence the child's functional performance "tomorrow."

"Tomorrow" can be the next day, the next year, or the next five years. The definition of "tomorrow" depends on the child's age and rate of growth and development.

How does a therapy guide meet these challenges? A therapy guide tries to understand the clients and families with whom he works through each client's life story. Since each client's life is unique, each decision must be unique. How, then, does a therapy guide determine which route is best for any particular client? Traditional educational systems teach students to look for the one "right answer." However, therapy guides who lead successful therapy expeditions learn to recognize many possible routes when mapping out the travel plan.

Your perceptions of the client's life story become your understanding of the truths within the situation. The phenomenon of how your perspective shapes your perception is illustrated in the following ancient Chinese story.

> Hui-tse said to Chuang-tse, "I have a large tree which no carpenter can cut into lumber. Its branches and trunk are crooked and tough, covered with bumps and depressions. No builder would turn his head to look at it." . . .
>
> Chuang-tse replied, "You complain that your tree is not valuable as lumber. But you could make use of the shade it provides, rest under its sheltering branches, and stroll beneath it, admiring its character and appearance. Since it would not be endangered by an axe, what could threaten its existence? It is useless to you only because you want to make it into something else and do not use it in its proper way."[18]

Hui-tse could not see any usefulness in the tree, while Chuang-tse saw the value of the tree because he viewed the tree from a different perspective. Therapy guides, like Chuang-tse, look beyond the boundaries established by their own perspective. Therapy guides stop, drop, and listen in order to understand the essence of what they see, hear, and feel. And because they know that appearances can at times be deceiving, as in the story of the tree, they listen for the message that may at times lie below the surface. Therapy guides actively search beyond the boundaries of their own perspective.

Understanding Paradigms

Each of us lives within psychological boundaries that frame the way we think and act as we go about our daily lives. The boundaries are formed by our values. Our values are those subjective bits of knowledge and feelings on which we base assumptions. Another name for a psychological boundary is *paradigm* (pronounced pair-a-dime).[19] Paradigms are responsible for shaping and defining our perceptions.

Let's begin to explore how paradigms influence our perception by considering the following scenario. Imagine for a moment that you and a roommate have returned home from attending your high school reunion. You had a wonderful time. You enjoyed the surf-and-turf entrée and visited with old friends you had not seen in years. Your roommate, however, does not like large gatherings and attended the affair only out of a sense of obligation to you. Your roommate is a vegetarian, and so she had ordered a special menu in advance. Her plate arrived late, when everyone else was halfway through the meal.

In the scenario, you and your roommate were operating under very different paradigms. And because of those differences, your perspectives of the alumni event were very different. Now consider a real experience you have had.

REFLECTIVE JOURNAL ENTRY 3.18

Complete the following thoughts:

1. *A time when I remember learning that my perception of a particular event was very different from someone else's was . . .*

(continued)

2. My personal paradigm filtered my perception of the event by . . .

3. In retrospect, I might have broadened my perspective of the event had I . . .

When a therapist works with a client to increase his function, the therapist needs to recognize the client's psychological boundaries or paradigms. Understanding the concept of paradigms is important to therapy decision making because at various times, you may be guiding clients toward making decisions that are beyond their paradigms. Therefore, to help a client search beyond his own paradigms, you must first understand your own paradigms. Understanding the limits of your paradigms will enhance your effectiveness as a therapy guide.

The word *paradigm* comes from the Greek root *paradeigma*, meaning "model, or pattern." In current jargon, paradigm refers to the rules and regulations that make up your mental model of the world.[20] Your paradigms include the beliefs that govern your thoughts on the rightness and wrongness of a given situation. You use your paradigms to navigate through every day of your life.

The recreational games you play are governed by paradigms. If you are wondering, "How do recreational games fit into this discussion about paradigms?" think about all of the games you have played since you were a young child. Each one had a set of rules. Once you learned the rules, you understood how to play the game. The rules established the boundaries—the paradigm. They told you "what to do to be successful within those boundaries."[21]

Imagine you are with a group of friends who begin playing a game for which you have no prior knowledge. Since you do not know the rules, you lack the mental model necessary to play the game and consequently decide to observe from the sidelines. If you closely watch those playing the game and ask questions, most likely within a short time you would pick up patterns that would reveal the rules that are operating. Games provide a useful analogy for understanding paradigms. They are played according to rules, and rules reflect the need for boundaries to help you determine whether you are playing the "right way." In life rules are established by a set of paradigms. Those rules can be such things as dress codes, waiters' expectations of receiving tips, your habit of making your bed before leaving the house, or any number of other invisible, yet powerful rules that guide your life actions. Paradigms are like the air you breathe. And like the act of breathing, you rarely give much thought to what paradigms are directing your thinking.

Another useful anology for understanding paradigms is to think of them as a pair of sunglasses through which you view the world. If you have ever worn tinted lenses for a while, you know that when you remove them, everything looks slightly different until your unshaded eyes readjust to the light. Paradigms, like wearing sunglasses, become the accepted way to view the world.

Paradigms shape history. Recall the time when people's lives were bound by the paradigm that the earth was flat. Columbus challenged the flat earth paradigm by setting sail to India. According to another paradigm, the *Titanic* was unsinkable. Because of this paradigm, life boats were not supplied for all the people on the boat and hundreds drowned. Paradigms are so powerful, they can even influence people's thinking in matters of life and death.

You use your paradigms to explain the "world" to yourself as you perceive it. This world is your personal, individual reality. Problems can occur when one person's paradigm clashes with another person's paradigm. Consider the following scenario.

Your friend invites you for the first time to a brunch at a local country club. He adds that dress is casual. You put on your new jeans and sweater (your paradigm for casual dress). You feel confident that you look sharp as you drive up to the front door of the club. But, when you arrive at the brunch, you realize that you are the only guest wearing denim; you later learn that the country club has a dress code prohibiting its members or any guests from wearing any form of denim (the country club manager's paradigm). Your friend assumed that you knew not to wear jeans.

Your paradigm for casual dress was a mismatch for the prevailing one at the country club. Behaving according to your paradigm caused a problem for your friend whose paradigm was different from yours; he's the one who received the reprimand from the country club manager for not informing his guest about the proper restaurant attire.

As this scenario illustrates, paradigms are rules to live by. They are different for all of us. They shape, and are shaped by, our principles, routines, values, assumptions, traditions, and customs. And because paradigms vary from one person to another, perceptions and viewpoints vary from one person to another. Hence, there is almost always more than one right answer when solving problems. The parent or the caregiver of the child with whom you are working may shift your paradigm or perception of how a problem might be solved. Changing or shifting a paradigm alters perceptions. A paradigm shift occurs when there is a change to a new set of rules that drive one's perceptions and performance within a given situation.

In the following activity, explore in what ways your paradigms influence your daily decisions.

DIRECTIONS

1. In column A, list activities that are influenced by your paradigms. Note: Use rows 1–5 to model your responses.
2. In column B, record the origin of each paradigm listed in column A. Remember that paradigms operate on such an automatic level it may take several minutes of deep thinking to bring them to the surface. Note: Use rows 1–2 to model your responses.

Daily Activities Influenced by My Paradigms Worksheet

| A
Daily Activity | B
The paradigm for this activity originated from . . . |
| --- | --- |
| 1. How I manage my money | the habits I formed as a child when I received an allowance. |
| 2. How I clean my living space | watching my mother clean the house. |
| 3. The type of clothing and jewelry I wear | |
| 4. What kind of music I prefer to listen to | |
| 5. The way I fold laundry | |

Review your responses in columns A and B. Reflect on the origin of your responses and complete Reflective Journal Entry 3.19.

> **REFLECTIVE JOURNAL ENTRY 3.19**
>
> *Complete the following thoughts:*
>
> *1. When I review the list of my paradigms, I realize that in large part they originated from . . .*
>
> *2. The influence of my family on the development of my paradigms was . . .*
>
> *3. The influence of my peers and friends on the development of my paradigms was . . .*

Effective therapy guides are able to recognize their own paradigms. They are aware of the impact these paradigms have on their thinking and decision making. Read through the list of characteristics of paradigms. When you can identify your own paradigms, you will recognize the rules that influence your decision making. The more clearly you are able to define your personal paradigms, the better able you will be to identify the paradigms of others.[22]

Characteristics of Paradigms

◆ **Paradigms are common to the "community."** Certain rules provide the discipline in which all activity occurs; the operating paradigms direct all behavior, including the way problems are solved. There are set standards that give the practitioner a special vision, understanding, and specific methods for solving problems.

◆ **Paradigms are functional.** They are necessary rules that maintain order in a complex world; without paradigms we would live in chaos.

◆ **Paradigms can reverse the common sense relationship between seeing and believing.** Our realities of what we sense (see, hear, feel) are defined by our paradigms.

◆ **There is almost always more than one right paradigm.** Changing your paradigm changes your perception. Each individual paradigm provides access to different sets of information; each set of information has different, yet correct explanations of what is happening within the particular situation.

◆ **When paradigms are held too strongly, they can lead to "paradigm paralysis," a terminal disease of certainty.** Paradigm paralysis occurs when one's thinking patterns become entrenched in mental models; one's paradigm is so strong that it becomes the only way to frame information.

◆ **"Paradigm pliancy" supports better decision making in turbulent times.** Paradigm pliancy is the opposite to paradigm paralysis. A sign of paradigm pliancy is when someone says, "I never thought about it that way before. Tell me more."

◆ **Individuals control their paradigms and have the power to change them.** Seeking knowledge, being open-minded, taking risks, exploring new challenges, developing your tolerance for ambiguity, developing flexibility and empathy are some ways to change your paradigms.

Now let's relate our discussion of paradigms to the area of developmental disabilities. For many years two strong paradigms shaped attitudes toward people with Down Syndrome. First, it was a commonly held belief that all children with a diagnosis of Down

Syndrome were "trainable" and could attain only a certain level of cognitive development. The *Australian Journal of Mental Retardation* reported in 1971 that only 1.2 percent of children with Down Syndrome might reach a borderline IQ range of 68–85.[23] Second, the life expectancy of children with Down Syndrome was much lower than that of other children; the high incidence of congenital heart defects and depressed immunity to infections among individuals with Down Syndrome was blamed for the shorter life span.

Today, educators view children with Down Syndrome as students with special needs who have individual learning styles and different levels of intelligence. And thanks to advances in cardiac surgery and health care in general, children with Down Syndrome can expect to live beyond the ages of 50 and 60 years. The greatest improvements in their physical and mental development are attributed to their training in self-help and work skills.[24]

Another example relates to the medical model that operates out of a paradigm in which treatment is driven by the client's diagnosis. Occupational therapy has been shifting from a medical model to a health model since the early 1980s. The set of rules and regulations in 1960 that governed the practice boundaries of occupational therapists who worked with children are dramatically different than those that prevail in the late 1990s. A paradigm shift has occurred. There is a dramatic shift from the medical model in which therapists worked with children in hospitals and out-patient clinics to the model in which therapists see children in schools and day-care programs.

Shifting Paradigms to Reframe a Problem

When you think about a problem, it is only natural to define it in terms of your personal paradigms. Personal paradigms provide a psychological comfort zone within which you can view problems without much risk. Your comfort zone is relatively predictable. Rules are not challenged in the comfort zone because, after all, the purpose of your being in this zone is to feel safe.

As you journey through this field book you will be introduced to many thinking strategies. Each one is designed to s t r e t c h your thinking beyond the comfort zone, beyond the place where your creative, imaginative self resides. You will be challenged to restructure or reframe problems in as many ways possible. When you reframe a problem, you look at it from a different perspective. To do this, you need to shift your paradigm and leave your comfort zone. A paradigm shift, to review, occurs when there is a change in the assumptions that underlie an event.

Cartoonists are masters at using paradigm shifts. Read the following scene and identify how the writer uses a paradigm shift.

> Two therapists were walking through the jungle when a lion appears on the path ahead of them. One of the two starts putting on a pair of running shoes.
>
> "Why bother with the running shoes?" says the first. "There's no way you can outrun a lion."
>
> "Who said anything about outrunning a lion?" says the second. "I just want to outrun you."[25]

The creator of this story set up a situation in which the reader assumes that the therapist is preparing to outrun the lion. Then, bang! A shift occurs in the last line when the reader learns that one therapist wants only to outrun the other therapist, leaving the latter therapist for lion bait. A paradigm shift is a change to a new game plan with a different set of rules.

The 20 visuals in Figure 3.2 will give you practice shifting your paradigms. To solve the puzzles, you must shift your paradigms between literal interpretations and abstract perspectives. Each of the visuals represents an expression or phrase. Your task is to figure out the expression embedded in these creative word problems. For example: the second item in the list of word problems has the word *man* printed over the word *board*. The expression is "Man overboard."

Practice S T R E T C H I N G your mind on the remainder of these word problems. Then compare your responses to the list in Appendix A.

Figure 3.2. *Creative Word Problems*

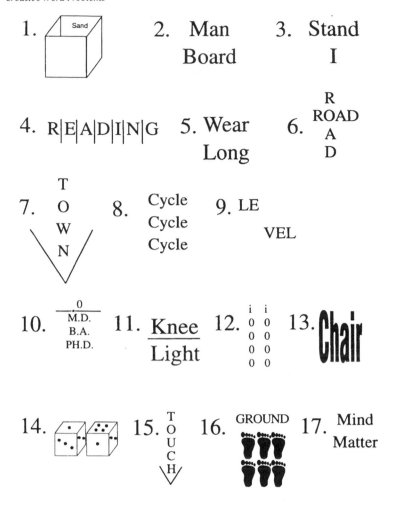

1. [box labeled "Sand"]   2. Man / Board   3. Stand / I

4. R|E|A|D|I|N|G   5. Wear / Long   6. R ROAD A D

7. T O W N (in V shape)   8. Cycle Cycle Cycle   9. LE / VEL

10. 0 / M.D. / B.A. / PH.D.   11. Knee / Light   12. i i / 0 0 / 0 0 / 0 0 / 0 0   13. **Chair**

14. [two dice]   15. T O U C H (in V shape)   16. GROUND [feet]   17. Mind / Matter

18. He's/Himself   19. ECNALG   20. DEATH LIFE

New Points of View

When you shift your paradigm you let go of the rules and assumptions with which you filtered your initial thoughts about a situation or problem. Shifting your paradigm allows you to reframe the problem and change your perception of the information surrounding it. Two Thinking Keys can help you reframe a problem.

The first is the **"Consider Other Viewpoints" Thinking Key.** When you consider other viewpoints, you cross over and view the problem from another person's viewpoint. To explore how this Thinking Key works, imagine yourself in the following scenario.

You depend on your car for transportation between home and work. One day the transmission on your car fails. You are suddenly faced with a problem that you perceive to be major. "How will I get to work? How will I arrange to get my car fixed?" you think.

You strongly dislike taking public transportation. Taking a bus to work, therefore, is not a viable solution to your problem—from your perspective. You call Alexis, your supervisor at work, to tell her about your "major" problem. And you learn that Alexis takes public transportation to work. She doesn't even own a car. She sees your absence from work as a bigger problem than that of your issues related to getting your car fixed. You suddenly decide to look for a bus schedule and deal with the car situation after work.

Use the "Consider Other Viewpoints" Field Organizer to analyze this scenario.

DIRECTIONS

1. Read the statements in column A, rows 1–3.
2. At the top of column B, record the name of the other person whose point of view you are considering.
3. Complete column B, rows 2–3, by identifying the viewpoint of the other person. Note: Use row 1 to model your responses.

FIELD ORGANIZER

"Consider Other Viewpoints"

A **I believe that . . .**	**B** **On the other hand, _____ believes that . . .**
1. *I cannot go to work because I have no transportation.*	*I should be at work regardless of my transportation problems.*
2. *I cannot use public transportation.*	
3. *I cannot go to work when my car needs to be taken in to be fixed.*	

Using the "Consider Other Viewpoints" Thinking Key directs your thoughts to consciously distinguish your perception of a situation from the perceptions of others. The ability to view problems from different viewpoints, especially from a positive perspective, is a necessary skill for a therapy guide.

The word *problem* is defined as a source of difficulty or trouble. Many people tend to describe a problem using negative wording. Wording a problem in the negative can strongly bias you to think about the problem from a negative perspective. But wording a problem in the positive can help you generate useful ideas for solving the problem. Reframing the problem by thinking positive is a principle of CPS. The **"Think Positive" Thinking Key** is an extremely valuable tool. Wording statements in the positive can be difficult at times, especially if you are accustomed to thinking in terms of, "This won't work because . . ." But by stating the problem in the positive, you can strongly influence your ability to generate ideas that will lead to new possibilities and actions.

Consider the following scenario with Mark, a school therapist.

Mark is the only occupational therapist working in a public school system. He has referrals for more students than he can possibly handle in the six hours that he is assigned to the school program. The students range in age from 8 years to 12 years and have a variety of therapy needs. Mark must make a decision regarding how to deliver therapy services to all of the students on his list. So the first thing that he does is make a schedule of the times he has available to slot in students.

He feels overwhelmed with the number of children that he must see in a day, because, in the past, he has always seen students individually. In the past, his paradigm for seeing children in school was, "The only way to achieve individual goals is to treat the children one on one." Unfortunately, in his current situation, there is not enough time in the school day to schedule students for individual sessions.

Maintaining a positive outlook, Mark decides to frame his problem in the positive. His old paradigm, that good quality therapy service can occur only one on one, no longer supports a successful therapy program in this context. Mark begins to focus on alternatives. He asks himself, "How can I schedule all the students so that they can benefit from therapy sessions?"

He decides that the only way to schedule all the students in one day is to see them in small groups. He arrives at this decision by forming a new paradigm that is triggered by his willingness to reframe the problem in the positive.

Mark shifted his focus to the benefits of seeing the students in small groups. Rethinking the situation led him to realize that group sessions would give the children opportunities to share, take turns, and practice peer communication and social interaction skills. Thinking in the positive helped Mark shift his vision of how he might help the children. Practice using the "Think Positive" Thinking Key by completing the "Think Positive" Field Organizer.

DIRECTIONS

1. Read the following scenario and think about how you might deal with the following problem: You are given one day's notice in which to evaluate a student and have the report ready for the staffing. Your first thoughts are, "I don't have time to do an evaluation and write the report before tomorrow morning."
2. Use the "Think Positive" Field Organizer to frame your thinking in the negative and positive. Begin by reading the negatively worded statement in column A. It begins with "I can't . . ."
3. Create a positive statement by using the stem in column B, "In what ways might I" (abbreviated version: IWWMI). Assume that the complete statement in this example is, "In what ways might I evaluate the student and write the report by tomorrow morning?"
4. Generate as many positive ways as you can think of for doing an evaluation and writing the report by the next day. Consider all possibilities, including preparations before the evaluation and constructing charts. Write the possibilities in column B, rows 3–5. On a separate sheet of paper, add more rows if you can generate more than three options.

FIELD ORGANIZER

"Think Positive"

A I can't . . .	B IWWMI . . .
do an evaluation and write the report before tomorrow morning.	1. .focus in on a few specific performance areas and write the results of this structured observation.
	2. reschedule another child on my case load in order to free up some time to complete the evaluation.
	3.
	4.
	5.

Even if you do not have an immediate answer about how you will solve the problem, framing your thoughts with positive words will influence your actions toward the possible. Shifting your paradigm from an "I can't do it" thought to a "How might I do it?" can jump start the flow of your creative juices.

Shift your thought patterns by focusing your efforts on framing a situation in the positive. Positive thinking leads to more productive outcomes than does negative thinking. Use the "Think Positive" Thinking Key whenever you feel you are concentrating on the negative aspects of a problem.

How Context Influences the Paradigm in Which a Decision Is Made

Because very few decisions are absolute on a therapy expedition, therapy guides must learn to select the "better" idea among several options. To be able to select that "better" idea, the therapy guide needs to understand the influence that context has on the paradigms she uses to make decisions. The context within which you make a decision has a pervasive influence on your operating paradigms. To further understand the relationship between context and paradigms, use the **"What Paradigm Is Operating?" Thinking Key.**

DIRECTIONS

1. Respond to the questions in column A by circling Yes or No. Don't ponder exceptions or extenuating circumstances.
2. In column B, identify the paradigm that was operating when you answered the question. Use row 1 to model your responses.

FIELD ORGANIZER

"What Paradigm Is Operating?"

A Record a behavior to be analyzed.	B Identify the operating paradigm that could explain the behavior described in column A.
1. *Would you go to the supermarket with shampoo in your hair?* Yes (No)	*Socially acceptable behavior dictates that I look respectable when I go outside.*
2. *Would you go outside wearing only a bathing suit in freezing weather?* Yes No	
3. *Would you eat a raw egg?* Yes No	

If your answer to any of the questions in the "What Paradigm Is Operating?" Thinking Key is no, consider under what circumstances or in what context you would respond yes to the question. Complete the sentences below in column A by writing your response in column B.

Context Can Cause a Paradigm Shift Worksheet

A	B
1. I would go to the supermarket with shampoo in my hair if . . .	
2. I would go outside wearing only a bathing suit in freezing weather if . . .	
3. I would eat a raw egg if . . .	

If you were able to identify circumstances under which you would execute any one of the behaviors you rejected in the What Paradigm Is Operating worksheet, you understand how circumstances or context can cause you to shift your paradigm.

Consider the following scenario:

You said that you would go to the supermarket with shampoo in your hair if you were paid one million dollars, tax free, and in cash. The monetary reward changes the circumstances under which you would act. Your anticipated receipt of the money is the criteria that frames the way you might consider doing an otherwise "unthinkable" act.

Consider another situation that is not quite as outlandish as going to the supermarket with a shampoo head.

You must decide what to wear to a job interview. You have been called back for a second interview for the position of senior occupational therapist at a privately funded special school. You will be meeting with the program director and the departing senior occupational therapist.

You were told that you may be asked to demonstrate your therapy skills as part of this interview. You want to make a favorable impression on the staff. Therefore you believe that the outward impression created by your dress is extremely important.

REFLECTIVE JOURNAL ENTRY 3.21

Complete the following thought:

For this second interview I will wear . . .

As you decided what to wear, perhaps you had one or more of the following thoughts: "I will wear a dark, tailored suit for the interview. I want to look neat and professional. I want the interviewer to think that I'm serious about wanting the position. I don't want to wear anything that might be construed as too casual or as weekend wear."

On the other hand, your thoughts might have been something like this: "This facility must really like me because they called me back for a second interview. What I wear isn't as important as the treatment skills that I demonstrate. Since I may be demonstrating my therapy skills with the children in the school, I will wear something casual that won't restrict my movements when I work with the children."

Context helps define the paradigm you use to make decisions within a particular situation. For you to best understand something, it must make sense to your personal frame of reference. Your frame of reference is shaped by your paradigms. Imposing on others the paradigms that guide your life choices can be a roadblock, however, to fully understanding the issues presented by others. After all, the perceptions that are formed by your paradigm are unique to you alone. Using your paradigms to view new information presented by others can deeply impair your ability to benefit from any new information that passes your way. It takes a conscious effort to *avoid* viewing new information from the perspective of your personal paradigms because your paradigms are so much a part of your thinking and their use is so automatic.

As a therapy guide your role is to seek to understand the paradigms of the clients with whom you work, in order to help them define their problems. Asking questions in a nonjudgmental manner can help you understand the client's paradigms. Practice being sensitive enough to understand clients whose behaviors reveal paradigms different from your own. Practice keeping an open mind. Defer judgment. When a client has a different perspective from yours, think about what questions you might ask in order to gain a greater understanding of his perspective.

If, for example, a client or a client's parent does not have the same attitude as you do toward a piece of equipment or treatment strategy, rather than judge his perspective as wrong, explore why your perspectives differ. Your wondering might be as simple as:

- I wonder why that parent thinks this way.
- How does he think he will be able to do that?
- Why would this child say that?

Once a therapy guide understands that a client's perspective of the therapy process is different from his, he can say to himself, "Oh, she sees the problem that way because that is her paradigm." A therapy guide uses empathy when solving problems creatively in order to build bridges of understanding between himself and the client.

Intuition as the Therapy Guide's Compass

To help you promote understanding on your therapy expeditions, use your intuition as a compass. A compass is a tool that helps you to determine the direction you are going. When the needle on the compass moves, it is cueing you about the direction you are headed. Then it is up to you to determine whether the direction indicated by the compass needle is the "right" direction for your journey. We all have an internal compass. It is called intuition.

Intuition is from the Latin "to watch over." Intuition is an internal guidance system that watches over all your actions. Have you ever said to yourself or perhaps heard someone else say, "Oh, I just knew that was going to happen!" or "I just had a weird feeling about that!" These thoughts reflect an individual's internal compass, his inner sense of knowing. Intuition occurs when you feel that you know something but don't know exactly how you know about it. "Intuition is increasingly recognized as a natural mental faculty, an important element in discovery, problem solving, and decision making, a generator of creative ideas, a revealer of truth."[26] Use your intuition to assess the "rightness" or "wrongness" of an idea when you solve problems creatively.

Intuition is a source of knowledge that exists at the most basic level. "We know it is from within because it is usually accompanied by a strong physical, visual and/or emotional sensation." Intuition is not limited to the occasional flash of insight. You can develop your intuition "into a source of insight reliable enough for you to call upon when you need it."[27]

Intuition is like a muscle; it can be exercised. Learning to listen to what your intuition is saying takes practice because it is not necessarily verbal or rational. To hear what your intuition is saying requires you to develop a certain sensitivity to how you sense events that occur in you. Research on intuition shows that intuition speaks to people in the following three primary ways: through images and symbols, through feelings and emotions, and, through physical sensations.[28]

REFLECTIVE JOURNAL ENTRY 3.22

Complete the following thoughts:

1. *I remember making a "good" decision based on my intuition rather than my intellect the time that . . .*

2. *I recall making a "bad" decision because I didn't listen to my intuiton the time that . . .*

You can cultivate your inner way of knowing by routinely asking yourself such questions as, "How did I feel about that situation?" "Did I listen to my intuition that time?" "What am I sensing about this situation?" Learning to listen to your intuition can deepen your insights regarding a problem and, many times, will lead you to a smoother, more direct route to solving a problem.[29]

Journaling is one way to help you to get in touch with your intuition. By committing to paper your thoughts and feelings about a situation either at the time of occurrence or soon after, you can reflect on your sensitivities and determine the role that your feelings had on the decisions that you made. Journaling is a tool with which you can reflect on your past decisions and rate their level of success. This commitment to reflection can help you develop a mentoring relationship with yourself. You are, afterall, your best mentor. Only you know what you have learned from your past decisions. When you examine the realities of past decisions you have made, you can learn more from those experiences than from listening to the advice of any other person.[30]

Create a Mind Map of Section

3

Mind Map Guidelines

1. Place the section's main concept in the center of the space using pictures or words or both.
2. Radiate ideas from the central thought.
   - Use images (be sure to use color).
   - Headline text—one or two words per line.
   - Print text (for easy reading).
3. Link the main concepts and generate more ideas from the linkages.
4. Have fun!

Section 3
SELF-ASSESSMENT

Now that I have completed the third part of my journey, I can:

○ compare the therapy process to an expedition.

○ use the "What's Next? Question Series" Thinking Key to project a therapy idea into the future.

○ use the "If–Then" Thinking Key to create a hypothesis statement.

○ identify the mindset of a therapy guide.

○ use the "What If . . . ? Question Series" Thinking Key to anticipate possible outcomes.

○ explain how questions support a therapy guide's quest for knowledge.

○ use the "Stop, Drop, and Listen" Thinking Key to enhance my empathy.

○ use the "Watch for Cues and Look for Patterns" Thinking Key to analyze a story for relevant information.

○ explain why a therapy guide needs to understand paradigms.

○ use the "Consider Other Viewpoints" Thinking Key to reframe a problem.

○ use the "Think Positive" Thinking Key to frame a problem.

○ use the "What Paradigm Is Operating?" Thinking Key.

○ describe how intuition helps a therapy guide make decisions.

NOTES

1. Sidney J. Parnes, *Visionizing* (Buffalo, N.Y.: Creative Education Foundation Press, 1992); S. Covey, *The 7 Habits of Highly Effective People* (New York: Simon & Schuster, 1989).
2. D. Loye, *The Sphinx and the Rainbow* (Boulder, Colo.: Shambhala, 1983). Loye is co-director of the Institute for Future Forecasting in northern California. In this book he synthesizes brain/mind sciences using research on neurophysiology, psychology, parapsychology, and theoretical physics to show how we depend on the mind's ability to forecast the future, for economic and personal survival.
3. Frank Smith, *To Think* (New York: Teachers College Press, 1990).
4. C. Mattingly and M. H. Fleming, *Clinical Reasoning* (Philadelphia: F. A. Davis, 1993).
5. D. Markova, *The Art of the Possible: A Compassionate Approach to Understanding the Way People Think, Learn, and Communicate* (Berkeley, Calif.: Conari Press, 1991).
6. Roger von Oech, *A Kick in the Seat of the Pants* (New York: Harper & Row, 1986).
7. S. Johnson, *"Yes" or "No": The Guide to Better Decisions* (New York: HarperCollins, 1992), 65.
8. E. de Bono, *Six Thinking Hats* (New York: Penguin Books, 1985). De Bono's thinking structure attempts to obliterate the ego by having the individuals involved in the decision making process metaphorically wear hats. There are six different colored hats. Each hat represents a different thinking operation. For example, the yellow hat is bright like the sun; it represents positive thoughts about the target of the decision. When one wears the yellow hat, one focuses on generating constructive, positive thoughts about the situation. The black hat is the color of a judge's robe; it represents judgment or critical thinking. When one wears the black hat, one is allowed to express critical or negative thoughts about the situation. De Bono postulates that it is easier to ask someone to "remove" the black hat than to say, "Stop being so negative." The rules of the game are respected by all involved in the discussion and the ego remains intact.
9. D. Goleman, *Emotional Intelligence* (New York: Bantam Books, 1995).
10. Mary Ann Gidewell, "The Other Side of the Mirror," *Occupational Therapy Forum* 11, no. 11 (March 18, 1987): 1–6.

11. C. B. Royeen, "A Problem-Based Learning Curriculum for Occupational Therapy Education," *AJOT* 49, no. 12 (1995): 338–46.
12. B. Hoff, *The Tao of Pooh* (New York: Penguin Books, 1982), 115.
13. J. Hyams, *Zen in the Martial Arts* (New York: Bantam Books, 1979), 10–11.
14. Mattingly and Fleming, *Clinical Reasoning.*
15. E. de Bono, *Lateral Thinking: Creativity Step by Step* (New York: Harper & Row, 1970), 27–28.
16. Mattingly and Fleming, *Clinical Reasoning.*
17. von Oech, *Kick in the Seat of the Pants.*
18. Hoff, *Tao of Pooh*, 15.
19. T. Kuhn, *The Structure of Scientific Revolutions* (Chicago: University of Chicago Press, 1962). Kuhn introduced the concept of paradigm to the scientific community. A major point in his publication was that at a fundamental level, the basic assumptions of a discipline shape the research and results of research in that discipline. When evidence starts to challenge certain commonly held assumptions, conflicts occur. These conflicts lead to new assumptions and result in a shift in the way one perceives the event. When the conflicting knowledge becomes accepted by the community, a dramatic shift occurs. He labeled this shift "paradigm shift." Since that time, much has been written about the influence of paradigms in various fields.
20. J. Barker, *Discovering the Future: The Business of Paradigms* (New York: HarperCollins, 1993). Barker's work is based on Kuhn's (*Structure of Scientific Revolutions*); he applied the concept of paradigms to business.
21. Barker, *Discovering the Future*, 13.
22. Ibid.
23. Judith Dey, "Intelligence in Down's Syndrome," *Australian Journal of Mental Retardation* 1 (1971): 154. Dey's conclusions were based on a study of 465 subjects with Down Syndrome. See also J. Blackman, *Medical Aspects of Developmental Disabilities in Children Birth to Three*, rev. ed. (Rockville, Md.: Aspen Systems Corp., 1984).
24. Blackman, *Medical Aspects.*
25. Ichak Adizes, *Corporate Lifecycles: How and Why Corporations Grow and Die and What to Do About It* (New York: Prentice Hall, 1988).
26. Philip Goldberg, *The Intuitive Edge* (New York: Jeremy P. Tarcher, 1983), 15.
27. N. Rosanoff, *Intuition Workout: A Practical Guide to Discovering and Developing Your Inner Knowing* (Santa Rosa, Calif.: Aslan Publishing, 1988), 16, 15.
28. Goldberg, *Intuitive Edge.*
29. Ibid.
30. G. Caine, R. Caine, and S. Crowell, *Mindshifts: A Brain-Based Process for Restructuring Schools and Renewing Education* (Tucson, Ariz.: Zephyr Press, 1994). The authors present their perspective of brain-based learning, the manner in which humans take in new information and translate it for later use. The authors are educators who provide valuable insights that can be applied to therapy-related decision making, teaching new skills to others, teaching by doing rather than teaching about something. The authors ascribe to the philosophy that every experience is a learning experience. Everything that you experience operates within the learner's larger context of life and therefore must be relevant.

The Paradigm of Occupational Therapy: Performance Areas, Components, and Contexts

Itinerary #4

At the end of the fourth section of your journey, you will be able to:

✓ describe how occupational performance shapes the way a therapy guide views a client's behavior

✓ describe how context influences occupational performance

✓ explain the relationship between occupational performance and performance components

✓ describe the role of Uniform Terminology in occupational therapy

✓ play with Uniform Terminology by completing puzzles and writing stories that incorporate the terms of Performance Areas, Performance Components, and Performance Contexts

How Occupational Performance Shapes a Therapy Guide's Views

Effective occupational therapy expeditions begin with the therapy guide looking at ways to view the client's problem in an occupational therapy frame of reference. A frame of reference (see Section 3) is a set of guiding principles through which one views the world. It is a paradigm. Whether the therapy guide works with children or adults, in mental health or developmental disabilities, occupation, made manifest by one's occupational performance, is the paradigm that unifies all areas of occupational therapy practice.

Kathlyn Reed, an occupational therapy educator and historian who researched the roots of occupational therapy, notes that occupation has been central to humanity probably since the beginning of time. "Occupational therapy," she goes on to say, "is woven into the fabric of human existence, but the tapestry became rich in the 19th and early 20th centuries." The concept of wellness became connected with occupation when society began to recognize its important contribution to one's health and well-being.[1] "Occupation" is a guiding principle in occupational therapy.

Occupation encompasses three broad categories of activity in which everyone engages. These three categories of occupational performance are referred to as performance areas. The performance areas include activities of daily living, work and productive activities, and play and leisure activities. An individual's physical and mental development influence how much and how well (i.e., quantity and quality) he or she engages in each performance area. To capture the total picture of a client, a therapy guide must assess the client in all three performance areas at the beginning of the therapy expedition.

The following scenario of Gabrielle, a seven-year-old, demonstrates why a therapy guide must look at all performance areas of each client.

Gabrielle's teacher requested occupational therapy services because Gabrielle was having difficulty writing her name on written assignments. In addition to the handwriting problems, the teacher also noted that Gabrielle had trouble managing her papers and other materials such as scissors and glue sticks during classroom art activities. The referral information about Gabrielle was in the area of work and productive activities.

Upon receipt of the referral, Lydia, the school occupational therapist, arranged to meet Gabrielle and evaluate her handwriting performance. On the day of the evaluation, Gabrielle wore a pullover sweater. During the evaluation, Gabrielle tried, unsuccessfully, to remove her sweater. Observing the child's struggle, Lydia refrained from assisting her because she thought that Gabrielle would eventually remove the sweater by herself. Unfortunately for Gabrielle, the longer she tried to remove her arms from the sleeves, the more tangled up she became. Finally, in apparent frustration, she began to cry.

Watching Gabrielle struggle, Lydia began to consider possible causes for her difficulties with removing the sweater. She questioned Gabrielle's ability to mentally plan the movement patterns necessary to remove her sweater. She also made mental notes about the way Gabrielle approached the task. Lydia then began to wonder how Gabrielle managed other self-care activities at home. And the thoughts of self-care led her to wonder about how Gabrielle spent her leisure time and the quality of her social activities.

Lydia's thinking was framed by the paradigm of occupational performance. This frame of reference directed her to look at Gabrielle's handwriting problem within the broader scope of life as a seven-year-old child.

How Context Influences Occupational Performance

The context of every situation has a corresponding set of assumptions that frame your thoughts and actions within that particular situation. Consequently, the context has an important effect on how the performance occurs. Consider, for example, how context affects the way you might eat baked chicken. When you pack a basket for a picnic at the beach, most likely you do not even consider bringing forks and knives. The finger-feeding strategy you learned as a toddler will work just fine. When you are attending a catered formal affair, however, you expect a set-up of the proper eating utensils.

REFLECTIVE JOURNAL ENTRY 4.1

Think of an activity and how you perform the activity differently in two different contexts. Then complete the following thoughts:

1. An example of an activity I do differently depending on where I am or who is nearby is . . .

2. The reason I perform the activity described above differently in different contexts is because . . .

Your response in the Reflective Journal Entry 4.1 most likely demonstrates the powerful influence that context has on a person's occupational performance. Context is one of the most significant variables that helps us to remember isolated pieces of information. Context solidifies the content of the experience for storage in memory and later recall when needed.[2] Consider the following scenario:

Imagine that you receive a referral on Vinnie, a four-year-old-child who is unable to feed himself. He cannot hold a cup to drink or use a spoon to feed himself cereal. Before initiating a therapy program, you need to be able to determine whether occupational therapy intervention might help Vinnie acquire the skills to learn how to feed himself.

You begin the assessment process by framing your observations with your paradigm of occupational performance. First you draw on knowledge of normal development to identify the self-feeding competencies of a four-year-old child. Next, you try to figure out what might be preventing Vinnie from feeding himself.

Before meeting Vinnie to evaluate his eating performance, you decide to interview his parents. From the parent interview you learn that Vinnie is the youngest of 12 children, all of whom live at home. You also find out that Vinnie is regularly fed by one of his older brothers or sisters. Through a process of asking the parents open-ended questions, you discover that Vinnie takes twice as long as everyone else in the family to eat a meal. Because Vinnie eats so slowly his siblings would rather feed him than teach him how to feed himself. At this point you mentally note that Vinnie's feeding problems may be more related to the context in which he eats than to limitations in motor or cognitive capabilities.

Finding out about Vinnie's home life has influenced the way you view his independence in self-feeding. You also start to ponder, "In what ways might I encourage Vinnie's siblings to help him develop more mature self-help skills?" After all, you silently reason, "If I can work on self-feeding with Vinnie only one day of the week, and his family continues to feed him between the therapy appointments, are occupational therapy services appropriate in this situation?"

Now consider a slightly different scenario. Suppose Vinnie's family expressed interest in following a home program. You might instead ask yourself different questions, beginning with: "In what ways can I work with Vinnie's family to capitalize on their eagerness to help Vinnie learn how to feed himself independently?"

In each scenario, the context (of Vinnie's family circumstance) influences the way you would view the client's occupational performance and whether you felt occupational therapy services might be appropriate.

Now consider a scenario in which a problem that is solved under one set of circumstances (context) becomes a new problem when the context changes.

Tabetha is a five-year-old child who spent six weeks in a rehabilitation hospital recovering from a traumatic brain injury. During the last two weeks of her inpatient stay, Tabetha dressed herself without any help, including putting on her shoes and socks, in preparation for her full day of therapies. She was a star performer according to her therapy guide. Tabetha had successfully met all of her therapy goals the day before she was discharged home.

Unfortunately, six weeks later when Tabetha returned to the outpatient clinic for her recheck, her mother reported that Tabetha was no longer dressing herself.

Did Tabetha lose the ability to dress herself when she went home? What do you think happened?

REFLECTIVE JOURNAL ENTRY 4.2

Complete the following thought:

When Tabetha went home, perhaps Tabetha . . .

If you surmised that Tabetha had no real need to dress herself at home, you are correct. Her mother dressed her. Tabetha did not lose skills; the context changed. Since "context" is the frame of reference that provides meaning to any situation, a change in the context can produce a change in a person's occupational performance.[3] In Tabetha's situation, the demands and expectations are what changed, not her physical or perceptual abilities.

When Tabetha was in the hospital, she did not have the one-on-one help that her mother gave her at home. In the hospital, Tabetha knew that if she was not dressed when she went to breakfast each morning, she would be late to her therapy play group. She enjoyed play group more than any other activity in her busy rehabilitation program. When she returned home, the context was different. She no longer had the same incentive to get up and dress as she had at the hospital.

The more attuned a therapy guide is to the context that supports a client's optimal performance, the more likely the guide is to understand a client's occupational performance. Successful therapy expeditions depend on the therapy guide's ability to provide the client with opportunities to perform in noncontrived, real-life situations.

The Relationship Between Occupational Performance and Performance Components

A therapy guide's first level of thinking is to determine whether the referral is appropriate. The referral is deemed appropriate if the client's reason for referral falls within one or more of the three categories of occupational performance (activities of daily living; work and productive activities; play and leisure). If a referral is found to be appropriate, the therapy guide evaluates the performance components of the performance area or areas.

In Vinnie's situation (above), the occupational performance area that brought him to occupational therapy was activities of daily living, specifically feeding and eating. Hence, the evaluation process would address the following components of feeding and eating:

1. The coordination of eyes with hands required to reach out for a cup,
2. The figure ground perception required to accurately reach out in space for objects placed in front of one,
3. The muscle tone and strength needed to manage a cup and utensils, and
4. The ability to plan the oral movements necessary to chew a variety of food textures and sizes.

The performance components listed above are only a few of the components that a therapy guide would assess during the evaluation process.

Uniform Terminology: The Language of Occupational Therapy

Therapy guides on therapy expeditions use a uniform system of communication that was created by the American Occupational Therapy Association (AOTA). The system is called Uniform Terminology. Turn to page 147 for a list of the Uniform Terminology terms you will learn.

Uniform Terminology defines the paradigm of occupational therapy. It is the language with which occupational therapy practitioners communicate goals of therapy, client progress, and all other documentation related to occupational therapy practice.[4] Uniform Terminology is organized into Performance Areas, Performance Components, and Performance Contexts. These three domains constitute the major territory of occupational therapy practitioners. Practitioners focus on these domains when delivering occupational therapy services.

Performance Areas

The domain of Performance Areas includes the three broad categories encompassed by occupation: activities of daily living, work and productive activities, and play or leisure activities. Each category can be further defined by subcategories of typical activities in which one might engage. A therapy guide may choose to place a client's occupational performance in one or two or all three Performance Areas. The chosen category depends on the meaning the activity holds for the client. For example, for a young child, a therapy guide might consider socialization a daily living activity because socialization is part of a child's normal development. In contrast, for an adult client, the guide might consider socialization a play and leisure activity.

Performance Components

Performance Components are fundamental human abilities that all individuals demonstrate when they engage in the Performance Areas. The Performance Components fall into three categories: sensorimotor components, cognitive integration and cognitive components, and psychosocial skills and psychological components.

Performance Contexts

Performance Contexts are the situations in which an individual performs. Performance Contexts profoundly influence the quality of one's performance. Performance Contexts are divided into two categories: temporal aspects and environment. The temporal aspects include the individual's chronological age, developmental age (e.g., place within the life cycle), and health status. The environment context includes physical, social, and cultural considerations.

The therapy guide looks at the interrelationships between the three main domains of Performance Areas, Performance Components, and Performance Contexts when performing an assessment and planning a client's treatment. Uniform Terminology defines the territory you will travel through during the therapy expedition. The specific route that you take, however, is a function of your creativity.

Playing with Uniform Terminology

In the remainder of Section 4, you will be introduced to the three domains of Uniform Terminology in detail, one at a time. You will have an opportunity to play with the terminology that defines the three domains in a variety of ways that will help you become immersed in the language of occupational therapy. Once you are familiar with the language of occupational therapy, you will be able to use the concepts to frame your thinking about the stories that follow. The activities for each domain appear in the following sequence:

1. An **organizational chart** showing the domain and its categories and subcategories
2. A **concept map** for each category with a graphic representing each subcategory
3. A **picture dictionary** in which you will be asked first to generate definitions prompted by graphics and then to compare your definitions to the definitions from AOTA's Uniform Terminology
4. **Games** that include a word search and crossword puzzle
5. **Story writing** related to scenes depicting individuals interacting in community settings (such as on a picnic, in a park or playground, or at school)

For the story-writing activities, you will look at each of the Uniform Terminology terms individually, as isolated words with definitions. The next step will be to create a story to help you gain a deeper feel for the terminology so that you will be able to apply it to occupational therapy practice. "Stories are powerful because they bind information and understanding."[5] They help you make meaning from relatively isolated pieces of information. And they are an effective way to stimulate your memory.

Altogether, you will write nine short stories, each one based on a different scene. Each scene depicts individuals engaging in a variety of occupational performance activities. The ideas for the story content will generate from the scene.

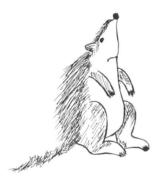

Note that each scene has one or more porcupines. Porcupines are highly sensitive to what is happening in their environment. A porcupine's response to what is happening around it can be observed in the position of the quills. Therapy guides on a therapy expedition need to have sharp observation skills, like porcupines. Hence, you will see a porcupine lurking in each of the scenes, reminding you to sharpen your sensitivities to what is occurring within the scene.

Have fun writing your stories. Be creative. Let your imagination go wild. Name the characters. Describe how they are relating to each other. Incorporate the Uniform Terminology into stories with mystery, intrigue, romance, humor, or just plain nonsense. You are the author. The only rule is that each story must have a beginning, a middle, and an ending.

You will go through the five-step sequence, described above, three times. First, you will go through the sequence learning about the Performance Areas. Next, you will play with Performance Components. And last, you will explore the domain of Performance Contexts.

Performance Areas

Begin your immersion into the language of occupational therapy by learning the meanings of terms that describe the activities in Performance Areas.

DIRECTIONS

1. Look at Figure 4.1 and familiarize yourself with the three main domains of Uniform Terminology and their respective categories.
2. Turn to Figure 4.2 and familiarize yourself with the categories and subcategories of the Performance Areas domain. Note that the subcategories of Work and Productive Activities are broken down further into sub-subcategories.
3. Next, turn to the concept maps for each Performance Areas category (Figures 4.3, 4.4, and 4.5) and note that each term is represented by a picture.

(Turn to page 92 for the continuation of the Directions.)

Figure 4.1. *The Three Domains of Uniform Terminology and Their Respective Categories*

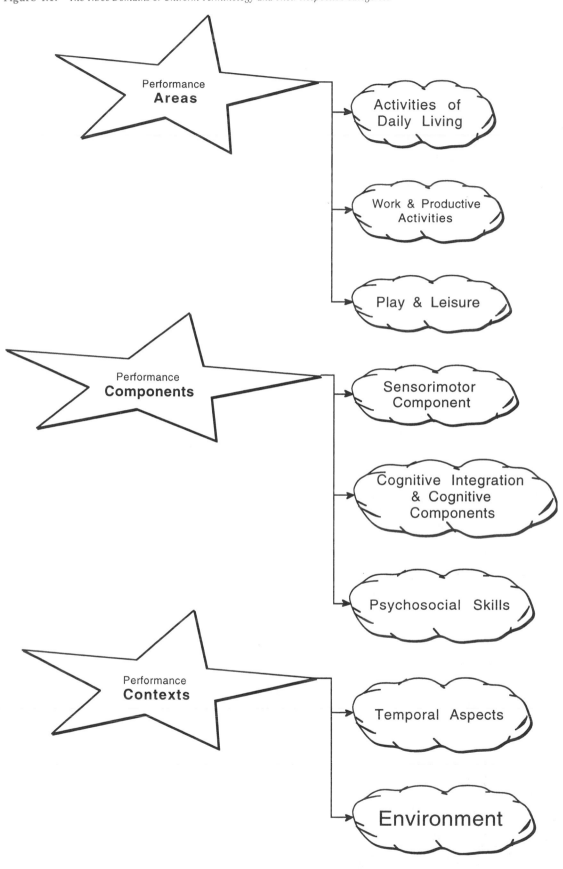

Figure 4.2. *Categories and Subcategories of the Uniform Terminology Domain Performance Areas*

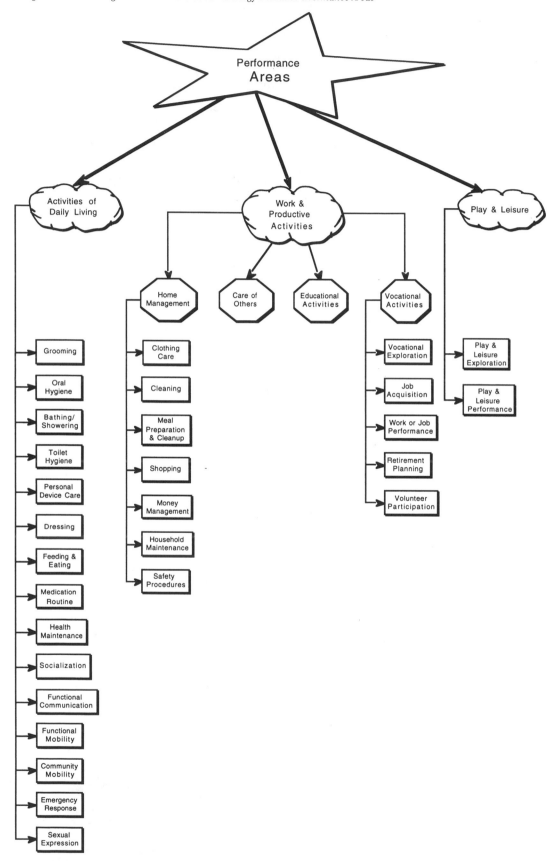

Figure 4.3. *Activities of Daily Living Concept Map*

Figure 4.3. *Activities of Daily Living Concept Map*

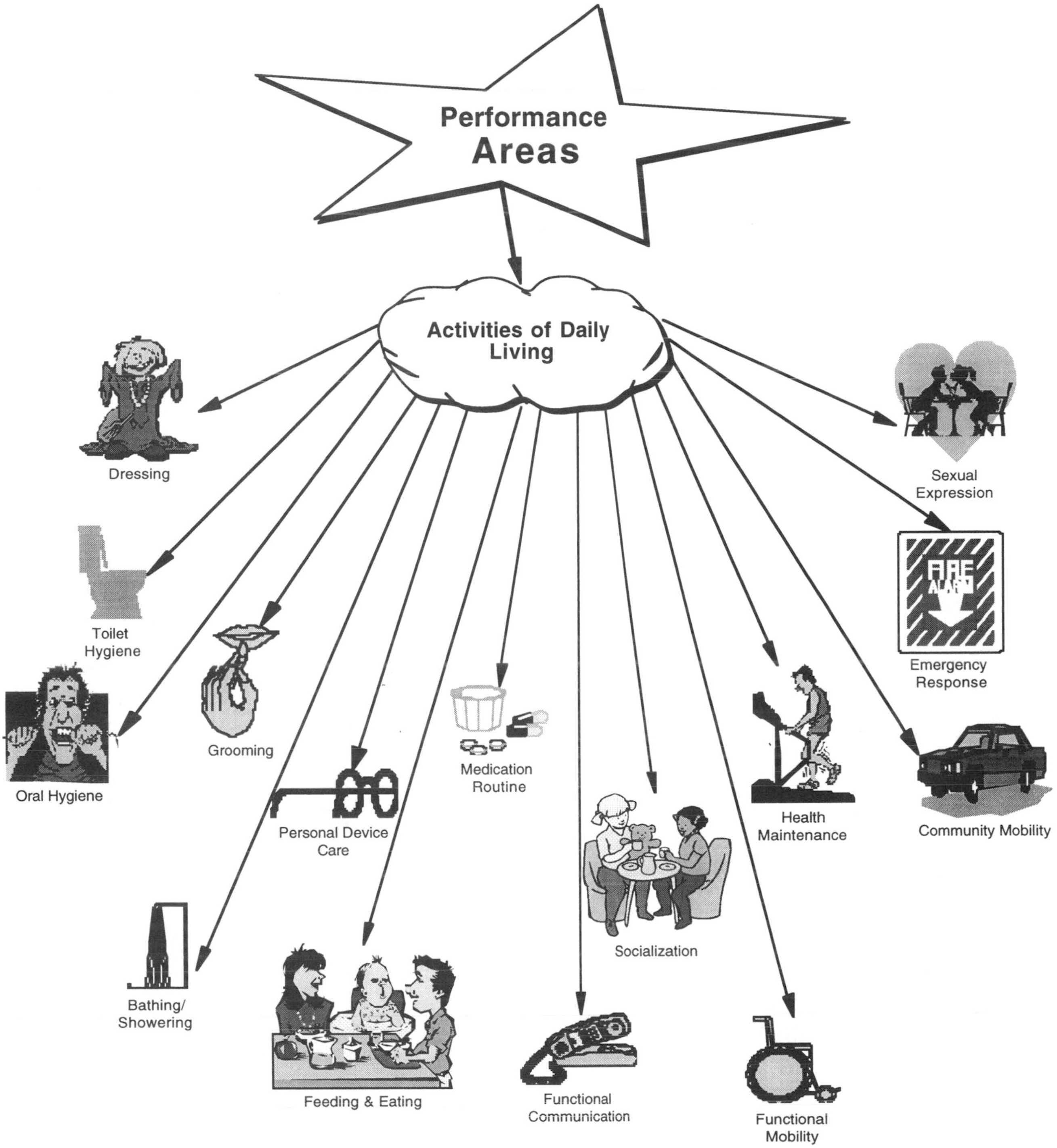

Figure 4.4. *Work and Productive Activities Concept Map*

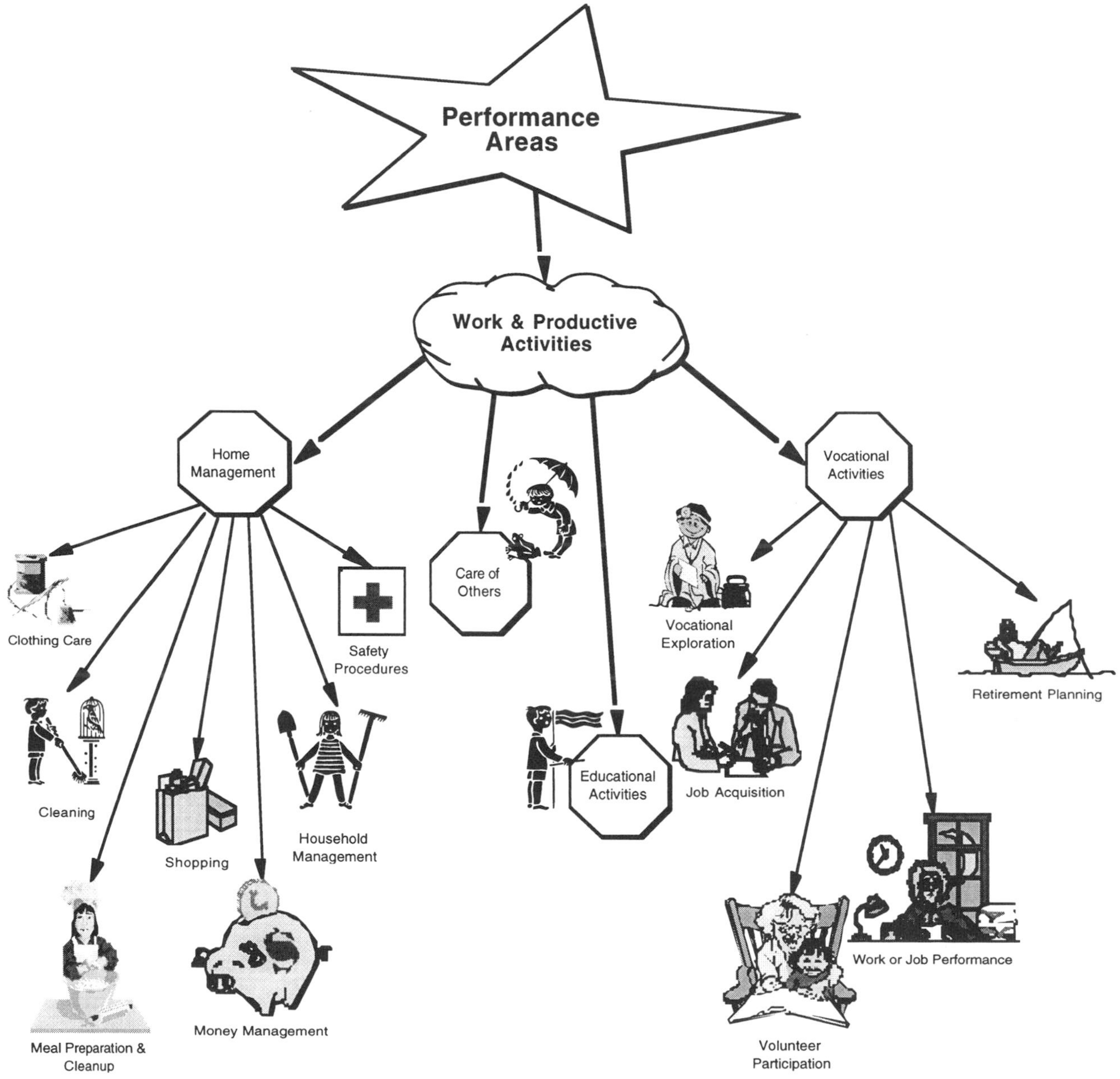

Figure 4.5. *Play and Leisure Concept Map*

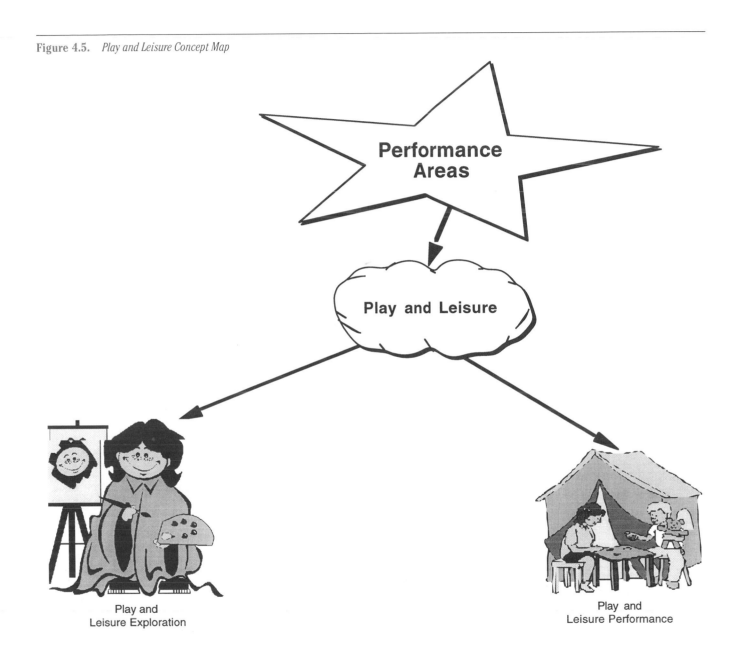

Play and
Leisure Exploration

Play and
Leisure Performance

I. Performance Areas:

A. ACTIVITES OF DAILY LIVING
Self—maintenance tasks

1. grooming
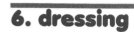

2. oral hygiene
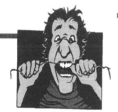

3. bathing/showering

4. toilet hygiene
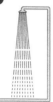

5. personal device care
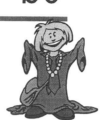

6. dressing

7. feeding and eating

8. medication routine

9. health maintenance

10. socialization

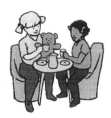

B. WORK AND PRODUCTIVE ACTIVITIES

Purposeful activities for self–development, social contribution and livelihood.

1. HOME MANAGEMENT

Obtaining and maintaining personal and household possessions and environment.

a. clothing care

11. functional communication

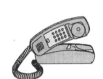

b. cleaning

12. functional mobility

13. community mobility

c. meal preparation and cleanup

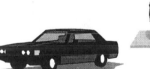

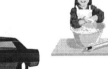

14. emergency response

d. shopping

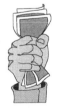

15. sexual expression

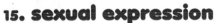

e. money management

f. household maintenance

g. safety procedures

2. care of others

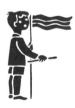

3. educational activities

4. vocational activities

Participating in work-related activities.

a. vocational exploration

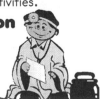

b. job acquisition

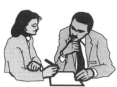

c. work or job performance

d. retirement planning

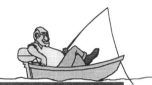

e. volunteer participation

C. PLAY AND LEISURE

Intrinsically motivating activities for amusement, relaxation, spontaneous enjoyment, or self expression.

1. play and leisure exploration

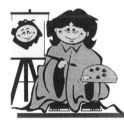

2. play and leisure performance

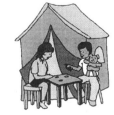

I. Performance Areas:

A. ACTIVITIES OF DAILY LIVING

Self-maintenance tasks

1. grooming

Obtaining and using supplies; removing body hair (use of razors, tweezers, lotions, etc.); applying and removing cosmetics; washing, drying, combing, styling, and brushing hair; caring for nails (hands and feet), caring for skin, ears, and eyes; and applying deodorant.

2. oral hygiene

Obtaining and using supplies; cleaning mouth; brushing and flossing teeth; or removing, cleaning, and reinserting dental orthotics and prosthetics.

3. bathing/showering

Obtaining and using supplies; soaping, rinsing, and drying body parts; maintaining bathing position; and transforming to and from bathing positions.

4. toilet hygiene

Obtaining and using supplies; clothing management; maintaining toileting position; cleaning body; and caring for menstrual and continence needs (including catheters, colostomies, and suppository management).

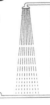

5. personal device care

Cleaning and maintaining personal care items, such as hearing aids, contact lenses, glasses, orthotics, prosthetics, adaptive equipment, and contraceptive and sexual devices.

6. dressing

Selecting clothing and accessories appropriate to time of day, weather, and occasion; obtaining clothing from storage area; dressing and undressing in a sequential fashion; fastening and adjusting clothing and shoes; and applying and removing personal devices, protheses, or orthoses.

7. feeding and eating

Setting up food; selecting and using appropriate utensils and tableware; bringing food or drink to mouth; cleaning face, hands, and clothing; sucking, masticating, coughing, and swallowing; and management of alternative methods of nourishment.

8. medication routine

Obtaining medication, opening and closing containers, following prescribed schedules, taking correct quantities, reporting problems and adverse effects, and administering correct quantities by using prescribed methods.

9. health maintenance

Developing and maintaining routines for illness prevention and wellness promotion, such as physical fitness, nutrition, and decreasing health risk behaviors.

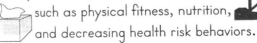

10. socialization

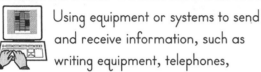

Accessing opportunities and interacting with other people in appropriate contextual and cultural ways to meet emotional and physical needs.

11. functional communication

Using equipment or systems to send and receive information, such as writing equipment, telephones, typewriters, computers, communication boards, call lights, emergency systems, Braille writers, telecommunication devices for the deaf, and augmentative communication systems.

12. functional mobility

Moving from one position or place to another, such as in-bed mobility, wheelchair mobility, transfers (wheelchair, bed, car, tub, toilet, tub/shower, chair, floor).

13. community mobility

Moving self in the community and using public or private transportation, such as driving, or accessing buses, taxi cabs, or other public transportation systems.

14. emergency response

Recognizing sudden, unexpected hazardous situations, and initiating action to reduce the threat to health and safety.

15. sexual expression

Engaging in desired sexual and intimate activities.

B. WORK AND PRODUCTIVE ACTIVITIES
Purposeful activities for self-development, social contribution and livelihood.

1. HOME MANAGEMENT
Obtaining and maintaining personal and household possessions and environment.

a. clothing care

Obtaining and using supplies; sorting, laundering (hand, machine, and dry clean); folding; ironing; storing; and mending.

b. cleaning

Obtaining and using supplies; picking up; putting away; vacuuming; sweeping and mopping floors; dusting; polishing; scrubbing; washing windows; cleaning mirrors; making beds; and removing trash and recyclables.

c. meal preparation and cleanup

Planning nutritious meals; preparing and serving food; opening and closing containers, cabinets and drawers; using kitchen utensils and appliances; cleaning up and storing food safely.

d. shopping

Preparing shopping lists (grocery and other); selecting and purchasing items; selecting methods of payment; and completing money transactions.

e. money management

Budgeting, paying bills, and using bank systems.

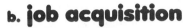

f. household maintenance

Maintaining home, yard, garden, appliances, vehicles, and household items.

g. safety procedures

Knowing and performing preventive and emergency procedures to maintain a safe environment and to prevent injuries.

2. care of others

Providing for children, spouse, parents, pets, or others, such as giving physical care, nurturing, communicating, and using age-appropriate activities.

3. educational activities

Participating in a learning environment through school, community, or work-sponsored activities, such as exploring educational interests, attending to instruction, managing assignments, and contributing to group experiences.

4. vocational activities

Participating in work-related activities.

a. vocational exploration

Determining aptitudes; developing interests and skills, and selecting appropriate vocational pursuits.

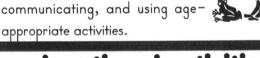

b. job acquisition

Identifying and selecting work opportunities, and completing application and interview processes.

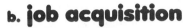

c. work or job performance

Performing job tasks in a timely and effective manner; incorporating necessary work behaviors.

d. retirement planning

Determining aptitudes; developing interests and skills; and selecting appropriate avocational pursuits.

e. volunteer participation

Performing unpaid activities for the benefit of selected individuals, groups, or causes.

C. PLAY AND LEISURE

Intrinsically motivating activities for amusement, relaxation, spontaneous enjoyment, or self expression.

1. play and leisure exploration

Identifying interests, skills and opportunities, and appropriate play or leisure activities.

2. play and leisure performance

Planning and participating in play or leisure activities. Maintaining a balance of play or leisure activities with work and productive activities, and activities of daily living. Obtaining, utilizing, and maintaining equipment and supplies.

4. Create your own definition for each term (i.e., each subcategory and sub-subcategory) by reflecting on the picture paired with the term. Before recording your definitions, note that the pages that follow contain two versions of a dictionary of AOTA's Uniform Terminology. The first version has blank spaces for your definitions; the second version shows the AOTA definitions.
5. Record your definitions in the blank spaces of the first AOTA dictionary.
6. When you have recorded all your definitions for the Performance Areas terms, turn to the second version of the AOTA Uniform Terminology dictionary and underline the words or phrases in each definition that relate to the graphic.

Example:

6. dressing

Selecting clothing and accessories appropriate to time of day, weather, and occasion; obtaining clothing from storage area; dressing and undressing in a sequential fashion; fastening and adjusting clothing and shoes; and applying and removing personal devices, protheses, or orthoses.

7. Go back to your definitions and see how closely each one matches the AOTA definition. Use the following criteria to score your work. Record the score in the margin next to each definition.

   2 points   Your definition has at least *two elements* included in AOTA's definition.
   1 point   Your definition has at least *one element* included in AOTA's definition.

8. Determine your total score by adding up your points. Record your score in the box below.

Score

If you scored

   ◆ 53–62 points: You're off and running.
   ◆ 44–52 points: You have a solid start.
   ◆ 43 points or below: Now you know what to work on.

Complete the Activities of Daily Living word search and crossword puzzle (see Appendix A for answers).

Performance Areas
- **Activities of Daily Living**

Directions: The terms related to Activities of Daily Living are hidden in the grid of letters. Look across, back, down, up, and diagonally. (The way each term is written in the list below is exactly the way it appears in the grid. Circle each term you discover. The word GROOMING has been circled as an example. Some terms have been abbreviated. For example, FunctCommunication is an abbreviation for "Functional Communication.")

TERMS
ADL
Grooming
OralHygiene
BathingShowering
ToiletHygiene
PersonalDeviceCare
Dressing
FeedingandEating
MedicationRoutine
HealthMaintenance
Socialization
FunctCommunication
FunctionalMobility
EmergencyResponse
SexualExpression
CommunityMobility

S	O	C	I	A	L	I	Z	A	T	I	O	N	P	A	K	M	F	N	F
F	U	N	C	T	I	O	N	A	L	M	O	B	I	L	I	T	Y	U	E
N	O	I	T	A	C	I	N	U	M	M	O	C	T	C	N	U	F	J	E
S	X	E	M	E	R	G	E	N	C	Y	R	E	S	P	O	N	S	E	D
S	E	X	U	A	L	E	X	P	R	E	S	S	I	O	N	R	S	L	I
C	O	M	M	U	N	I	T	Y	M	O	B	I	L	I	T	Y	A	F	N
Y	N	F	G	Q	D	G	I	S	A	Y	T	W	Q	G	Q	W	G	S	G
I	B	M	R	X	G	N	M	W	I	D	F	D	J	F	L	V	N	V	A
K	W	S	O	Q	P	Y	L	N	J	I	A	Z	L	E	E	N	P	I	N
I	E	L	O	G	F	S	F	F	L	U	V	G	A	N	I	C	S	G	D
J	N	W	M	H	A	D	L	G	N	I	S	S	E	R	D	C	L	J	E
M	V	A	I	X	F	Q	D	G	P	Q	V	V	E	F	Q	L	O	C	A
J	S	N	U	W	C	R	O	S	L	V	U	K	V	Q	Q	L	F	T	
G	M	Q	G	B	D	B	S	W	Z	R	Y	J	O	Q	Y	Y	L	P	I
B	A	T	H	I	N	G	S	H	O	W	E	R	I	N	G	W	K	H	N
V	E	R	A	C	E	C	I	V	E	D	L	A	N	O	S	R	E	P	G
M	E	D	I	C	A	T	I	O	N	R	O	U	T	I	N	E	Q	X	P
T	O	I	L	E	T	H	Y	G	I	E	N	E	K	M	E	D	M	S	Z
H	E	A	L	T	H	M	A	I	N	T	E	N	A	N	C	E	S	Z	R
O	R	A	L	H	Y	G	I	E	N	E	S	J	C	B	A	O	Z	I	V

CROSSWORD PUZZLE

Performance Areas
• **Activities of Daily Living**

Directions: Test your Activities of Daily Living vocabulary by completing the crossword puzzle. The answer key is in Appendix A.

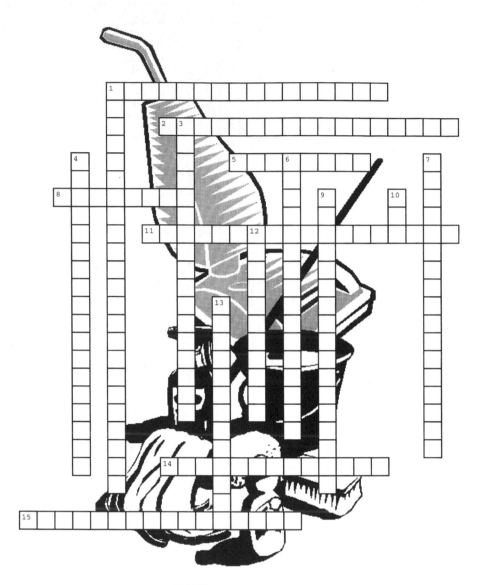

ACROSS

1. Setting up food; selecting and using appropriate utensils and tableware; bringing food or drink to mouth . . . (3 words)
2. Obtaining medication, opening and closing containers, following prescribed schedules . . . (2 words)
5. Selecting clothing and accessories appropriate to time of day, weather, and occasion . . .
8. Obtaining and using supplies; removing body hair; applying and removing cosmetics . . .
11. Moving from one position or place to another, such as in-bed mobility, wheelchair mobility . . . (2 words)
14. Accessing opportunities and interacting with other people in appropriate contextual and cultural ways . . .
15. Obtaining and using supplies; soaping, rinsing, and drying body parts . . . (2 words)

DOWN

1. Using equipment or systems to send and receive information, such as writing equipment, telephones . . . (2 words)
3. Recognizing sudden, unexpected hazardous situations, and initiating action to reduce the threat to health and safety (2 words)
4. Cleaning and maintaining personal care items, such as hearing aids, contact lenses . . . (3 words)
6. Engaging in desired sexual and intimate activities (2 words)
7. Developing and maintaining routines for illness prevention and wellness promotion . . . (2 words)
9. Moving self in the community and using public or private transportation, such as driving, or accessing buses, taxi cabs . . . (2 words)
10. Self-maintenance tasks (phrase: use first letter of each main word)
12. Obtaining and using supplies; cleaning mouth; brushing and flossing teeth . . . (2 words)
13. Obtaining and using supplies; clothing management; maintaining toileting position . . . (2 words)

Story Writing

The next activity is story writing. You will need a yellow, a green, and a blue crayon and a pen or pencil. Follow the directions below for each story.

DIRECTIONS

1. Review the list of terms that appears in the left margin of the story-writing page; then look at the scene for a visual representation of each term.
2. Create a story incorporating all of the terms within the designated section of Uniform Terminology.
3. Begin by completing the lead-in sentence that follows the list of terms. This sentence will be the first sentence of your story.
4. As you write the story do the following:
   a. Cross out the term from the list as you use it in the story.
   b. Underline the term in your story.
   c. Using the color associated with the domain you are working on (refer to the color code described below), lightly shade each area of the scene after it becomes part of the story. To help you remember the terminology, you will use the following colors to anchor your thinking about each domain of the Uniform Terminology.

Yellow for Performance Areas. Yellow is associated with the warmth of the sun and symbolizes happiness and well-being. Occupational therapy practitioners help others achieve satisfaction within their daily occupational performance.

Green for Performance Components. Green is the color of vegetation; it symbolizes growth and change. Therapy guides work to bring about change in the various Performance Components.

Blue for Performance Contexts. Blue is the color associated with the sky and the air below. Like sky and air, context is all inclusive. It gives each experience its unique set of memories, biases, predispositions, expectations, fears, reactions, knowledge, and meanings. Therapy guides always take the Performance Context into consideration when planning the route of a successful therapy expedition.

Figure 4.6. *The See-Through Apartment*

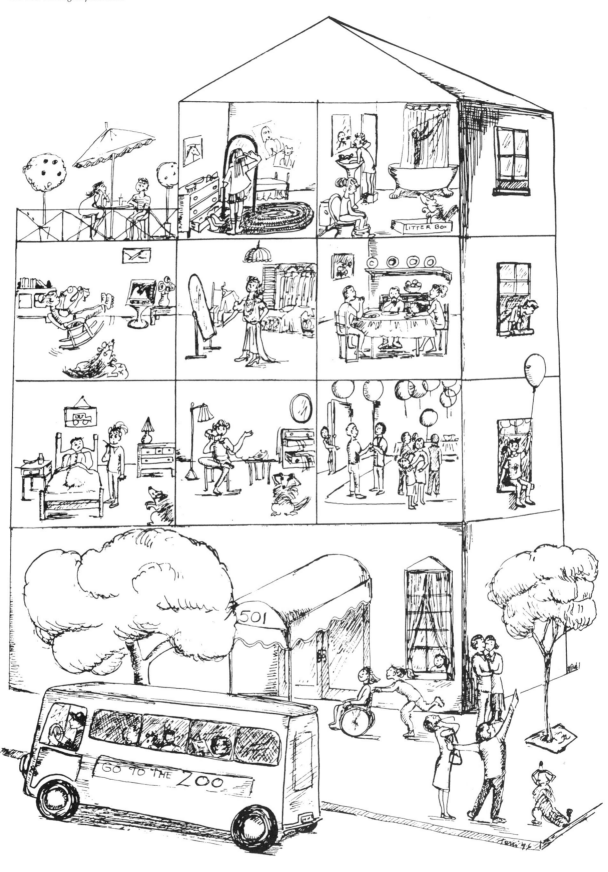

STORY WRITING

Performance Areas
- **Activities of Daily Living**

Directions: The activities represented by the 15 terms of Performance Areas, Activities of Daily Living, listed below, are hidden in Figure 4.6, "The See-Through Apartment." Can you write a story that incorporates all 15 terms? Cross out the term in the list as you use it and color that portion of the picture *yellow*. Parts of the scene fit more than one term. Try, however, to use a different part of the picture for each term that you include in your story. Begin your story by completing the sentence provided. Your story must have a beginning, a middle, and an ending.

TERMS
grooming
oral hygiene
bathing/showering
toilet hygiene
personal device care
dressing
feeding and eating
medication routine
health maintenance
socialization
functional communication
functional mobility
community mobility
emergency response
sexual expression

On a warm, sunny day as Kathy was being wheeled to the bus, she suddenly realized . . .

Continue your immersion in the Performance Areas terminology by completing the Work and Productive Activities/Play and Leisure word search, crossword puzzle, and story writing.

WORD SEARCH

Performance Areas
• **Work and Productive Activities**
• **Play and Leisure**

Directions: The terms related to Work and Productive Activities and Play and Leisure are hidden in the grid of letters. Look across, back, down, up, and diagonally. Circle each term you discover. The word CLEANING has been circled as an example.

TERMS

HomeManagement
ClothingCare
Cleaning
MealPrepCleanup
Shopping
MoneyManagement
HouseholdMaintenance
SafetyProcedures
CareOfOthers
EduActivities
VocActivities
VocExploration
JobAcquisition
WorkPerformance
RetirementPlan
Volunteer
PlayLeisureExpl
PlayLeisurePerf

T	Y	A	Q	C	L	I	C	N	M	S	N	W	S	M	N	L	F	A	X
T	N	E	T	W	M	W	L	O	E	E	O	O	H	O	A	P	R	T	G
B	P	W	N	R	Z	P	O	I	A	I	I	R	O	N	L	X	E	M	P
X	B	W	C	N	P	A	T	T	L	T	T	K	P	E	P	E	P	K	M
F	N	U	J	S	X	R	H	A	P	I	I	P	P	Y	T	E	E	S	L
A	F	Y	N	F	Q	D	I	R	R	V	S	E	I	M	N	R	R	G	I
C	S	A	Y	T	W	Q	N	O	E	I	I	R	N	A	E	U	U	G	Q
W	L	G	S	I	B	M	G	L	P	T	U	F	G	N	M	S	S	X	G
N	M	E	W	I	D	F	C	P	C	C	Q	O	D	A	E	I	I	J	F
L	V	N	A	V	K	W	A	X	L	A	C	R	S	G	R	E	E	Q	P
Y	L	N	J	N	I	A	R	E	E	C	A	M	Z	E	I	L	L	L	E
E	N	P	I	I	I	E	E	C	A	O	B	A	L	M	T	Y	Y	G	F
S	F	F	L	U	V	N	G	O	N	V	O	N	A	E	E	A	A	N	I
C	S	G	J	N	W	H	G	V	U	C	J	C	L	N	R	L	L	J	M
R	E	E	T	N	U	L	O	V	P	V	A	E	X	T	F	P	P	Q	D
H	O	U	S	E	H	O	L	D	M	A	I	N	T	E	N	A	N	C	E
G	P	Q	S	A	F	E	T	Y	P	R	O	C	E	D	U	R	E	S	V
C	A	R	E	O	F	O	T	H	E	R	S	V	E	F	Q	L	O	C	J
E	D	U	A	C	T	I	V	I	T	I	E	S	S	N	U	W	C	R	O
H	O	M	E	M	A	N	A	G	E	M	E	N	T	S	L	V	U	K	V

CROSSWORD PUZZLE

Directions: Test your Work and Productive Activities and Play and Leisure vocabulary by completing the crossword puzzle. The answer key is in Appendix A.

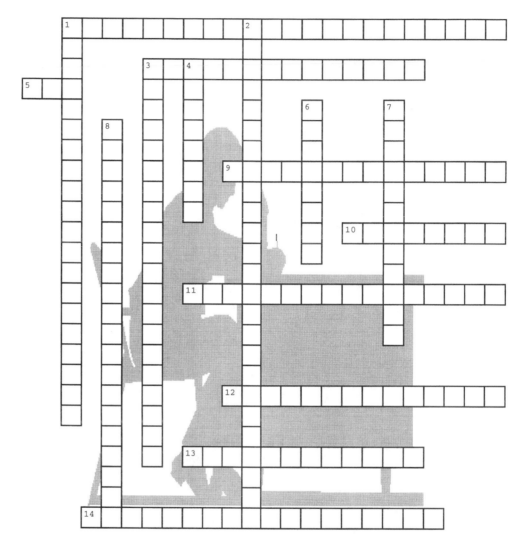

ACROSS

1. Performing unpaid activities for the benefit of individuals, groups, or causes (2 words)
3. Obtaining and maintaining personal and household possessions and environment (2 words)
5. Purposeful activities for self-development, social contribution, and livelihood (Phrase; use first letter of each main word)
9. Intrinsically motivating activities for amusement, relaxation, enjoyment, or self-expression (3 words)
10. Preparing shopping lists; selecting and purchasing items
11. Knowing and performing preventive and emergency procedures to maintain a safe environment . . . (2 words)
12. Identifying and selecting work opportunities, and completing application and interview processes (2 words)
13. Obtaining and using supplies; sorting, laundering, folding; ironing; storing; and mending
14. Determining aptitudes; developing interests and skills; selecting avocational pursuits (2 words)

DOWN

1. Participating in work-related activities (2 words)
2. Identifying interests, skills, and opportunities, and appropriate play or leisure activities (4 words)
3. Maintaining home, yard, garden, appliances . . . (2 words)
4. Planning meals; preparing and serving food (first 2 words of 4-word phrase; shortened term)
6. Obtaining and using supplies; picking up; putting away; vacuuming; sweeping and mopping floors . . .
7. Providing for children, spouse, parents, pets or others and using age-appropriate activities (3 words)
8. Performing job tasks in a timely and effective manner . . . (4 words)

Figure 4.7. *The Community Center*

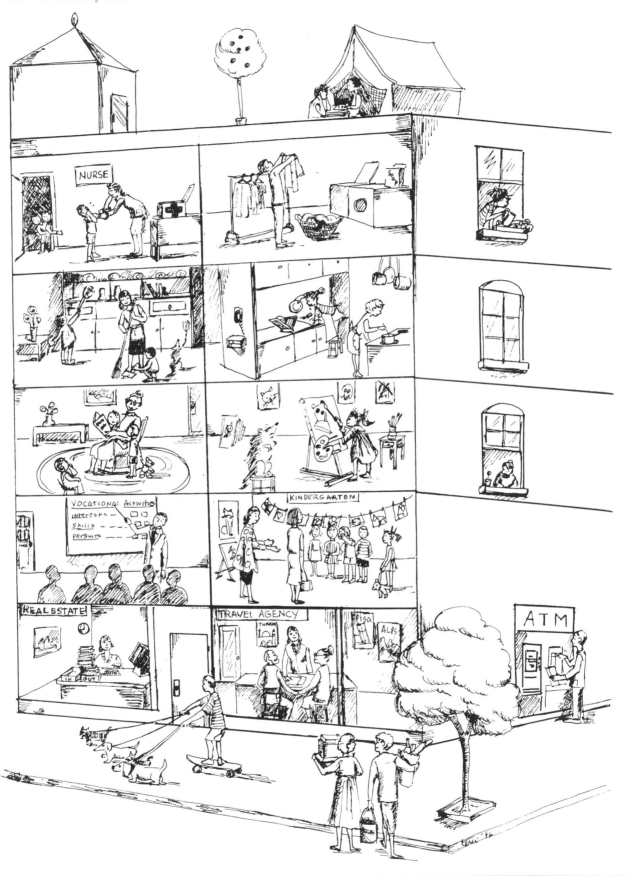

STORY WRITING

Performance Areas
- **Work and Productive Activities**
- **Play and Leisure**

Directions: The activities represented by the 18 terms of Performance Areas, Work and Productive Activities and Play and Leisure, listed below, are hidden in Figure 4.7, "The Community Center." Can you write a story that incorporates all 18 terms? Cross out the term in the list as you use it in the story and color that portion of the picture *yellow*. Parts of the scene fit more than one term. Try, however, to use a different part of the picture for each term that you include in your story. Begin your story by completing the sentence provided.

TERMS

home management
clothing care
cleaning
meal preparation and cleanup
shopping
money management
household maintenance
safety procedures
care of others
educational activities
vocational activities
vocational exploration
job acquisition
work or job performance
retirement planning
volunteer participation
play and leisure exploration
play and leisure performance

Jose was on his way to school, riding a skate board pulled by his trusty pack of "wiener dogs," when he thought about . . .

You have completed your work on the Performance Areas. You will now learn about Performance Components.

Performance Components

The Performance Components are capabilities that individuals must master in order to successfully engage in Performance Areas. Continue your immersion into the language of occupational therapy by learning the meanings of terms that describe aspects of Performance Components.

DIRECTIONS

1. Look at Figure 4.8 and familiarize yourself with the categories and subcategories of the Performance Components domain.
2. Next, turn to the concept maps of the Performance Components (Figures 4.9 through 4.14). Can you see the relationship between each graphic and its respective term?
3. Create your own definition for each term by reflecting on the picture paired with the term. Before recording your definitions, locate the two versions of the AOTA dictionary. The first version has blanks for your definitions; the second version shows the AOTA definitions.
4. Record your definitions in the blank spaces of the first AOTA dictionary.
5. When you have recorded all your definitions for the Performance Components terms, turn to the second version of the AOTA Uniform Terminology dictionary and underline the words or phrases in each definition that relate to the graphic.

   Example:

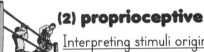

(2) proprioceptive
Interpreting stimuli originating in muscles, joints, and other internal tissues that give information about the position of one body part in relation to another.

6. Go back to your definitions and see how closely each one matches the AOTA definition. Use the following criteria to score your work. Record the score in the margin next to each definition.

   2 points Your definition has at least *two elements* included in AOTA's definition.
   1 point   Your definition has at least *one element* included in AOTA's definition.

7. Determine your total score by adding up your points. Record your score in the box below.

Score

If you scored

- ◆ 108–126 points: You're off and running.
- ◆ 88–107 points: You have a solid start.
- ◆ 87 points or below: Now you know what to work on.

Complete the Performance Components word searches and crossword puzzles (see Appendix A for answers). Pause along the way to study the scenes and write stories using the terms you are learning.

Figure 4.8. *Categories and Subcategories of the Uniform Terminology Domain Performance Components*

Performance **Components**

Sensorimotor Component

Sensory
- Sensory Awareness
- Sensory Processing
  - Tactile
  - Proprioceptive
  - Vestibular
  - Visual
  - Auditory
  - Gustatory
  - Olfactory
- Perceptual Processing
  - Stereognosis
  - Kinesthesia
  - Pain Response
  - Body Scheme
  - Right-Left Discrimination
  - Form Constancy
  - Position in Space
  - Visual-Closure
  - Figure Ground
  - Depth Perception
  - Spatial Relations
  - Topographical Orientation

Neuromusculo-skeletal
- Reflex
- Range of Motion
- Muscle Tone
- Strength
- Endurance
- Postural Control
- Postural Alignment
- Soft Tissue Integrity

Motor
- Gross Coordination
- Crossing Midline
- Laterality
- Bilateral Integration
- Motor Control
- Praxis
- Fine Coordination/Dexterity
- Visual-Motor Integration
- Oral-Motor Control

Psychosocial Skills

Psychological
- Values
- Interests
- Self-concept

Social
- Role Performance
- Social Conduct
- Interpersonal Skills
- Self-Expression

Self-Management
- Coping Skills
- Time Management
- Self-Control

Cognitive Integration & Cognitive Components
- Level of Arousal
- Orientation
- Recognition
- Attention Span
- Initiation of Activity
- Termination of Activity
- Memory
- Sequencing
- Categorization
- Concept Formation
- Spatial Operations
- Problem Solving
- Learning
- Generalization

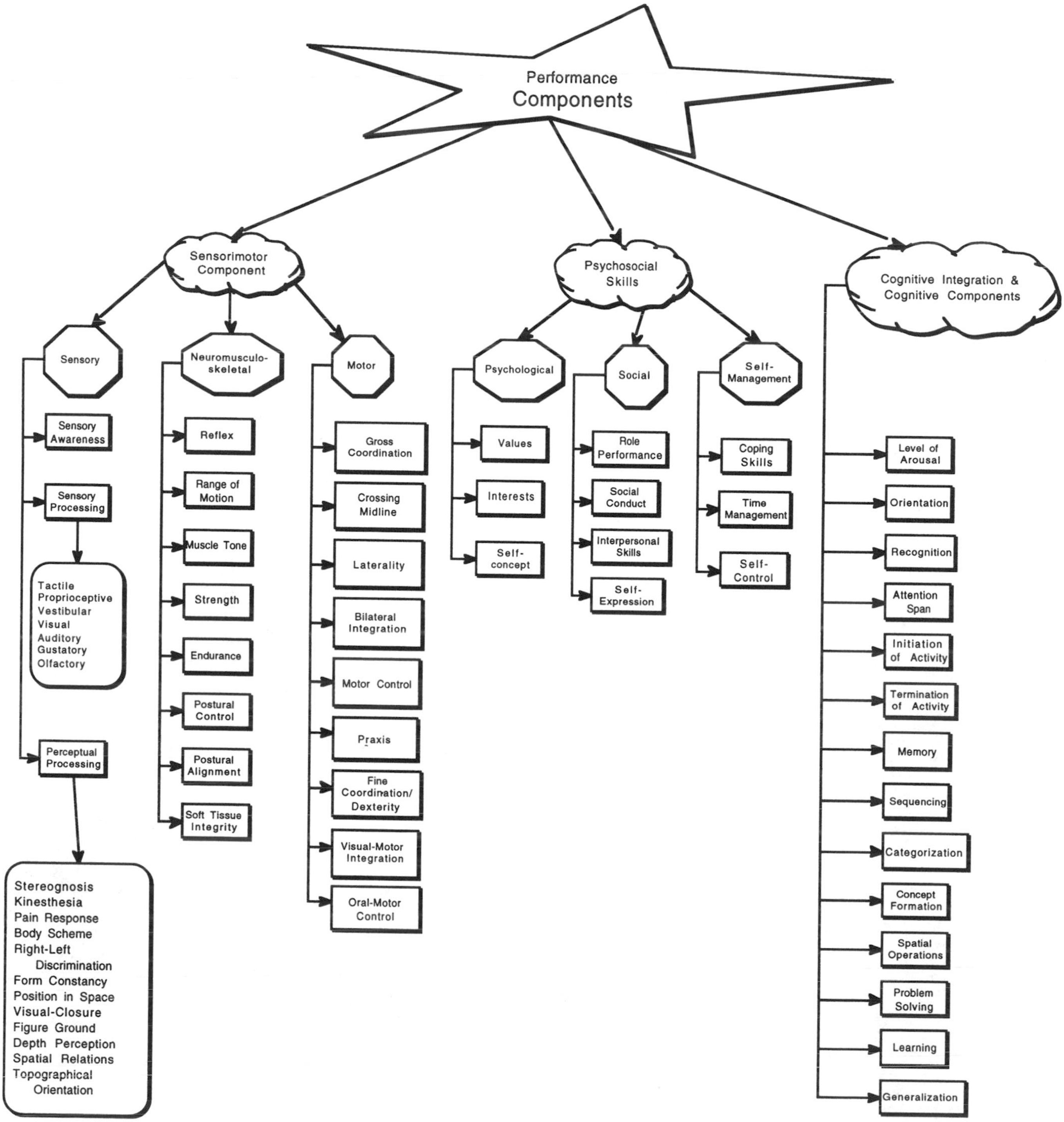

Figure 4.9. *Sensorimotor Component and Sensory and Sensory Processing Concept Map*

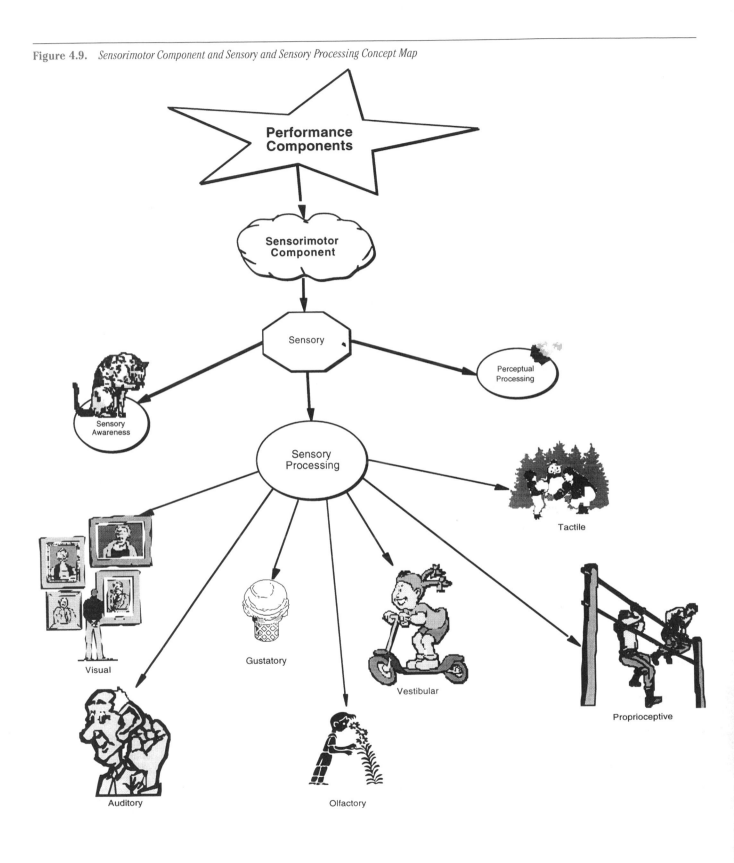

Figure 4.10. *Sensorimotor Component and Sensory and Perceptual Processing Concept Map*

Performance Components
Sensorimotor Component
Sensory
Stereognosis
Spatial Relations
Kinesthesia
Perceptual Processing
Topographical Orientation
Pain Response
Depth Perception
Body Scheme
KEEP
RIGHT
Right-Left Discrimination
Visual-Closure
Position in Space
Form Constancy
Figure Ground

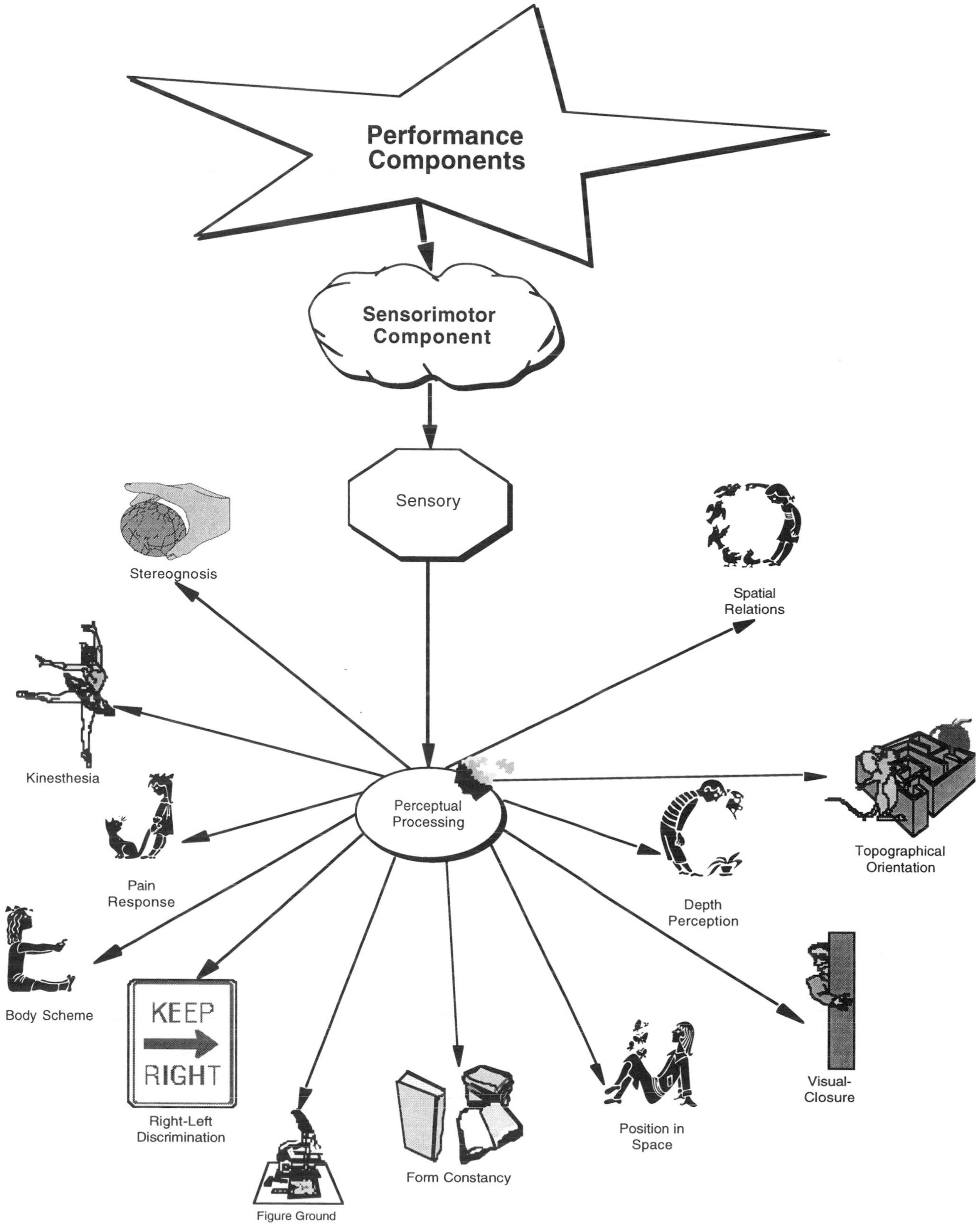

Figure 4.11. *Sensorimotor Component and Neuromusculoskeletal Concept Map*

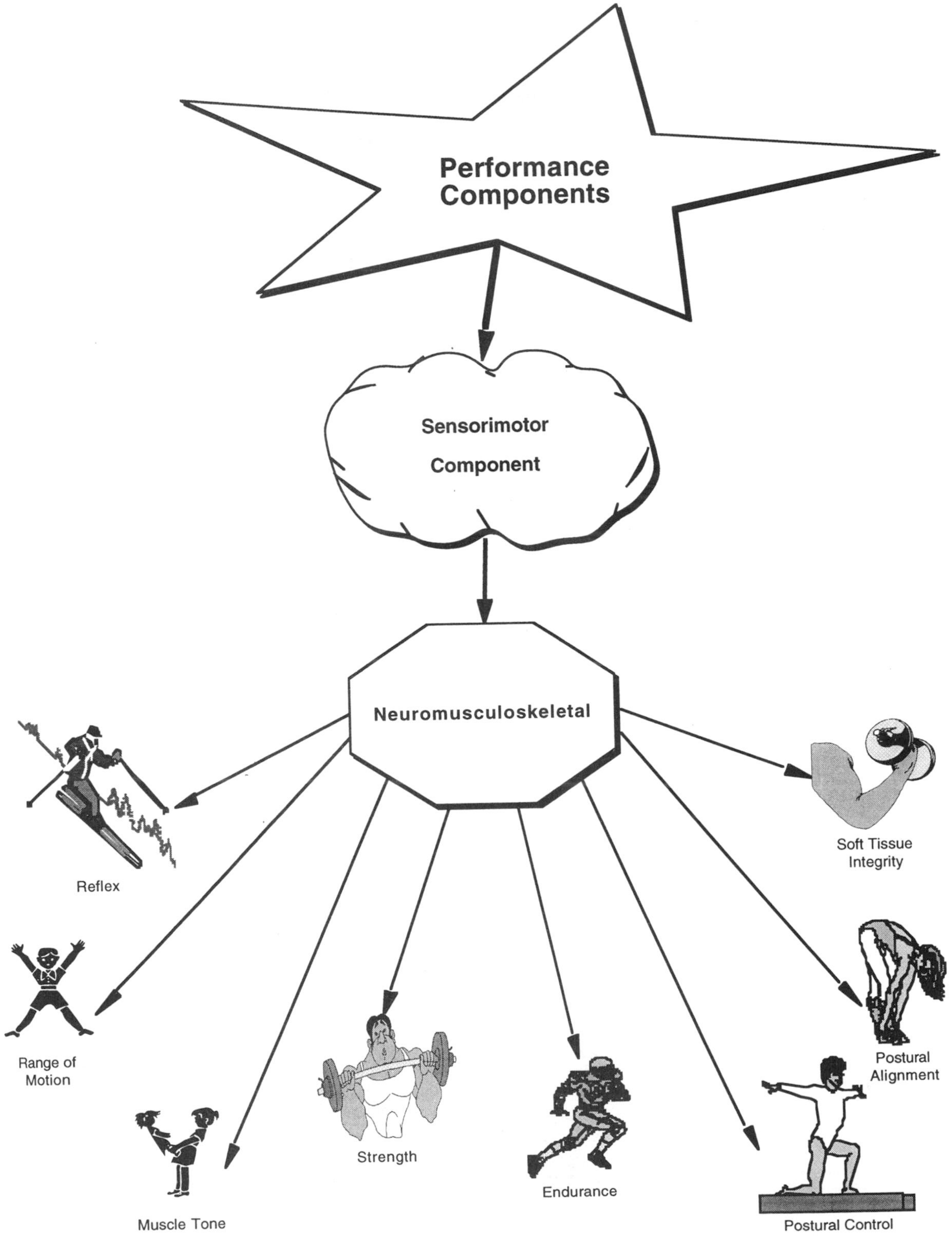

Performance Components

Sensorimotor Component

Neuromusculoskeletal

Reflex

Range of Motion

Muscle Tone

Strength

Endurance

Postural Control

Postural Alignment

Soft Tissue Integrity

Figure 4.12. *Sensorimotor Component and Motor Concept Map*

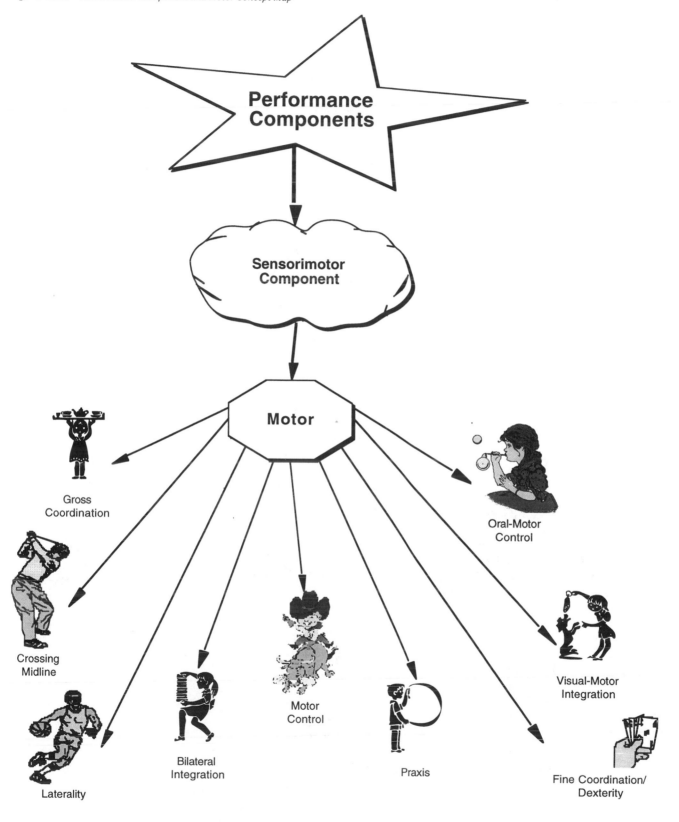

Figure 4.13. *Cognitive Integration and Cognitive Components Concept Map*

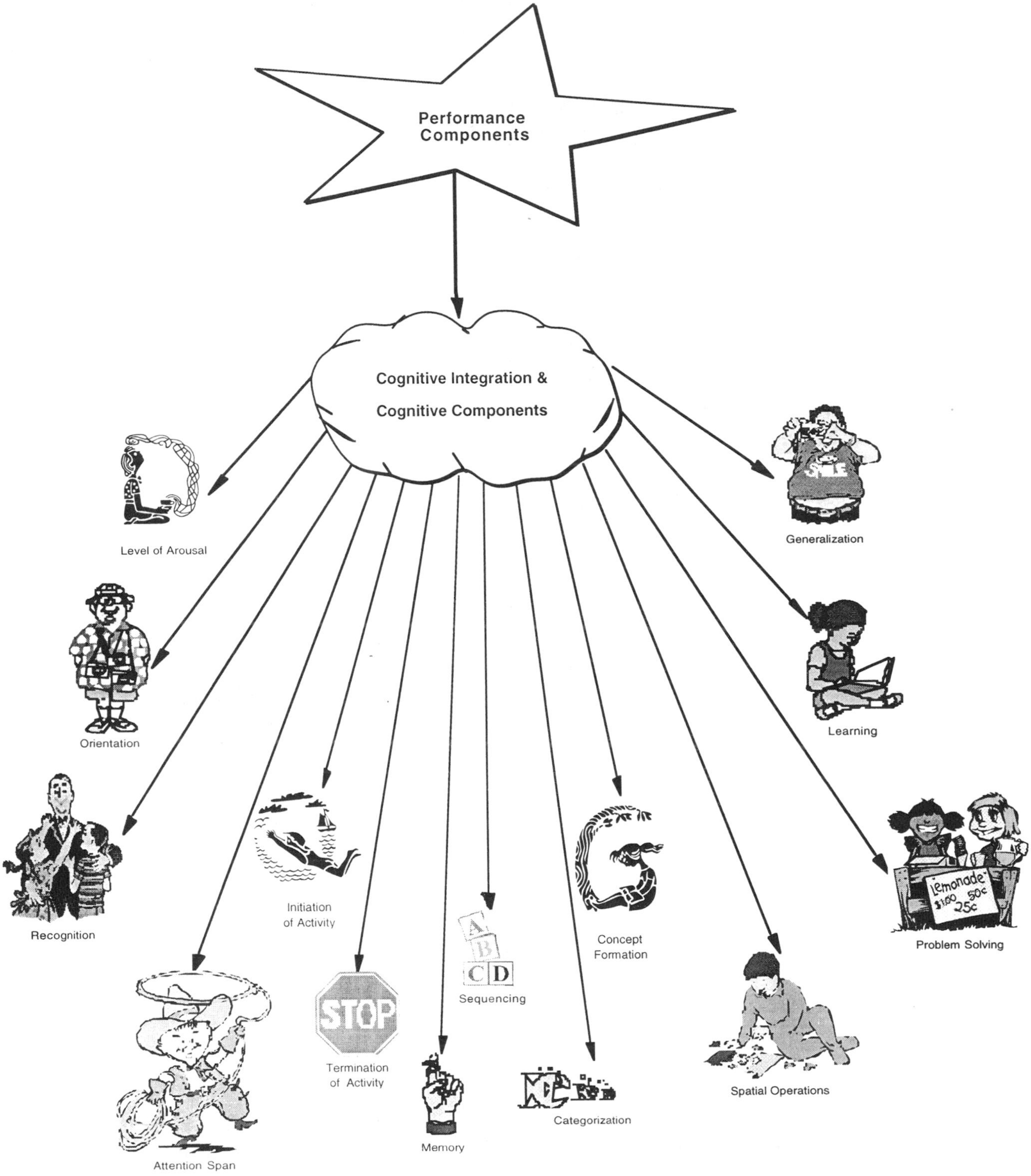
Performance Components
Cognitive Integration & Cognitive Components
Level of Arousal
Orientation
Recognition
Attention Span
Initiation of Activity
STOP
Termination of Activity
A
B
C D
Sequencing
Memory
Categorization
Concept Formation
Spatial Operations
Generalization
Learning
Lemonade
$1.00
50¢
25¢
Problem Solving

Figure 4.14. *Psychosocial Skills Concept Map*

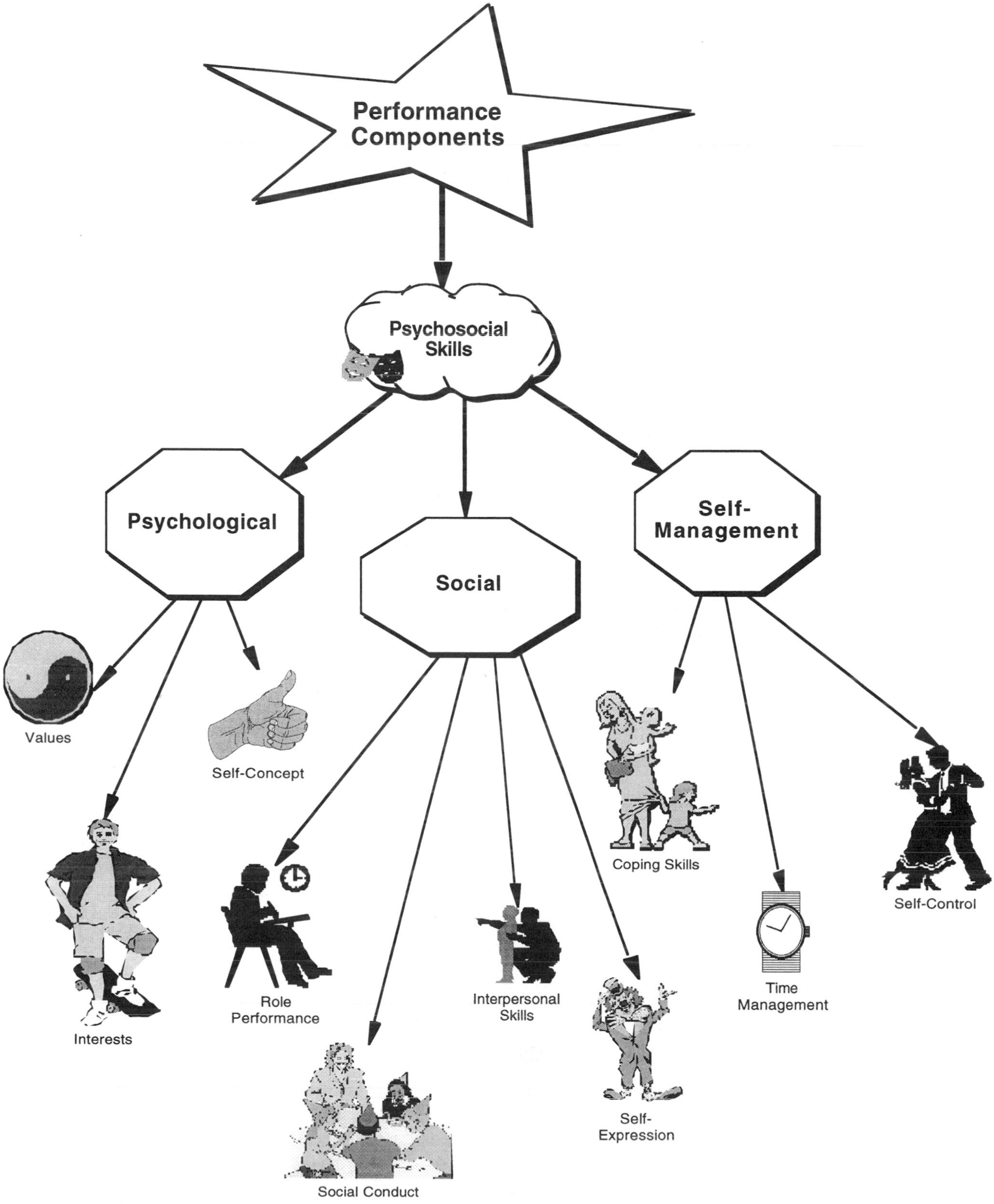

Performance Components

Psychosocial Skills

Psychological

Social

Self-Management

Values

Self-Concept

Interests

Role Performance

Social Conduct

Interpersonal Skills

Self-Expression

Coping Skills

Time Management

Self-Control

II. Performance Components:

A. SENSORIMOTOR COMPONENT

The ability to receive input, process information, and produce output.

1. Sensory

a. sensory awareness

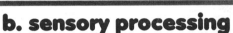

b. sensory processing

Interpreting sensory stimuli:

(1) **tactile**

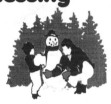

(2) **proprioceptive**

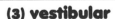

(3) **vestibular**

(4) **visual**

(5) **auditory**

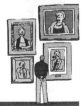

(6) **gustatory**

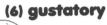

(7) **olfactory**

c. perceptual processing

Organizing sensory input into meaningful patterns:

(1) **stereognosis**

(2) **kinesthesia**

(3) **pain response**

(4) **body scheme**

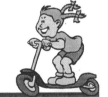

(5) **right - left discrimination**

(6) **form constancy**

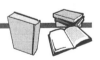

(7) **position in space**

(8) visual – closure

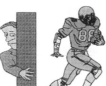

e. endurance

(9) figure ground

f. postural control

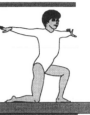

(10) depth perception

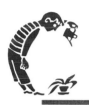

g. postural alignment

(11) spatial relations

h. soft tissue integrity

(12) topographical orientation

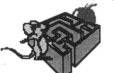

3. Motor
   a. gross coordination

2. Neuromusculoskeletal
a. reflex

b. crossing midline

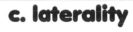

b. range of motion

c. laterality

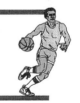

c. muscle tone

d. bilateral integration

d. strength

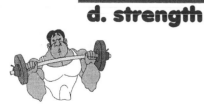

e. motor control

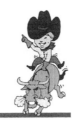

4. attention span

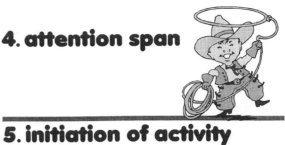

f. praxis

5. initiation of activity

g. fine coordination/dexterity

6. termination of activity

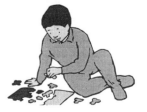

h. visual – motor integration

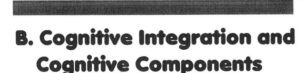

7. memory

8. sequencing

i. oral – motor control

9. categorization

B. Cognitive Integration and Cognitive Components

The ability to use higher brain functions.

1. level of arousal

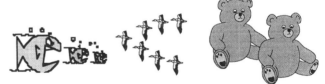

10. concept formation

2. orientation

11. spatial operations

3. recognition

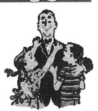

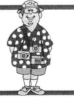

12. problem solving

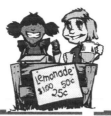

b. social conduct

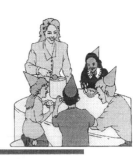

13. learning

c. interpersonal skills

14. generalization

d. self - expression

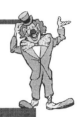

C. Psychosocial Skills

The ability to interact in society and to process emotions.

1. psychological
a. **values**

Forces of Creation
Positive & Negative

3. self - management
a. **coping skills**

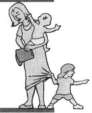

b. **interests**

b. time management

c. self - concept

c. self - control

2. social
a. **role performance**

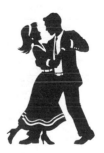

II. Performance Components:

A. SENSORIMOTOR COMPONENT

The ability to receive input, process information, and produce output.

1. Sensory

a. sensory awareness

Receiving and differentiating sensory stimuli

b. sensory processing

Interpreting sensory stimuli:

(1) tactile

Interpreting light touch, pressure, temperature, pain, and vibration through skin contact/receptors.

(2) proprioceptive

Interpreting stimuli originating in muscles, joints, and other internal tissues that give information about the position of one body part in relation to another.

(3) vestibular

Interpreting stimuli from the inner ear receptors regarding head position and movement.

(4) visual

Interpreting stimuli through the eyes, including peripheral vision and acuity, and awareness of color and pattern.

(5) auditory

Interpreting and localizing sounds, and discriminating background sounds.

(6) gustatory

Interpreting tastes.

(7) olfactory

Interpreting odors.

c. perceptual processing

Organizing sensory input into meaningful patterns:

(1) stereognosis

Identifying objects through proprioception, cognition, and the sense of touch.

(2) kinesthesia

Identifying the excursion and direction of joint movement.

(3) pain response

Interpreting noxious stimuli.

(4) body scheme

Acquiring an internal awareness of the body and the relationship of the body parts to each other.

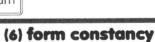 **(5) right – left discrimination**

Differentiating one side from the other.

(6) form constancy

Recognizing forms and objects as the same in various environments, positions, and sizes.

(7) position in space

Determining the spatial relationship of figures and objects to self or other forms and objects.

(8) visual - closure
Identifying forms or objects from incomplete presentations.

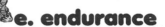

(9) figure ground
Differentiating between foreground and background forms and objects.

(10) depth perception
Determining the relative distance between objects, figures, or landmarks and the observer, and changes in planes of surfaces.

(11) spatial relations
Determining the position of objects relative to each other.

(12) topographical orientation
Determining the location of objects and settings and the route to the location.

2. Neuromusculoskeletal
a. reflex
Eliciting an involuntary muscle response to sensory input.

b. range of motion
Moving body parts through an arc.

c. muscle tone
Demonstrating a degree of tension or resistance in a muscle at rest and in response to stretch.

d. strength
Demonstrating a degree of muscle power when movement is resisted, as with objects of gravity.

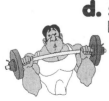

e. endurance
Sustaining cardiac, pulmonary, and musculoskeletal exertion over time.

f. postural control
Using righting and equilibrium adjustments to maintain balance during functional movements.

g. postural alignment
Maintaining biomechanical integrity among body parts.

h. soft tissue integrity
Maintaining anatomical and physiological condition on interstitial tissue and skin.

3. Motor
a. gross coordination
Using large muscle groups for controlled, goal-directed movements.

b. crossing midline
Moving limbs and eyes across the midsagittal plane of the body.

c. laterality
Using a preferred unilateral body part for activities requiring a high level of skill.

d. bilateral integration
Coordinating both body sides during activity.

e. motor control

Using the body in functional and versatile movement patterns.

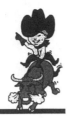

f. praxis

Conceiving and planning a new motor act in response to an environmental demand.

g. fine coordination/dexterity

Using small muscle groups for controlled movements, particularly in object manipulation.

h. visual – motor integration

Coordinating the interaction of information from the eyes with body movement during activity.

i. oral – motor control

Coordinating oropharyngeal musculature for controlled movement

B. Cognitive Integration and Cognitive Components

The ability to use higher brain functions.

1. level of arousal

Demonstrating alertness and responsiveness to environmental stimuli.

2. orientation

Identifying person, place, time, and situation.

3. recognition

Identifying familiar faces, objects, and other previously presented materials.

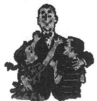

4. attention span

Focusing on a task over time.

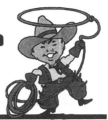

5. initiation of activity

Starting a physical or mental activity.

6. termination of activity

Stopping an activity at an appropriate time.

7. memory

Recalling information after brief or long periods of time.

8. sequencing

Placing information, concepts, and actions in order.

9. categorization

Identifying similarities of and differences among pieces of environmental information.

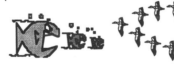

10. concept formation

Organizing a variety of information to form thoughts and ideas.

11. spatial operations

Mentally manipulating the position of objects in various relationships.

12. problem solving

Recognizing a problem, defining a problem, identifying alternative plans, selecting a plan, organizing steps in a plan, implementing a plan, and evaluating the outcome.

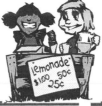

13. learning

Acquiring new concepts and behaviors.

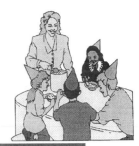

14. generalization

Applying previously learned concepts and behaviors to a variety of new situations.

C. Psychosocial Skills

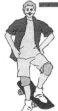

The ability to interact in society and to process emotions.

1. psychological
a. values

Identifying ideas or beliefs that are important to self and others.

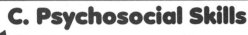
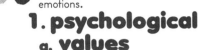

Forces of Creation
Positive & Negative

b. interests

Identifying mental or physical activities that create pleasure and maintain attention.

c. self - concept

Developing the value of the physical, emotional, and sexual self.

2. social
a. role performance

Identifying, maintaining, and balancing functions one assumes or acquires in society (e.g., work, student, parent, friend, religious participant).

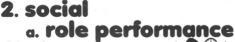

b. social conduct

Interacting by using manners, personal space, eye contact, gestures, active listening, and self–expression appropriate to one's environment.

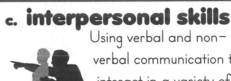

c. interpersonal skills

Using verbal and non–verbal communication to interact in a variety of settings.

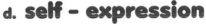

d. self - expression

Using a variety of styles and skills to express thoughts, feelings, and needs.

3. self - management
a. coping skills

Identifying and managing stress and related factors.

b. time management

Planning and participating in a balance of self–care, work, leisure, and rest activities to promote satisfaction and health.

c. self - control

Modifying one's own behavior in response to environmental needs, demands, constraints, personal aspirations, and feedback from others.

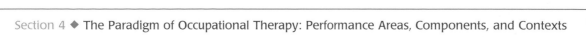

WORD SEARCH

Performance Components
- **Sensorimotor Component**
  - **Sensory**
    - **Sensory Awareness**
    - **Sensory Processing**

Directions: The terms related to Sensory Awareness and Sensory Processing are hidden in the grid of letters. Look across, back, down, up, and diagonally. You will find the terms on the grid exactly as you see them listed below. Circle each term you discover. The word SENSORYPROCESSING has been circled as an example.

TERMS

Sensorimotor
SensoryAwareness
SensoryProcessing
Tactile
Proprioceptive
Vestibular
Visual
Auditory
Gustatory
Olfactory

R	P	Z	S	D	L	G	S	Z	M	Y	Q	P	A	E	G	R	O	M	O
D	P	R	E	W	D	U	Y	N	G	R	Y	T	U	C	F	Y	Q	F	J
J	E	T	N	G	J	S	C	Z	T	Q	K	C	D	C	K	U	V	V	J
O	W	R	S	X	X	T	K	V	C	K	P	A	I	M	A	Q	A	Z	B
K	T	E	O	O	J	A	Z	K	S	A	L	R	T	T	A	I	N	F	K
J	U	N	R	S	Y	T	S	F	K	H	B	P	O	Z	A	Q	U	E	Y
D	W	N	Y	H	P	O	H	Q	W	H	G	P	R	W	K	P	P	G	K
D	P	B	A	L	X	R	Y	V	H	M	G	E	Y	B	L	N	I	H	I
V	V	T	W	I	D	Y	B	M	S	E	R	D	W	D	G	A	T	O	L
S	C	D	A	J	C	H	Q	J	W	B	K	D	A	V	Y	Z	H	X	H
O	V	Z	R	L	S	E	N	S	O	R	I	M	O	T	O	R	J	R	X
J	W	E	E	A	L	A	U	S	I	V	G	P	W	K	R	F	U	D	J
U	L	Q	N	M	F	C	S	K	J	L	E	N	O	H	J	H	R	W	T
E	K	T	E	R	A	L	U	B	I	T	S	E	V	A	H	F	C	M	Q
L	Y	O	S	T	A	C	T	I	L	E	U	V	A	B	Y	F	O	T	B
U	I	F	S	T	B	O	L	F	A	C	T	O	R	Y	E	Q	N	R	K
J	B	V	A	F	N	G	K	U	V	W	N	O	J	D	R	I	P	O	W
P	R	O	P	R	I	O	C	E	P	T	I	V	E	F	R	G	V	A	O
Q	C	C	D	N	U	O	D	W	O	R	V	U	P	X	Q	A	V	R	Q
S	E	N	S	O	R	Y	P	R	O	C	E	S	S	I	N	G	L	K	H

CROSSWORD PUZZLE

Performance Components
- **Sensorimotor Component**
  - **Sensory**
    - **Sensory Awareness**
    - **Sensory Processing**

Directions: Test your Sensory Awareness and Sensory Processing vocabulary by completing the crossword puzzle below. The answer key is in Appendix A.

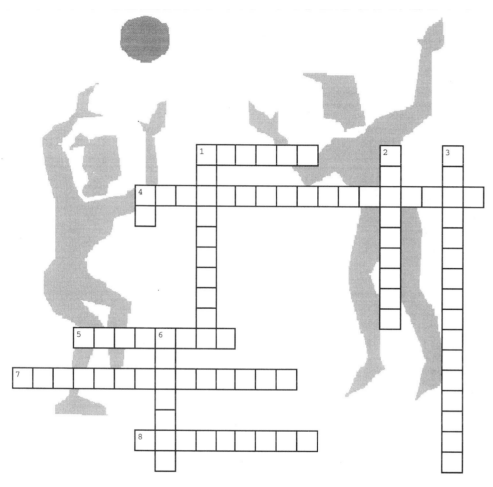

ACROSS

1. Interpreting stimuli through the eyes . . .
4. Interpreting sensory stimuli (2 words)
5. Interpreting and localizing sounds, and discriminating background sounds
7. Interpreting stimuli originating in muscles, joints and other internal tissues that give information about the position of one body part in relation to another
8. Interpreting odors

DOWN

1. Interpreting stimuli from the inner ear receptors regarding head position and movement
2. Interpreting tastes
3. Receiving and differentiating sensory stimuli (2 words)
4. The ability to receive input, process information, and produce output (two words; abbrev.)
6. Interpreting light touch, pressure, temperature, pain, and vibration through skin contact

Figure 4.15. *Day at the Park*

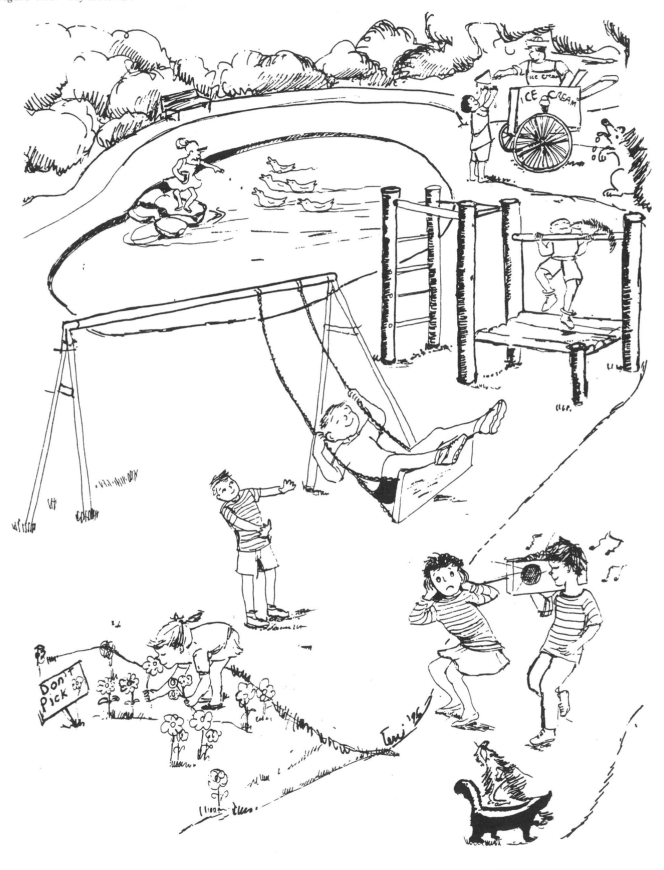

STORY WRITING

Mr. Hy Scream was just about to hand Darryl a dripping popsicle when all of a sudden . . .

Performance Components
- **Sensorimotor Component**
  - **Sensory**
    - **Sensory Awareness**
    - **Sensory Processing**

Directions: The concepts and sensory systems represented by the 9 terms of Performance Components, Sensorimotor Component, Sensory Awareness and Sensory Processing subcategories, listed below, are hidden in Figure 4.15, "Day at the Park." Can you write a story that incorporates all 9 terms? Cross out the term in the list as you use it in the story and color that portion of the picture *green*. Parts of the scene fit more than one term. Try, however, to use a different part of the picture for each term that you include in your story. Begin your story by completing the sentence provided.

TERMS
sensory awareness
sensory processing
tactile
proprioceptive
vestibular
visual
auditory
gustatory
olfactory

Performance Components
- **Sensorimotor Component**
  - **Sensory**
    - **Perceptual Processing**

Directions: The terms related to Perceptual Processing are hidden in the grid of letters. Look across, back, down, up, and diagonally. Circle each term you discover. The word KINESTHESIA has been circled as an example.

TERMS

PerceptualProcessing
Stereognosis
Kinesthesia
PainResponse
BodyScheme
RightLeftDiscriminat
FormConstancy
PositionInSpace
VisualClosure
FigureGround
DepthPerception
SpatialRelations
TopographicalOrienta

P	O	S	I	T	I	O	N	I	N	S	P	A	C	E	S	F	F	L	U
T	O	P	O	G	R	A	P	H	I	C	A	L	O	R	I	E	N	T	A
V	G	A	N	I	C	S	G	J	N	W	H	C	L	J	M	V	A	X	F
Q	D	G	P	Q	V	V	E	F	Q	L	O	C	J	S	N	U	W	C	R
O	S	L	V	U	K	V	Q	Q	L	F	G	M	Q	B	D	B	S	W	Z
R	Y	J	O	Q	Y	Y	L	P	W	K	H	V	Q	X	P	K	M	E	D
M	S	Z	S	T	E	R	E	O	G	N	O	S	I	S	S	Z	R	S	J
C	B	A	O	Z	I	V	D	J	U	C	T	N	E	W	Y	J	N	D	W
V	Q	Z	Z	N	D	H	N	W	T	T	H	P	C	K	D	P	N	H	X
R	U	Y	U	J	O	J	U	T	Q	G	V	A	M	L	M	I	G	L	K
P	E	R	C	E	P	T	U	A	L	P	R	O	C	E	S	S	I	N	G
X	W	N	F	X	Y	C	N	A	T	S	N	O	C	M	R	O	F	E	E
S	N	O	I	T	A	L	E	R	L	A	I	T	A	P	S	T	W	V	V
T	A	N	I	M	I	R	C	S	I	D	T	F	E	L	T	H	G	I	R
P	A	I	N	R	E	S	P	O	N	S	E	Y	J	Y	I	R	W	L	R
G	B	K	Q	K	T	V	I	S	U	A	L	C	L	O	S	U	R	E	B
O	K	A	O	Z	X	F	I	G	U	R	E	G	R	O	U	N	D	V	T
Z	T	W	U	W	J	C	E	H	B	O	D	Y	S	C	H	E	M	E	O
D	E	P	T	H	P	E	R	C	E	P	T	I	O	N	S	J	M	L	S
K	I	N	E	S	T	H	E	S	I	A	S	B	E	U	H	V	N	X	D

Performance Components
- **Sensorimotor Component**
  - **Sensory**
    - **Perceptual Processing**

Directions: Test your Perceptual Processing vocabulary by completing the crossword puzzle. The answer key is in Appendix A.

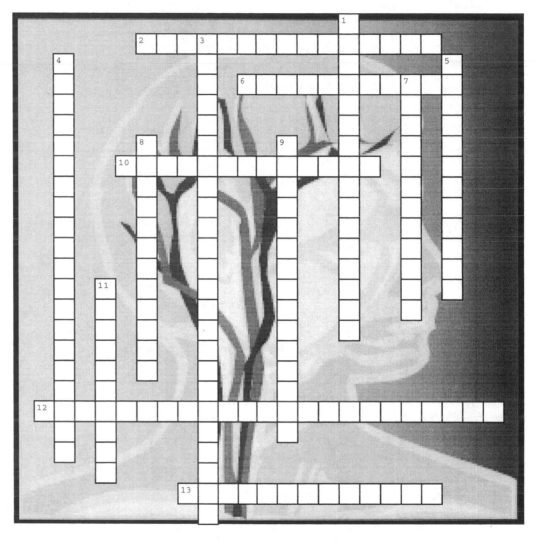

ACROSS

2. Determining the relative distance between objects, figures, or landmarks and the observer, and changes in planes of surfaces (2 words)
6. Identifying the excursion and direction of joint movement
10. Identifying forms or objects from incomplete presentations (2 words)
12. Differentiating one side from the other (3 words)
13. Recognizing forms and objects as the same in various environments, positions, and sizes (2 words)

DOWN

1. Determining the position of objects relative to each other (2 words)
3. Determining the location of objects and settings and the route to the location (2 words)
4. Organizing sensory input into meaningful patterns (2 words)
5. Interpreting noxious stimuli (2 words)
7. Identifying objects through proprioception, cognition, and the sense of touch
8. Differentiating between foreground and background forms and objects (2 words)
9. Determining the spatial relationship of figures and objects to self of other forms and objects (3 words)
11. Acquiring an internal awareness of the body and the relationship of the body parts to each other (2 words)

Figure 4.16. *Camp Fun*

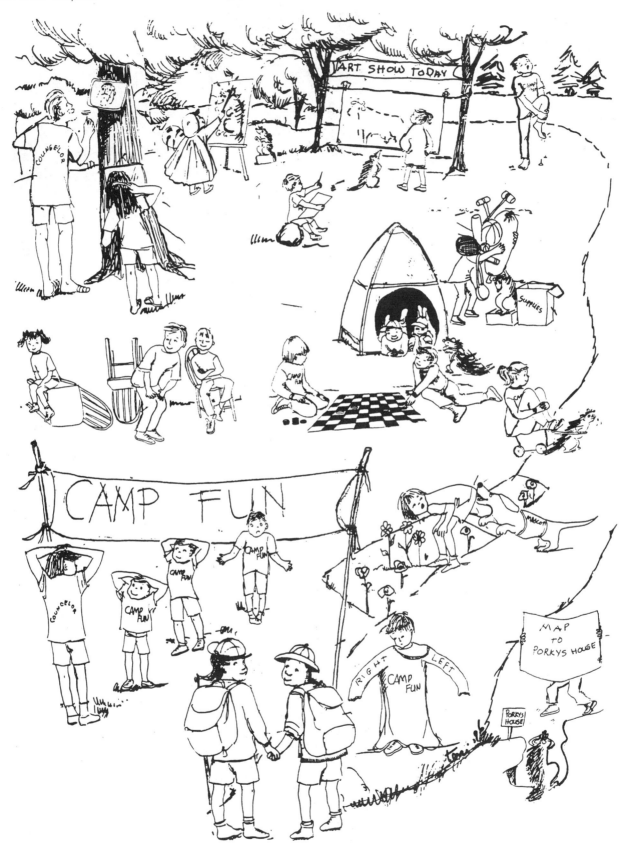

STORY WRITING

Performance Components
- **Sensorimotor Component**
  - **Sensory**
    - **Perceptual Processing**

Little Big Foot had just arrived at Camp Fun when someone . . .

Directions: The perceptual concepts represented by the 12 terms of Performance Components, Sensorimotor Component, Perceptual Processing subcategory, listed below, are hidden in Figure 4.16, "Camp Fun." Can you write a story that incorporates all 12 terms? Cross out the term in the list as you use it in the story and color that portion of the picture *green*. Parts of the scene fit more than one term. Try, however, to use a different part of the picture for each term that you include in your story. Begin your story by completing the sentence provided.

TERMS

stereognosis
kinesthesia
pain response
body scheme
right-left discrimination
form constancy
position in space
visual-closure
figure ground
depth perception
spatial relations
topographical orientation

WORD SEARCH

Directions: The terms related to Neuromusculoskeletal are hidden in the grid of letters. Look across, back, down, up, and diagonally. Circle each term you discover. The word REFLEX has been circled as an example.

TERMS
Reflex
ROM
MuscleTone
Strength
Endurance
PosturalControl
SoftTissueIntegrity
PosturalAlignment

C	D	A	T	Y	A	Q	C	L	I	A	X	T	N	E	T	W	M	W	P
T	G	B	P	W	N	R	Z	P	M	P	X	B	W	C	N	P	A	K	O
M	F	N	U	J	S	X	R	S	L	A	F	Y	N	F	Q	D	G	I	S
S	A	Y	T	W	Q	G	Q	W	G	S	I	B	M	X	G	N	M	W	T
I	D	F	D	J	F	L	V	N	V	K	W	S	Q	P	Y	L	N	J	U
I	A	Z	L	E	E	N	P	I	I	E	L	G	F	S	F	F	L	U	R
V	G	A	R	N	I	C	S	G	J	N	W	H	C	L	J	M	V	A	A
X	F	Q	O	D	G	P	Q	V	V	E	F	Q	L	O	C	J	S	N	L
U	W	C	M	R	O	S	L	V	U	K	V	Q	Q	L	F	G	M	Q	A
B	D	B	S	W	Z	R	Y	J	O	Q	Y	Y	L	P	W	K	H	V	L
Q	X	P	K	M	R	E	F	L	E	X	E	D	M	S	Z	S	Z	R	I
Y	T	I	R	G	E	T	N	I	E	U	S	S	I	T	T	F	O	S	G
S	J	C	B	A	O	Z	I	V	D	J	U	C	T	N	E	W	Y	J	N
N	L	O	R	T	N	O	C	L	A	R	U	T	S	O	P	D	W	V	M
S	T	R	E	N	G	T	H	Q	Z	Z	N	D	H	N	W	T	T	H	E
P	C	K	D	P	N	H	X	R	U	Y	U	J	O	J	U	T	Q	G	N
V	A	M	L	M	I	G	L	K	X	W	N	F	X	E	E	T	W	V	T
V	Y	J	Y	I	R	W	L	R	E	N	D	U	R	A	N	C	E	G	B
K	Q	K	T	B	O	K	A	O	Z	X	V	T	Z	T	W	U	W	J	C
M	U	S	C	L	E	T	O	N	E	E	H	O	S	J	M	L	S	S	B

CROSSWORD PUZZLE

Directions: Test your Neuro-musculoskeletal vocabulary by completing the crossword puzzle below. The answer key is in Appendix A.

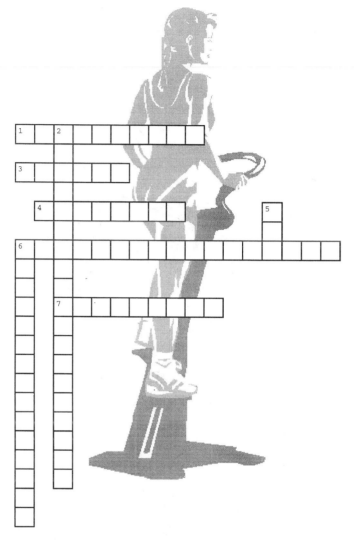

ACROSS

1. Demonstrating a degree of tension or resistance in a muscle at rest and in response to stretch (2 words)
3. Eliciting an involuntary muscle response to sensory input
4. Demonstrating a degree of muscle power when movement is resisted, as with objects of gravity
6. Maintaining biochemical integrity among body parts (2 words)
7. Sustaining cardiac, pulmonary, and musculoskeletal exertion over time

DOWN

2. Maintaining anatomical and physiological condition on interstitial tissue and skin (3 words)
5. Moving body parts through an arc (abbrev.)
6. Using righting and equilibrium adjustments to maintain balance during functional movements (2 words)

Figure 4.17. *The Beach*

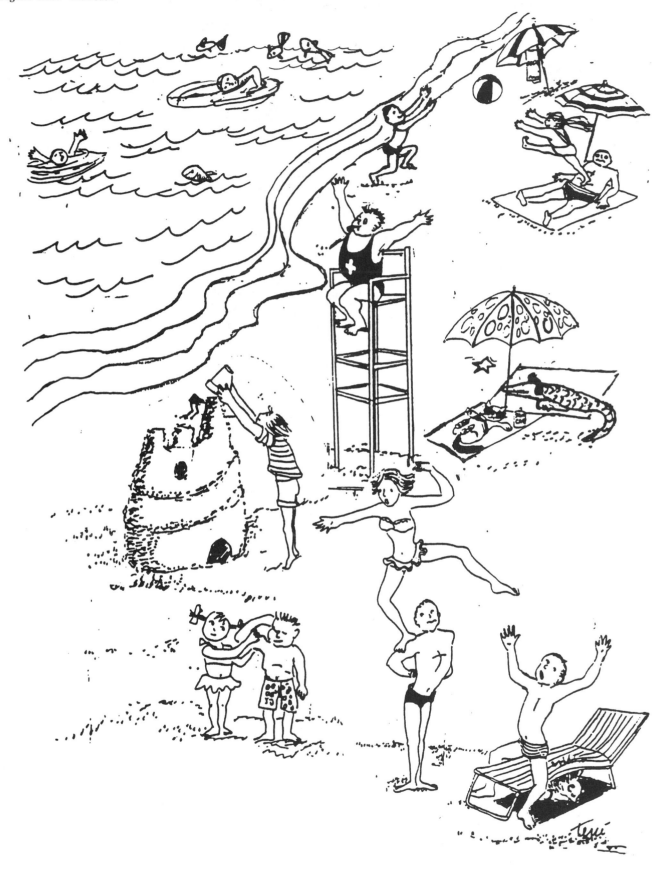

STORY WRITING

Directions: The concepts represented by the 8 terms of Performance Components, Sensorimotor Component, Neuromusculoskeletal subcategory, listed below, are hidden in Figure 4.17, "The Beach." Can you write a story that incorporates all 8 terms? Cross out the term in the list as you use it in the story and color that portion of the picture *green*. There is ambiguity among the actions representing terms. For example, muscle tone is visually represented in more than one place within the scene. Try, however, to use a different part of the picture for each term that you include in your story. Begin your story by completing the sentence provided.

TERMS

reflex
range of motion
muscle tone
strength
endurance
postural control
postural alignment
soft tissue integrity

Mr. Crock O. Dile and Ms. Kit Eee wished to have a peaceful day at the beach, but . . .

WORD SEARCH

Performance Components
- **Sensorimotor**
  Component
  - **Motor**

Directions: The terms related to Motor are hidden in the grid of letters. Look across, back, down, up, and diagonally in the letters. Circle each term you discover. The word LATERALITY has been circled as an example.

TERMS

GrossCoordination
CrossingMidline
Laterality
BilateralIntegration
MotorControl
Praxis
FineCoordinationDext
VisualMotorInteg
OralMotorControl

B	I	L	A	T	E	R	A	L	I	N	T	E	G	R	A	T	I	O	N
Q	Z	Z	N	D	H	N	W	T	T	H	P	C	K	D	P	N	H	X	R
F	I	N	E	C	O	O	R	D	I	N	A	T	I	O	N	D	E	X	T
U	Y	M	O	T	O	R	C	O	N	T	R	O	L	U	J	O	J	U	T
Q	G	V	A	M	L	M	I	G	L	K	X	W	N	F	X	E	E	T	W
V	V	Y	J	Y	C	R	O	S	S	I	N	G	M	I	D	L	I	N	E
I	R	W	L	R	G	B	K	Q	K	T	B	O	K	A	O	Z	X	V	T
O	R	A	L	M	O	T	O	R	C	O	N	T	R	O	L	Z	T	W	U
W	J	C	E	H	O	S	J	M	L	S	S	B	E	U	H	V	N	X	D
A	T	B	S	P	L	I	Q	X	L	Y	T	M	C	S	R	C	E	M	O
G	R	Y	O	Y	R	T	A	Y	Q	A	V	G	A	F	W	N	L	I	I
A	I	T	C	H	V	T	J	U	T	U	T	U	C	W	N	V	C	G	J
M	F	A	A	V	N	Q	H	N	W	P	I	E	R	P	H	S	Y	R	P
A	V	P	R	A	X	I	S	S	U	B	W	A	R	P	V	Q	X	K	Q
G	I	H	G	W	M	M	B	T	A	C	Z	J	P	A	N	R	L	Q	Q
D	J	R	N	U	L	O	Y	O	T	O	T	U	E	T	L	P	T	F	U
Q	D	Z	K	Y	Y	G	Q	S	G	A	I	U	S	D	V	I	W	I	P
G	R	O	S	S	C	O	O	R	D	I	N	A	T	I	O	N	T	I	K
Z	K	Q	D	S	W	K	Y	E	X	E	V	S	Z	X	H	Z	Z	Y	E
A	V	I	S	U	A	L	M	O	T	O	R	I	N	T	E	G	U	J	J

CROSSWORD PUZZLE

Performance Components
- **Sensorimotor Component**
  - **Motor**

Directions: Test your Motor vocabulary by completing the crossword puzzle below. The answer key is in Appendix A.

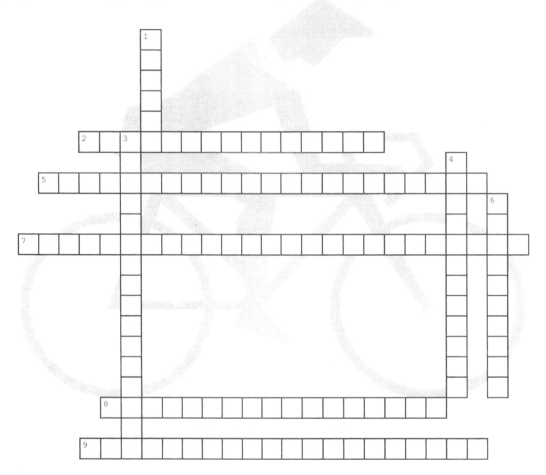

ACROSS

2. Moving limbs and eyes across the midsagittal plane of the body (2 words)
5. Coordinating the interaction of information from the eyes with body movement during activity (3 words)
7. Using small muscle groups for controlled movements, particularly in object manipulation
8. Using large muscle groups for controlled, goal-directed movements (2 words)
9. Coordinating both body sides during activity (2 words)

DOWN

1. Using the body in functional and versatile movement patterns
3. Coordinating oropharyngeal musculature for controlled movements (3 words)
4. Using the body in functional and versatile movement patterns (2 words)
6. Using a preferred unilateral body part for activities requiring a high level of skill

Figure 4.18. *Porky's Picnic*

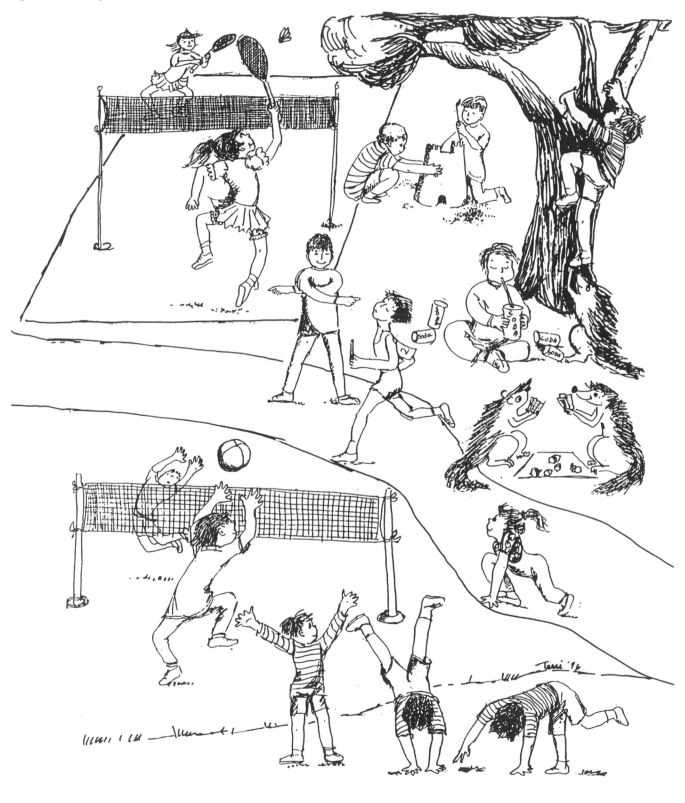

STORY WRITING

Directions: The concepts represented by the 9 terms of Performance Components, Sensorimotor Component, Motor subcategory, listed below, are hidden in Figure 4.18, "Porky's Picnic." Can you write a story that incorporates all 9 terms? Cross out the term in the list as you use it in the story and color that portion of the picture *green*. There is ambiguity among the actions representing terms. One term may be represented by more than one portion of the scene. Try, however, to use a different part of the picture for each term that you include in your story. Begin your story by completing the sentence provided.

TERMS

gross coordination
crossing midline
laterality
bilateral integration
motor control
praxis
fine coordination/dexterity
visual-motor integration
oral-motor control

It was a beautiful spring day and Porky Pine could hardly wait until . . .

WORD SEARCH

Performance Components
- **Cognitive Integration and Cognitive Components**

Directions: The terms related to Cognitive Integration and Cognitive Components are hidden in the grid of letters. Look across, back, down, up, and diagonally in the letters. Circle each term you discover. The word MEMORY has been circled as an example.

TERMS
LevelOfArousal
Orientation
Recognition
AttentionSpan
InitiatOfActivity
TerminOfActivity
Memory
Sequencing
Categorization
ConceptFormation
SpatialOperations
ProblemSolving
Learning
Generalization

S	H	C	L	J	M	V	A	X	F	Q	D	G	P	Q	V	V	E	F	C
N	S	E	Q	U	E	N	C	I	N	G	Q	L	O	C	J	S	N	U	A
O	W	C	R	O	S	L	V	U	K	V	Q	Q	L	F	G	M	Q	B	T
I	D	B	L	E	A	R	N	I	N	G	S	W	Z	R	Y	J	O	Q	E
T	Y	Y	L	P	W	K	H	V	Q	X	P	K	M	E	D	M	S	Z	G
A	O	R	I	E	N	T	A	T	I	O	N	S	Z	R	S	J	C	B	O
R	A	O	Z	I	V	D	J	U	C	T	N	E	W	Y	J	N	D	W	R
E	V	Q	Z	Z	N	D	H	N	W	T	T	H	P	C	K	D	P	N	I
P	H	X	R	U	Y	U	J	O	J	U	T	Q	G	V	A	M	L	M	Z
O	I	G	L	K	X	W	N	F	X	E	E	T	W	V	V	Y	J	Y	A
L	I	R	W	L	L	E	V	E	L	O	F	A	R	O	U	S	A	L	T
A	R	G	B	K	Y	R	O	M	E	M	Q	K	T	B	O	K	A	O	I
I	Z	X	V	G	N	I	V	L	O	S	M	E	L	B	O	R	P	T	O
T	Z	T	W	G	E	N	E	R	A	L	I	Z	A	T	I	O	N	U	N
A	A	T	T	E	N	T	I	O	N	S	P	A	N	W	J	C	E	H	O
P	S	J	M	C	O	N	C	E	P	T	F	O	R	M	A	T	I	O	N
S	L	S	S	T	E	R	M	I	N	O	F	A	C	T	I	V	I	T	Y
I	N	I	T	I	A	T	O	F	A	C	T	I	V	I	T	Y	B	E	U
H	V	N	X	D	A	T	B	S	P	L	I	Q	X	Y	T	M	C	S	R
R	E	C	O	G	N	I	T	I	O	N	C	E	M	O	G	R	Y	O	Y

CROSSWORD PUZZLE

Performance Components
- **Cognitive Integration and Cognitive Components**

Directions: Test your Cognitive Integration and Cognitive Components vocabulary by completing the crossword puzzle. The answer key is in Appendix A.

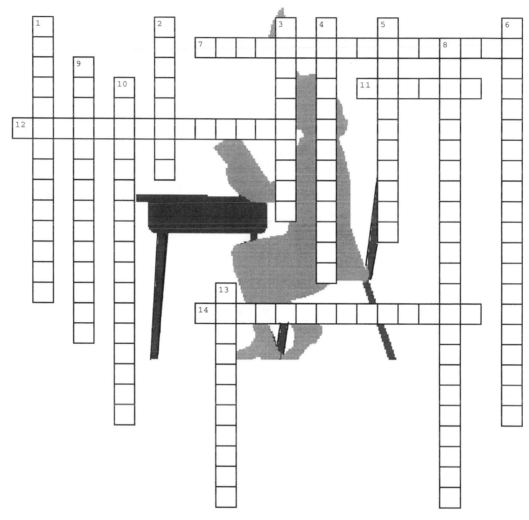

ACROSS

7. Organizing a variety of information to form thoughts and ideas (2 words)
11. Recalling information after brief or long periods of time
12. Applying previously learned concepts and behaviors to a variety of new situations
14. Demonstrating alertness and responsiveness to environmental stimuli (3 words)

DOWN

1. Recognizing a problem, defining a problem, identifying alternative plans . . . (2 words)
2. Acquiring new concepts and behaviors
3. Placing information, concepts, and actions in order
4. Focusing on a task over time (2 words)
5. Identifying person, place, time, and situation
6. Starting a physical or mental activity (3 words)
8. Stopping an activity at an appropriate time (3 words)
9. Identifying similarities of and differences among pieces of environmental information
10. Mentally manipulating the position of objects in various relationships (2 words)
13. Identifying familiar faces, objects, and other previously presented materials

Figure 4.19. *The See-Through School*

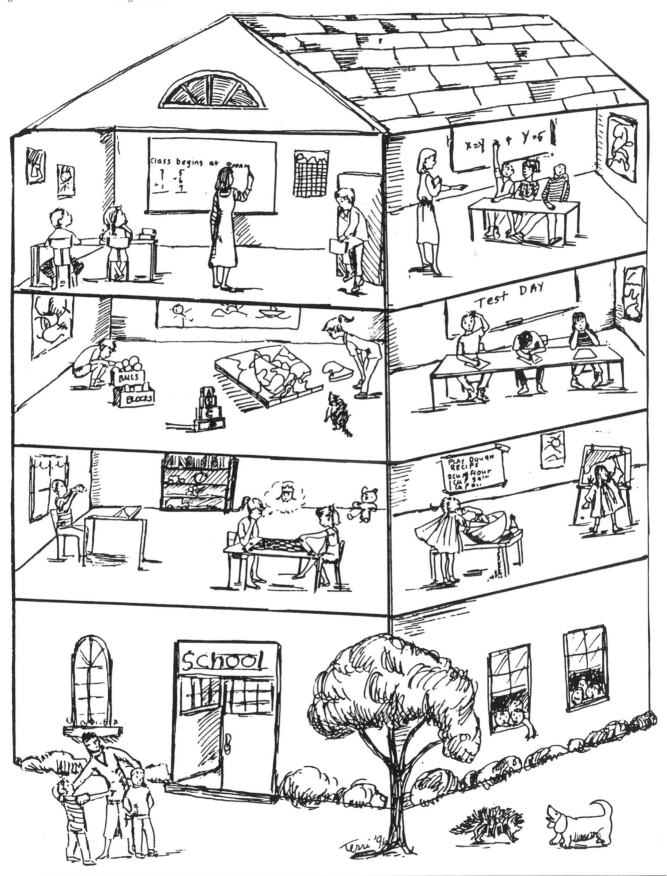

STORY WRITING

Performance Components
- **Cognitive Integration and Cognitive Components**

Directions: The concepts represented by the 14 terms of Performance Components, Cognitive Integration and Cognitive Components, listed below, are hidden in Figure 4.19, "The See-Through School." Can you write a story that incorporates all 14 terms? Cross out the term in the list as you use it in the story and color that portion of the picture *green*. There is ambiguity among the actions representing terms. Try, however, to use a different part of the picture for each term that you include in your story. Begin your story by completing the sentence above.

TERMS
level of arousal
orientation
recognition
attention span
initiation of activity
termination of activity
memory
sequencing
categorization
concept formation
spatial operations
problem solving
learning
generalization

It was the first day of school and Gerard was trying to quietly sneak into the class before . . .

WORD SEARCH

Performance Components
- **Psychosocial Skills**

Directions: The terms related to Psychosocial skills are hidden in the grid of letters. Look across, back, down, up, and diagonally in the letters. Circle each term you discover. The word INTERESTS has been circled as an example.

TERMS

PsychosocialSkills
Values
Interests
SelfConcept
RolePerformance
SocialConduct
InterpersonalSkills
SelfExpression
CopingSkills
TimeManagement
SelfControl

B	A	O	Z	I	V	D	J	U	C	T	N	E	W	Y	J	N	D	S	C
W	V	Q	Z	Z	N	D	H	N	W	T	T	H	P	C	K	D	P	E	O
N	H	X	R	U	Y	U	J	O	J	U	T	Q	G	V	A	M	L	L	P
M	I	G	L	K	X	W	N	F	X	E	E	T	W	V	V	Y	J	F	I
Y	I	R	W	L	R	G	B	K	Q	K	T	B	O	K	A	O	Z	E	N
X	V	T	Z	T	W	U	W	J	C	E	H	O	S	J	M	L	S	X	G
S	B	E	U	H	V	N	X	D	A	T	B	S	P	L	I	Q	X	P	S
Y	T	M	C	S	R	C	E	M	O	G	R	Y	O	Y	R	T	A	R	K
Y	Q	V	G	A	F	W	N	L	I	I	A	I	T	C	H	V	T	E	I
J	U	T	U	U	C	W	N	V	C	G	J	M	F	A	A	V	N	S	L
P	S	Y	C	H	O	S	O	C	I	A	L	S	K	I	L	L	S	S	L
Q	H	N	V	W	P	I	R	P	H	S	Y	R	P	A	V	S	U	I	S
B	W	A	A	P	V	Q	X	K	Q	G	I	H	G	W	M	M	B	O	T
A	C	Z	L	T	C	U	D	N	O	C	L	A	I	C	O	S	J	N	P
N	R	L	U	S	E	L	F	C	O	N	C	E	P	T	Q	Q	D	J	R
N	U	L	E	O	Y	T	I	M	E	M	A	N	A	G	E	M	E	N	T
O	T	O	S	T	U	E	T	P	S	E	L	F	C	O	N	T	R	O	L
R	O	L	E	P	E	R	F	O	R	M	A	N	C	E	T	F	U	Q	D
S	L	L	I	K	S	L	A	N	O	S	R	E	P	R	E	T	N	I	Z
I	N	T	E	R	E	S	T	S	K	Y	Y	G	Q	S	G	A	I	U	S

CROSSWORD PUZZLE

Performance Components
• **Psychosocial Skills**

Directions: Test your Psychosocial Skills vocabulary by completing the crossword puzzle below. The answer key is in Appendix A.

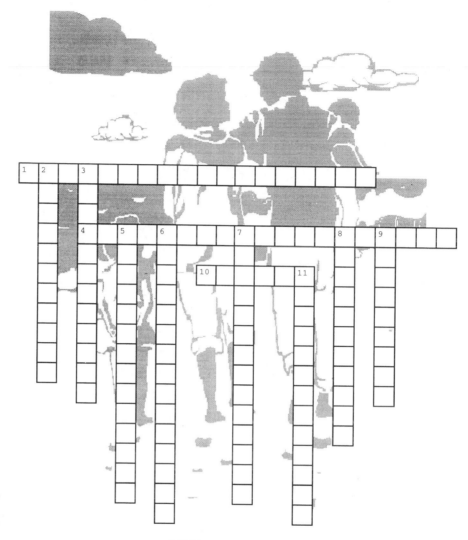

ACROSS

1. The ability to interact in society and to process emotions (2 words)
4. Using verbal and non-verbal communication to interact in a variety of settings (2 words)
10. Identifying ideas or beliefs that are important to self and others

DOWN

2. Modifying one's own behavior in response to environmental needs . . .
3. Identifying and managing stress and related factors (2 words)
5. Planning and participating in a balance of self-care, work, leisure, and rest activities to promote satisfaction and health (2 words)
6. Identifying, maintaining, and balancing functions one assumes or acquires in society (2 words)
7. Using a variety of styles and skills to express thoughts, feelings, and needs
8. Developing the value of the physical, emotional, and sexual self
9. Identifying mental or physical activities that create pleasure and maintain attention
11. Interacting by using manners, personal space, eye contact, gestures, active listening, and self-expression . . . (2 words)

Figure 4.20.   *The City Kids' Neighborhood*

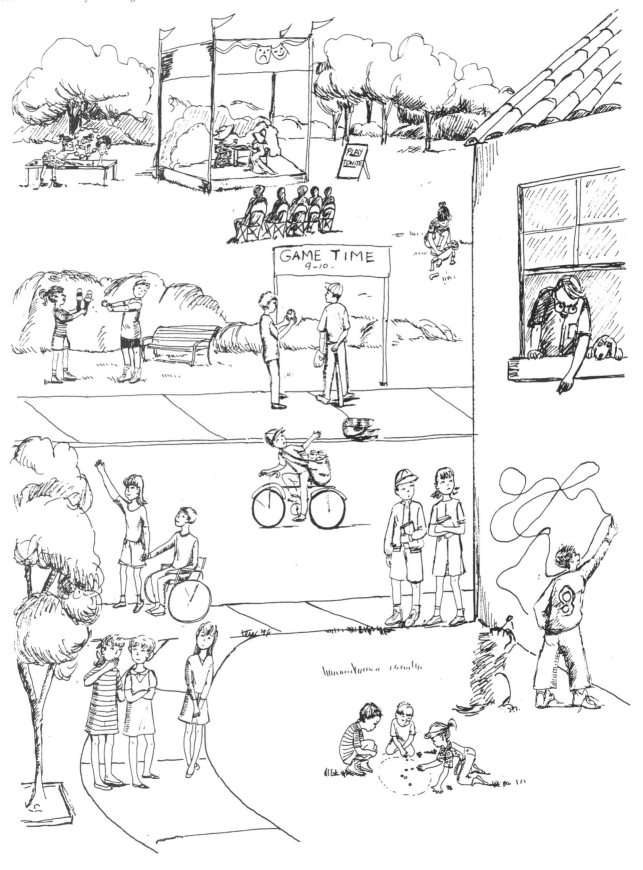

Performance Components
- **Psychosocial Skills**

Porky knew who had drawn on the wall, but . . .

Directions: The concepts represented by the 13 terms of Performance Components, Psychosocial Skills, listed below, are hidden in Figure 4.20, "The City Kids' Neighborhood." Can you write a story that incorporates all 13 terms? Cross out the term in the list as you use it in the story and color that portion of the picture *green*. There is ambiguity among the actions representing terms. Try, however, to use a different part of the picture for each term that you include in your story. Begin your story by completing the sentence provided.

TERMS
values
interests
self-concept
social
role performance
social conduct
interpersonal skills
self-expression
self-management
coping skills
time management
self-control
psychological

You have completed your work on the Performance Components. You will now learn about Performance Contexts.

Performance Contexts

The Performance Contexts are those situations or variables that play a role in engaging a desired and/or required response from an individual in any of the performance areas. Complete your immersion into the language of occupational therapy by learning the meanings of terms that describe aspects of Performance Contexts.

DIRECTIONS

1. Look at Figure 4.21 to familiarize yourself with the categories and subcategories of the Performance Contexts domain.
2. Next, turn to the concept map of the Performance Contexts (Figure 4.22). Can you see the relationship between each graphic and its respective term?
3. Create your own definition for each term by reflecting on the picture paired with the term.
4. Record your definitions in the blank spaces of the first AOTA dictionary.
5. When you have recorded all your definitions for the Performance Contexts terms, turn to the second version of the AOTA Uniform Terminology dictionary and underline the words or phrases in each definition that relates to the graphic.

Example:

4. disability status

Place in continuum of <u>disability</u>, such as acuteness of <u>injury</u>, chronicity of disability, or terminal nature of illness.

6. Go back to your definitions and see how closely each one matches the AOTA definition. Use the following criteria to score your work. Record the score in the margin next to each definition.

   2 points Your definition has at least *two elements* included in AOTA's definition.
   1 point   Your definition has at least *one element* included in AOTA's definition.

7. Determine your total score by adding up your points. Record your score in the box below.

Score

If you scored

◆ 12–14 points: You're off and running.
◆ 9–11 points: You have a solid start.
◆ 10 points or below: Now you know what to work on.

Complete the Performance Contexts word search and crossword puzzle (see Appendix A for answers). Then pause to study the scene in Figure 4.23 and write a story using the terms you have just learned.

Performance Contexts

Temporal Aspects
- Chronological
- Developmental
- Life Cycle
- Disability Status

Environment
- Physical
- Social
- Cultural

Figure 4.22. *Performance Contexts Concept Map*

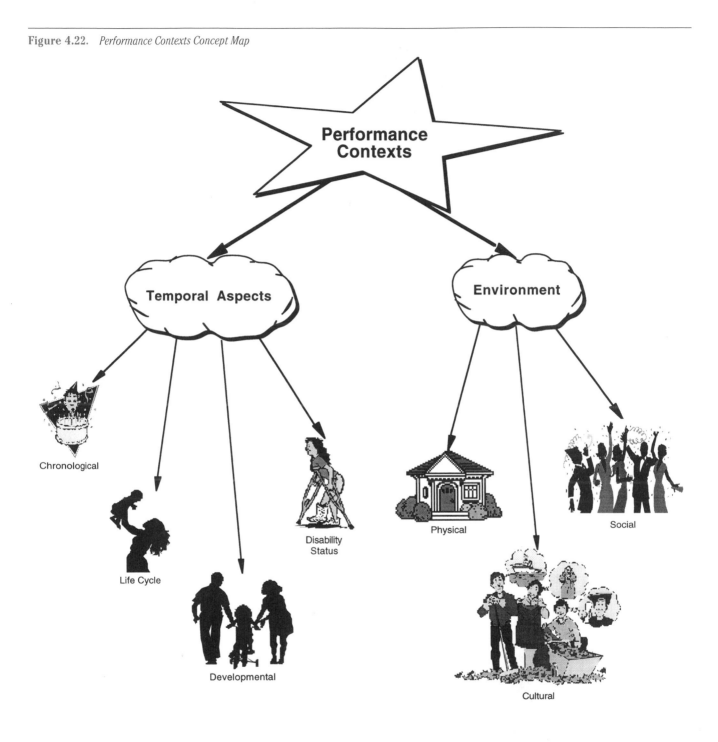

Performance Contexts

Temporal Aspects

Chronological

Life Cycle

Developmental

Disability Status

Environment

Physical

Cultural

Social

III. Performance Contexts:

Assessment of function in performance areas is greatly influenced by the contexts in which the individual must perform. Occupational therapy practitioners consider performance contexts when determining feasibility and appropriateness of interventions. Occupational therapy practitioners may choose interventions based on an understanding of contexts, or may choose interventions directly aimed at altering the contexts to improve performance.

A. Temporal Aspects
1. chronological

2. developmental

3. life cycle

4. disability status

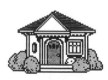

B. Environment
1. physical

2. social

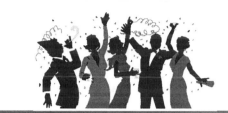

3. cultural

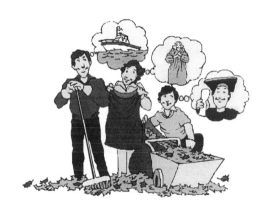

III. Performance Contexts:

Assessment of function in performance areas is greatly influenced by the contexts in which the individual must perform. Occupational therapy practitioners consider performance contexts when determining feasibility and appropriateness of interventions. Occupational therapy practitioners may choose interventions based on an understanding of contexts, or may choose interventions directly aimed at altering the contexts to improve performance.

A. Temporal Aspects
1. chronological

Individual's age.

2. developmental

Stage or phase of maturation.

3. life cycle

Place in important life phases, such as career cycle, parenting cycle, or educational process.

4. disability status

Place in continuum of disability, such as acuteness of injury, chronicity of disability, or terminal nature of illness.

B. Environment
1. physical

Nonhuman aspects of contexts. Includes the accessibility to and performance within environments having natural terrain, plants, animals, buildings, furniture, objects, tools, or devices.

2. social

Availability and expectations of significant individuals, such as spouse, friends, and caregivers. Also included larger social groups which are influential in establishing norms, role expectations, and social routines.

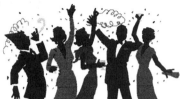

3. cultural

Customs, beliefs, activity patterns, behavior standards, and expectations accepted by the society of which the individual is a member. Includes political aspects, such as laws that affect access to resources and affirm personal rights. Also includes opportunities for education, employment, and economic support.

Uniform Terminology: The Language of Occupational Therapy

I. **Performance Areas**
  A. Activities of daily living
    1. Grooming
    2. Oral hygiene
    3. Bathing/showering
    4. Toilet hygiene
    5. Personal device care
    6. Dressing
    7. Feeding and eating
    8. Medication routine
    9. Health maintenance
    10. Socialization
    11. Functional communication
    12. Functional mobility
    13. Community mobility
    14. Emergency response
    15. Sexual expression
  B. Work and productive activities
    1. Home management
      a. Clothing care
      b. Cleaning
      c. Meal preparation and cleanup
      d. Shopping
      e. Money management
      f. Household maintenance
      g. Safety procedures
    2. Care of others
    3. Educational activities
    4. Vocational activities
      a. Vocational exploration
      b. Job acquisition
      c. Work or job performance
      d. Retirement planning
      e. Volunteer participation
  C. Play and leisure
    1. Play and leisure exploration
    2. Play and leisure performance

II. **Performance Components**
  A. Sensorimotor component
    1. Sensory
      a. Sensory awareness
      b. Sensory processing
        (1) Tactile
        (2) Proprioceptive
        (3) Vestibular
        (4) Visual
        (5) Auditory
        (6) Gustatory
        (7) Olfactory
      c. Perceptual processing
        (1) Stereognosis
        (2) Kinesthesia
        (3) Pain response
        (4) Body scheme
        (5) Right-left discrimination
        (6) Form constancy
        (7) Position in space
        (8) Visual-closure
        (9) Figure ground
        (10) Depth perception
        (11) Spatial relations
        (12) Topographical orientation
    2. Neuromusculoskeletal
      a. Reflex
      b. Range of motion
      c. Muscle tone
      d. Strength
      e. Endurance
      f. Postural control
      g. Postural alignment
      h. Soft tissue integrity
    3. Motor
      a. Gross coordination
      b. Crossing midline
      c. Laterality
      d. Bilateral integration
      e. Motor control
      f. Praxis
      g. Fine coordination/dexterity
      h. Visual-motor integration
      i. Oral-motor control
  B. Cognitive integration and cognitive components
    1. Leval of arousal
    2. Orientation
    3. Recognition
    4. Attention span
    5. Initiation of activity
    6. Termination of activity
    7. Memory
    8. Sequencing
    9. Categorization
    10. Concept formation
    11. Spatial operations
    12. Problem solving
    13. Learning
    14. Generalization
  C. Psychosocial skills
    1. Psychological
      a. Values
      b. Interests
      c. Self-concept
    2. Social
      a. Role performance
      b. Social conduct
      c. Interpersonal skills
      d. Self-expression
    3. Self-management
      a. Coping skills
      b. Time management
      c. Self-control

III. **Performance Contexts**
  A. Temporal aspects
    1. Chronological
    2. Developmental
    3. Life cycle
    4. Disability status
  B. Environmental
    1. Physical
    2. Social
    3. Cultural

Source: AOTA, "Uniform Terminology for Occupational Therapy—Third Edition," *American Journal of Occupational Therapy* 48, no. 11 (1994): 1047–54; AOTA, "Uniform Terminology—Third Edition: Application to Practice," *American Journal of Occupational Therapy* 48, no. 11 (1994): 1055–59. AOTA strongly recommends that these two documents be read in their entirety.

WORD SEARCH

Performance Contexts
- **Temporal Aspects**
- **Environment**

Directions: The terms related to Performance Contexts are hidden in the grid of letters. Look across, back, down, up, and diagonally. Circle each term you discover. The word CHRONOLOGICAL has been circled as an example.

TERMS

Chronological
Developmental
LifeCycle
DisabilityStatus
Physical
Social
Cultural

Y	O	Y	R	T	A	C	Y	Q	V	G	A	F	S	W	N	L	I	I	A
I	T	C	H	V	T	U	J	U	T	U	U	C	O	W	N	V	C	G	J
M	F	A	A	V	N	L	Q	H	N	W	P	I	C	R	P	H	S	Y	R
P	A	V	S	U	B	T	W	A	P	V	Q	X	I	K	Q	G	I	H	G
W	M	M	B	T	A	U	C	Z	J	P	N	R	A	L	Q	Q	D	J	R
N	U	L	O	Y	O	R	T	O	T	U	E	T	L	P	T	F	U	Q	D
Z	K	Y	D	Y	G	A	Q	S	G	A	I	U	S	D	V	W	I	P	I
K	Z	K	E	Q	D	L	S	W	K	Y	E	X	E	V	S	Z	X	H	Z
Z	E	A	V	U	J	J	D	N	B	J	H	U	T	L	S	N	Q	Q	C
E	F	Q	E	J	K	W	F	I	X	V	V	H	G	A	U	G	J	O	U
T	O	Z	L	J	C	H	R	O	N	O	L	O	G	I	C	A	L	X	D
S	M	O	O	W	L	A	C	I	S	Y	H	P	J	A	U	O	L	G	B
O	T	N	P	B	I	Y	B	G	Z	S	X	W	R	Z	G	W	Z	P	Y
J	W	O	M	N	U	X	J	H	W	A	C	P	E	Y	G	R	K	M	E
V	P	R	E	D	I	S	A	B	I	L	I	T	Y	S	T	A	T	U	S
F	Z	V	N	H	K	S	S	F	J	D	Z	G	S	A	K	T	F	V	R
K	C	J	T	E	B	S	F	N	M	P	Y	U	A	O	L	S	K	X	R
S	Y	R	A	Z	P	K	B	B	K	R	I	C	A	G	T	V	J	R	M
R	B	G	L	S	O	L	Z	P	Q	T	X	X	D	I	B	S	M	Q	Z
L	I	F	E	C	Y	C	L	E	S	B	X	H	Z	J	M	X	P	S	J

CROSSWORD PUZZLE

Performance Contexts
- **Temporal Aspects**
- **Environment**

Directions: Test your Performance Contexts vocabulary by completing the crossword puzzle below. The answer key is in Appendix A.

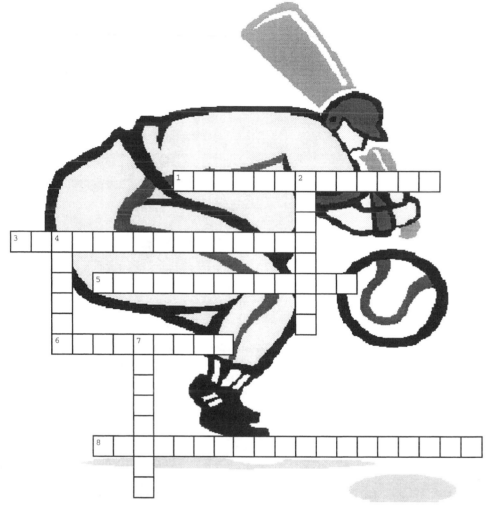

ACROSS
1. Stage or phase of maturation
3. Place in continuum of disability, such as acuteness of injury . . . (2 words)
5. Individual's age
6. Place in important life phases, such as career cycle, parenting cycle, or educational process (2 words)
8. The specific environment in which the performance occurs

DOWN
2. Nonhuman aspects of contexts, includes plants, animals, buildings, objects . . .
4. Availability and expectations of significant individuals . . .
7. Customs, beliefs, activity patterns, behavior standards, and expectations accepted by the society of which the individual is a member

Figure 4.23. *The Birthday Party*

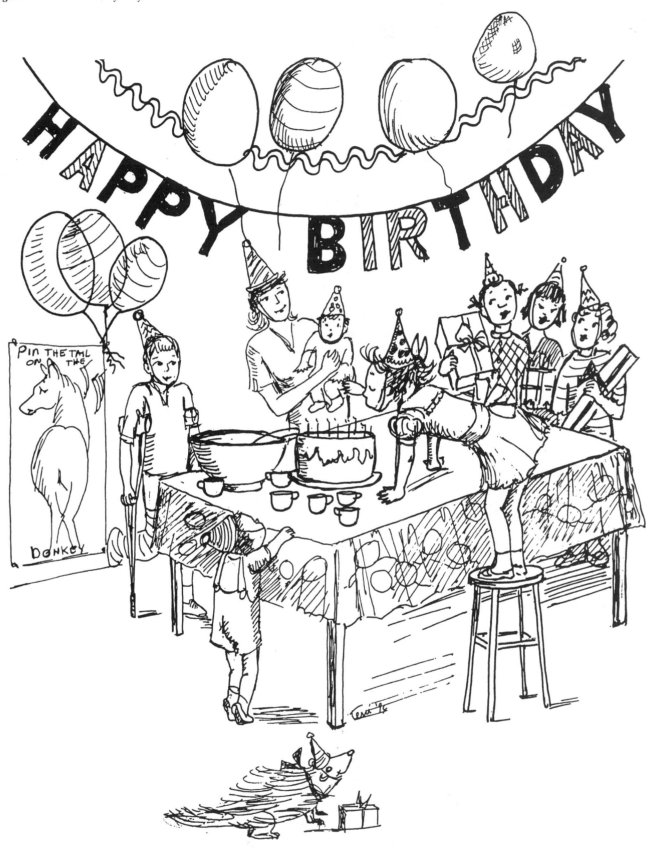

STORY WRITING

Performance Contexts
- **Temporal Aspects**
- **Environment**

Directions: The concepts and environments represented by the 7 terms of Performance Contexts, Temporal Aspects and Environment, listed below, are hidden in Figure 4.23, "The Birthday Party." Can you write a story that incorporates all 7 terms? Cross out the term in the list as you use it in the story and color that portion of the picture *blue*. Parts of the scene fit more than one term. Try, however, to use a different part of the picture for each term that you include in your story. Begin your story by completing the sentence provided.

TERMS

chronological
developmental
life cycle
disability status
physical environment
social environment
cultural environment

Just as Renee leaned on the table to blow out the candles . . .

You have completed your work on the Performance Contexts. Go on to the Section 4 Self-Assessment (there is no Mind Map activity for this section of your journey).

Section 4
SELF-ASSESSMENT

Now that I have completed the fourth part of my journey, I can:

○ describe how occupational performance shapes the way a therapy guide views a client's behavior.

○ describe how context influences occupational performance.

○ explain the relationship between occupational performance and performance components.

○ describe the role of Uniform Terminology in occupational therapy.

○ play with Uniform Terminology by completing puzzles and writing stories that incorporate the terms of Performance Areas, Performance Components, and Performance Contexts.

NOTES

1. Kathlyn Reed, "The Beginnings of Occupational Therapy," in Helen L. Hopkins and Helen D. Smith, eds., *Willard and Spackman's Occupational Therapy*, 8th ed. (Philadelphia: J. B. Lippincott, 1993), 27.
2. R. N. Caine and Geoffrey Caine, *Making Connections: Teaching and the Human Brain*. New York: Addison-Wesley, 1994.
3. J. Edward Clark, "The Search for a New Educational Paradigm," in A. Costa, J. Bellanca, and R. Fogarty, eds., *If Minds Matter: A Foreword to the Future* (Palatine, Ill.: Skylight Publishing, 1992), 1:25–40.
4. AOTA, "Uniform Terminology—Third Edition," *American Journal of Occupational Therapy* 48, no. 11 (1994): 1047–54, and AOTA, "Uniform Terminology—Third Edition: Application to Practice," *American Journal of Occupational Therapy* 48, no. 11 (1994): 1055–59 (AOTA strongly recommends that these two documents be read in their entirety). The Uniform Terminology dictionaries included in Section 4 are drawn from three sources authored by the AOTA: *Occupational Therapy Product Output Reporting System and Uniform Terminology for Reporting Occupational Therapy Services* (Rockville, Md.: AOTA, 1979); "Uniform Terminology for Occupational Therapy—Second Edition," *American Journal of Occupational Therapy* 43 (1989): 808–15; and "Association Policies: Definition of Occupational Therapy Practice for State Regulation (Policy 5.3.1)," *American Journal of Occupational Therapy* 47 (1993): 1117–21.
5. Caine and Caine, *Making Connections*, 121.

Preparing to Use CPS

Itinerary #5

At the end of the fifth part of your journey, you will be able to:

✓ distinguish among the seven Thinking Keys used to prepare for CPS

✓ describe how appreciating individual differences helps you understand a problem from the client's perspective

✓ explain the importance of establishing problem ownership when on a therapy expedition and identify the four criteria used to establish problem ownership

✓ explain why creating a shared vision enhances the client-therapist relationship

✓ distinguish between a well-structured and an ill-structured problem

✓ use the "PACC" to analyze data according to Performance Areas, Performance Components, and Performance Contexts

Four + Three Thinking Keys = Preparing for CPS

In Section 3, you were introduced to the "Watch for Cues and Look for Patterns," "Stop, Drop, and Listen," "What Paradigm Is Operating?" and "Consider Other Viewpoints" Thinking Keys. In this section you will learn three additional Thinking Keys to be used along with these first four. They are the "Problem Ownership Checklist," the "Well-Structured vs. Ill-Structured Problem Checklist," and the "PACC."[1]

These seven Thinking Keys are designed to help a therapy guide prepare to use Creative Problem Solving (CPS). Preparation to use CPS on a therapy expedition involves first surveying the territory to determine whether it is necessary to use CPS to solve the client's problem.

Recall the first four Thinking Keys. The "Watch for Cues and Look for Patterns" Thinking Key helps a guide first pick up relevant cues from the client and then cluster the cues into patterns in order to make sense of the data that has been gathered. "Stop, Drop, and Listen" helps a guide remain open to the information a client provides by reminding the guide to drop assumptions he or she might have made before meeting the client. "What Paradigm Is Operating?" reminds the guide to pay close attention to the paradigms that influence the client's actions in a given circumstance. "Consider Other Viewpoints" directs a guide to view a problem from more than one perspective.

Thinking Keys That Help Prepare for CPS

"Watch for Cues and Look for Patterns": Gather information and identify patterns in a client's behavior.

"Stop, Drop, and Listen": Remain open to what a client is communicating by dropping assumptions he or she might hold about the client.

"What Paradigm Is Operating?": Explore what paradigms influence a client's behavior.

"Consider Other Viewpoints": See a problem from different points of view.

"Problem Ownership Checklist": Examine the level of ownership of individuals on a therapy expedition.

"Well-Structured vs. Ill-Structured Problem Checklist": Determine whether a client's problem is well-structured or ill-structured.

"PACC": Seek to understand a client's problem through an occupational therapy paradigm.

You will find an icon like the one on the left on all Field Organizers that help a therapy guide prepare for CPS. This icon symbolizes framing the situation within an occupational therapy paradigm.

Preparing for CPS Involves Appreciating Individual Differences

John Dewey, a famous American educator, once said that a problem well defined is a problem half solved.[2] Defining the correct problem is the number one challenge therapists face when helping individuals seek a resolution to their therapy needs. Inherent in the process of "defining the correct problem" is understanding the role that individual differences play in the process of solving problems.

Individual differences are those traits that make each of us unique. No two people are exactly alike, not even twins. In addition to the obvious characteristics of hair, eyes, skin tone, body stature, and voice quality, our life experiences make us the individuals we are. According to Josephine C. Moore, an occupational therapist, anatomist, and educator in the neurosciences, our success as therapists lies in our understanding and treating each person as an individual. "We can neither standardize our treatment," says Moore, "nor categorize it to fit a given population." She affirms that "the whole field of rehabilitation is individualistic in nature, just as we are."[3]

Because of individual differences among clients, it is safe to say that you will never find two problems that are exactly alike. And it is equally safe to say that because of the uniqueness of each problem, you will never find a book entitled *A Therapy Guide's Complete List of Answers to Therapy Problems*. Each problem a therapy guide faces is unique because each client has a unique set of paradigms that influence how he perceives his problem and in turn his desire to solve that problem. Thoroughly understanding a problem from the client's perspective or the client's family's paradigm can be one of the most challenging tasks on a therapy expedition.

Problem Ownership

As you prepare for CPS, it is important that you consider what individuals will help solve the client's therapy-related problems. Identifying who will be part of the therapy expedition involves understanding who has a clear sense of ownership of the problem. To trigger your thoughts about who might share ownership of a problem consider the following six questions:[4]

1. How many people are involved in finding a solution to the problem?
2. Who is *not* currently involved but could be?
3. Who is interested in solving the problem?
4. Who is not interested in solving the problem?
5. Who has the time and the resources to help solve the problem?
6. Who will make working on this problem a priority?

 The **"Problem Ownership Checklist" Thinking Key** can help you determine who will participate in working on a solution to the problem. The "Problem Ownership Checklist" includes four criteria to help determine whether a person is a candidate to share in the ownership of a problem.

Criteria to Establish Ownership of a Problem

To share in the ownership of a problem a person must:

1. Be aware that there is a gap between what is and what should be
2. Be able to measure the gap
3. Need to solve the problem
4. Have access to the resources needed to solve the problem

To learn how to use the criteria in the "Problem Ownership Checklist" Thinking Key, read the scenario and complete a Reflective Journal Entry about how each of the criteria applies to the story. Then put the Thinking Key to work in a Field Organizer.

Imagine you are the occupational therapist in an early childhood education program in a community public school program. You receive two different referrals for therapy services. One referral is for Alonzo and the other for Sabrina, both four years old.

The referrals each state, "evaluate and treat as needed." As part of the evaluation, you seek information from the parents about their respective child's self-feeding behavior. Alonzo's mother describes her child's mealtime behavior as "messy and slow." Sabrina's mother describes her child's self-feeding behavior as "independent."

You evaluate Alonzo and find that his mother's comments about the way he eats matches your observations. Alonzo is a messy eater.

You have several ideas to discuss with his mother and teacher about how to make mealtime a neater experience for everyone involved. His mother and teacher are willing to support your therapy intervention efforts in the classroom and at home.

Refer to the four criteria in the "Problem Ownership Checklist" listed on p. 155 (and in boldface below) to consider whether Alonzo's mother and teacher, two of the key players in Alonzo's situation, share ownership of the identified problem.

1. To share in the ownership of a problem a person must **be aware that there is a gap** between what is and what should be. The gap causes the person to experience an emotional pull or tension between the present state (what is) and a future state (what should be). The person has an internal motivation to close the gap.

> ### REFLECTIVE JOURNAL ENTRY 5.1
>
> Complete the following thought:
>
> *In reference to Alonzo's messy eating, I feel that both Alonzo's mother and his teacher are aware that a gap exists between what is and what should be because . . .*

2. To share in the ownership of a problem a person must **be able to measure the gap.** Unless the person is able to measure the gap he or she will not perceive when the gap is closed. Anyone who shares in the ownership of a problem must be able to measure the difference between what is and what ought to be.

> ### REFLECTIVE JOURNAL ENTRY 5.2
>
> Complete the following thought:
>
> *One way I would help Alonzo's mother and teacher measure the gap between what is (Alonzo's messy eating behavior) and what should be (the changes she can expect to see as a result of therapy) is by . . .*

3. To share in the ownership of a problem a person must **need to solve the problem.** Without sufficient motivation to solve the problem, the person will not make a sincere effort to close the gap between what is and what should be.

> ### REFLECTIVE JOURNAL ENTRY 5.3
>
> Complete the following thought:
>
> *I speculate that Alonzo's mother and teacher are motivated to close the gap between the way Alonzo eats and the way they would like to see him eat because . . .*

4. To share in the ownership of a problem a person must **have access to the resources needed to solve the problem.** Resources can be in the form of time, information, money, or other people. The person must have sufficient time to use the resources to solve the problem.

REFLECTIVE JOURNAL ENTRY 5.4

Complete the following thought:

I feel that the resources most likely to be available to Alonzo's mother and teacher to help Alonzo close the gap between the way he eats and the way he might learn to improve his eating behavior are . . .

In the scenario Alonzo's mother and teacher supported your assessment that Alonzo could learn to become a neater eater. Alonzo's mother and teacher are key players who see that Alonzo has a problem. They each accept responsibility for working on a solution to the problem. In this scenario ownership of the problem is clearly established to be Alonzo's mother and his teacher. The scenario continues.

Next, you evaluate Sabrina and conclude that she, like Alonzo, is also a messy self-feeder. In addition she is slow because of the problems she has managing a spoon and fork. "What should I do?" you ponder to yourself.

Alonzo's mother supports your suggestions to work on developing neat and mature self-feeding behaviors during his therapy time. Sabrina's mother, however, has different expectations for her daughter. She values independence over neatness. Through her eyes, Sabrina does not have a self-feeding problem that warrants the help of a therapist. Sabrina's mother does not see the need for the occupational therapist to spend time working on feeding skills.

Use the "Problem Ownership Checklist" Thinking Key Field Organizer to consider whether Sabrina's mother shares ownership of the problem identified. Discuss your answers and the rationale for your selections with a classmate or colleague. Follow the directions below.

DIRECTIONS

1. Answer questions 2–4 in the Field Organizer with a check in the appropriate box.
2. Briefly describe your rationale in the space under the question. Use question 1 to model your answers.

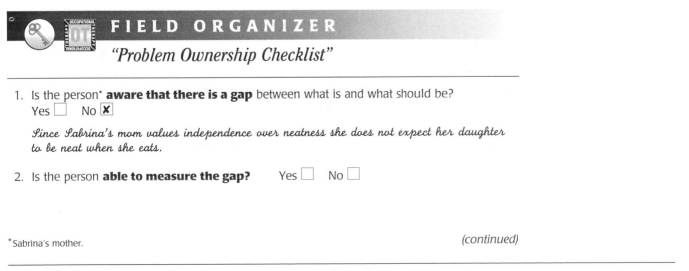

FIELD ORGANIZER
"Problem Ownership Checklist"

1. Is the person* **aware that there is a gap** between what is and what should be?
   Yes ☐   No ☒

   Since Sabrina's mom values independence over neatness she does not expect her daughter to be neat when she eats.

2. Is the person **able to measure the gap?**   Yes ☐   No ☐

---

*Sabrina's mother.

(continued)

3. Does the person **need to solve the problem?**   Yes ☐   No ☐

4. Does the person **have access to the resources** needed to solve the problem?
Yes ☐   No ☐?

To see the need for therapy services, Sabrina's mother must perceive a gap between the way Sabrina currently feeds herself and a future vision of Sabrina as a neat eater. If she does not view the situation as a problematic, there is no problem in which to share ownership. If you strongly believe that Sabrina has occupational therapy needs that center on her self-feeding behavior, your first strategy will be to understand in what ways Sabrina's mother feels that her daughter is an independent self-feeder.

In each therapy situation, ask yourself, "Is this a problem from the client's perspective or from my perspective?" Another way to phrase this question is to ask, "Whose problem is it?" The definition of a problem is "any situation in which a [psychological] gap is perceived to exist between what is and what should be."[5] Thus, there is no problem when the actual situation and the desired situation are perceived as the same.

In the above scenario, Alonzo's mother supports the therapist's assessment that Alonzo could learn to become a neater eater. Sabrina's mother, however, values independence over neatness in eating. She does not feel Sabrina needs the help of a therapist to work on self-feeding skills.

Creating a Shared Vision

Gathering information about the problem from the client's perspective is an important part of CPS. Once you perceive the client's point of view, you begin to develop a shared understanding of the problem. Out of that shared understanding a collaborative relationship begins to build. You and the client work as a team to identify the gap between what is and what ought to be. And out of that team collaboration a future vision for change will emerge.

In the following story imagine yourself as the therapist. There is a problem between what you perceive the child's therapy needs to be and what the parent sees as the goal of occupational therapy services.

> You work in an out-patient clinic. You receive referral for occupational therapy services for Shondra, a three-year-old. Shondra has a diagnosis of "delayed development." She is not yet walking. Her parents agreed with the pediatrician to begin a therapy program on one condition—the therapist will teach their child to walk.
>
> You are unaware of the parents' agreement with the pediatrician. After you evaluate Shondra, you perceive her primary needs to be in self-help and play behaviors.

The above scenario has the potential of becoming a sticky situation between the family and you. What should you do? You need to seek additional information from Shondra's parents about their perspective on the purpose of therapy services.

An important principle of CPS is to try to understand the client and the client's family. Drawing on the wisdom of business consultant Stephen Covey, "seek first to understand then to be understood."[6] Applying Covey's advice to this therapy situation, seek a mutual understanding by asking the following questions:

1. **What is the problem from your and the client's point of view?** Strive to listen to the parents so intently that you can express their perspective as well as or better than they can. Show the parents that you understand their perspective of the situation instead of trying to impose yours. Articulate back to the parents your interpretation of what brought them to therapy. Empathize with their feelings over their concern of having a toddler who is not yet walking. Give the parents an opportunity to correct any misperceptions that you might have.
2. **What are the key issues?** Look at the problem with the parents. Describe to them ways in which you can improve their life situation by anchoring what you know to what they understand.
3. **What outcome do you and the client see as an acceptable solution?** Discuss short-term and long-term solutions. Work to connect your understanding of the therapy process to their understanding of what they see as their vision. Go for a "win-win" solution in which both you and the client benefit and enjoy the therapy relationship.[7]

It is out of your compassion that you, as the therapist, are prepared to yield until you find an emotional and psychological point at which you intersect with the client. The therapeutic process is not a battle of wills but rather a journey of understanding.

Well-Structured and Ill-Structured Problems

In your journey to understand a client's problem it is important to consider the characteristics of the problem, or how the problem is structured. Problems fit two broad categories. They are either well-structured or ill-structured.[8]

A well-structured problem has at least one readily available answer. There is a predictable outcome. A well-structured problem may be solved with a ready-made solution. A ready-made solution is a solution that can be transferred from one problem to another. And because the solution is ready-made there are routine procedures for solving the problem.

In contrast, an ill-structured problem is more complex than a well-structured problem in the following three ways: First, ill-structured problems lack adequate information. You realize that something is wrong, but you need more information before you can develop a solution to the problem. Second, ill-structured problems have unpredictable outcomes. And third, ill-structured problems require custom-made solutions. Ill-structured problems require that you design solutions that match the unique nature of the situation because ready-made (routine) solutions cannot be readily transferred from other situations.

Well-structured problems are distinguished from ill-structured problems by three characteristics: information, outcome, and solution.

Well-Structured Versus Ill-Structured Problems

Characteristic	Well-Structured Problem	Ill-Structured Problem
Information	Sufficient	Insufficient
Outcome	Predictable	Unpredictable
Solution	Ready-made	Custom-made

When you apply your knowledge of how a problem is structured you will use the **"Well-Structured vs. Ill-Structured Problem Checklist" Thinking Key** Field Organizer. In this Field Organizer a small box appears to the left side of each characteristic. When you use this Field Organizer to analyze the structure of a problem, go through each characteristic and check the box that applies to the problem. If you check Sufficient information, Predictable outcome(s), and Ready-made solutions, you see that you have a well-structured problem. If you check the other three boxes, you see that you have an ill-structured problem.

Use the "Well-Structured vs. Ill-Structured Problem Checklist" Thinking Key Field Organizer to evaluate the following scenario: You lose your keys in your backpack.

DIRECTIONS

1. Check the appropriate box in rows 2–3.
2. Describe the rationale for your decisions in the areas below the checked boxes. Use row 1 as a model.

 FIELD ORGANIZER

"Well-Structured vs. Ill-Structured Problem Checklist"

Well-Structured	Ill-Structured
☒ Sufficient information	☐ Insufficient information
I have sufficient information to solve this problem because I know the keys are located somewhere in my backpack.	
☐ Predictable outcome(s)	☐ Unpredictable outcome(s)
☐ Ready-made solution(s)	☐ Custom-made solution(s)

If you concluded that losing your keys in your backpack is a "well-structured problem," you are correct. Rationale: You know where your keys are. You just can't put your hand on them immediately. You may be frustrated with the situation, especially if you are in the rain and the lost keys are your car keys. You know, however, that the keys are in your bag.

Drawing on prior experiences of losing small objects in a bag, you recall several strategies for solving this problem. First you may rummage through the bag feeling for the keys. If you still can't find your keys, you might remove items one-by-one or in handfuls until you see the keys. If that, too, fails, you may finally resort to a ready-made solution to solve the problem. You turn the bag upside-down, emptying all of the contents, including your keys.

REFLECTIVE JOURNAL ENTRY 5.5

Complete the following thought:

During the past week, I encountered the following well-structured problems . . .

Ill-structured problems lack obvious possible solutions. They need custom-made solutions. Now, let's create an ill-structured problem from the lost-key scenario.

You have just completed a full day of shopping in the city. As you return to your car, you reach into your pocket to retrieve your keys. This is when you discover that your keys are no longer there. You have no information about their whereabouts. You know only that your keys are missing.

REFLECTIVE JOURNAL ENTRY 5.6

Complete the following thought:

Discovering that my keys are missing after a long day of shopping is an ill-structured problem because . . .

Rationale: There is no readily available answer to where your keys might be. Knowing that the keys are missing is not enough information to tell you where to begin your search for them. There is no ready-made solution to this problem.

REFLECTIVE JOURNAL ENTRY 5.7

Complete the following thought:

During the past week, I encountered the following ill-structured problems . . .

Occupational therapists are faced with the challenges of solving both well-structured and ill-structured problems. Ill-structured problems are the most demanding and thought-provoking. The solutions to ill-structured problems cannot be found in textbooks and depend on the following two factors: the context in which the problem occurs and the person to whom the problem belongs.

Have you ever been in a situation where you thought you had a problem only because you were focusing on the wrong part of it? This can happen when you focus on the wrong information, simply because you lack sufficient knowledge that allows you to fully understand the complexities of the situation.[9] Consider the following scenario:

Bill is in the copy room at a new community center, trying, unsuccessfully, to turn on the photocopier. This is his first experience with this particular machine. His problem is that he cannot find the correct switch to start the machine. Bill looks all over the copier, pushing every button he can find.

REFLECTIVE JOURNAL ENTRY 5.8

Complete the following thought:

I think that Bill should . . .

In the midst of Bill's frustration, someone from the support staff walks into the room and offers to help. Before Bill can explain his frustration with the apparently malfunctioning machine, his helper points to the vacant electrical wall outlet and the plug attached to the electrical cord from the machine lying on the floor beside the outlet. The machine is unplugged. All of a sudden Bill's problem is solved.

Most likely Bill's search for the on switch is supported by the assumption that finding the correct button on the copier will activate it. Therefore the only option he considers is to focus on the buttons on the machine itself. Finding the correct copier switch is obviously not the key to solving this problem. Gaining the right information is.

REFLECTIVE JOURNAL ENTRY 5.9

Complete the following thought:

I focused on the wrong aspect of the problem one time when I . . .

PACC Your Bags for an Expedition

You will now read a story written by Louise Betteridge, an occupational therapist, about her experiences teaching a group of four- to six-year-old children how to blow their noses. For this field book, Louise's story has been renamed "The Nose Blowing Expedition." Through the Nose Blowing Expedition you will learn about the "PACC" Thinking Key (in this section) and all the Thinking Keys associated with the six stages of the CPS process (Sections 6–11). Before you begin to use the "PACC" Thinking Key, read the story.

Consider the following three questions to which you will respond in Reflective Journal Entry 5.10:

1. Was Louise's problem ill-structured or well-structured?
2. How was Louise like an explorer on a therapy expedition?
3. How did Louise demonstrate her creativity?

The Nose Blowing Expedition

E. Louise Betteridge, OTR

1 Several years ago I was employed as a contract occupational therapist in a local school for young deaf children. In the fall semester, I received a request from a teacher concerning the possibility of providing a motor program designed to teach her hearing impaired four to six-year-olds to blow their noses into a Kleenex. I became intrigued by her request, put together some information on the subject, and developed and implemented the program.

2 At the first meeting with the teacher and her aide, they described the problems that had prompted them to initiate the request for occupational therapy services. They were dreading the approaching winter head cold season, heralding a classroom filled with congested children wiping their noses on anything available, mostly their hands and clothing. They felt these practices were contributing to the spread of cold germs to other children and staff. They also spoke of the painful chapping and chafing the children suffered as a result of the constant need to wipe, and of the children's inability to manage any relief from their congestion by blowing.

3   Since I had been unable to find anything in the published literature which identified the appropriate age for developing the skill to blow through your nose on request, I visited local day care centers to observe normal children in this age group. After questioning the parents and teachers of many children in the two to five-year-old age group, I found the general consensus seemed to be that most children acquire this skill between the ages of three and four. At age four, approximately 95% of normal children seem to have accomplished the skill.

4   We began assessments on twelve children in the classroom and found that only two of them were able to blow through their noses on request, and surprisingly, only five of them could blow through their mouths on request! None of the others could combine the concept with the motor output and come up with a successful "blow." Many of the children attempted to manage the skill by using a quick, forward head snap, instead of using any blowing! We realized early in the planning that the program would have to begin with mouth blowing skills to establish the concept, since that skill appears to be mastered earlier than nose blowing. Our physician had checked the children for nasal obstructions prior to the assistants, and none of the children had been identified as having any oral motor deficits, so we are certain we were dealing with experimental developmental deficits.

5   The project was set up as a play group, which met twice weekly for one-half hour each time, and six children were chosen from the classroom to participate. We began with games that involved relay teams, blowing by mouth to move objects using light materials such as balloons, feathers, ping pong balls and cotton balls. We progressed the materials as the children improved in blowing abilities, from easier to move, to more difficult to move. We continued this general format for two weeks, varying the games and activities and learning ourselves as the children learned. We repeatedly gave enthusiastic signs for "blow" (at the mouth), using animated body language and signing "good work," "good try," helping each child finish the activity with feelings of accomplishment.

6   By the end of the second week, all six children were mouth blowing with vigor and enthusiasm, and we felt ready to move on to phase two—nose blowing. At the following session, the teacher, the aide and I each appeared with a piece of masking tape over our mouths, which fascinated the children. We encouraged them to accept their tape also, but decided to let them put it on their mouths themselves to permit more feeling of control. They were allowed to remove the tape at any time, but we indicated that the game was strictly a "tape" game—if you removed your tape you dropped out of the game until it was replaced. I had been uncertain of their tolerance for this very important step in the program, but it was never a problem. For this second phase of the program, a new set of games was introduced. These games had been scaled down to table top size but required the same kinds of blowing skills; this time the air had come from the nose instead of the mouth. About half the children immediately regressed to the old familiar head snapping movement without blowing, but we demonstrated the proper technique, giving the sign for "blow" as before, putting the hand sign at the nose this time. Gradually, the motor skills acquired during the mouth blowing were transferred to their noses and they began to grasp the similarities. By the end of the third week, four of the children were managing the task successfully, and by the fourth week all had mastered it. Each child was presented with a sticker and a Kleenex, and the parents were notified of their child's new skill so they could follow through at home.

7   The final test came when several of the children developed head colds. The teacher held a Kleenex to their noses, signed "blow" at the nose, and the children blew, and blew, performing like stars! The program was so successful that we repeated it with several new groups with similar results. The children were so enthusiastic about getting into a group that we wondered if we were creating a new elite class . . . those who could blow their noses in a socially appropriate manner.[10]

REFLECTIVE JOURNAL ENTRY 5.10

Complete the following thoughts:

1. *I feel Louise was dealing with an ill-structured/well-structured* (circle one) *problem because . . .*

2. I feel Louise was like an explorer on a therapy expedition when she . . .

3. I feel Louise was creative when she . . .

You are correct if you said that Louise was dealing with an ill-structured problem because, from the beginning, the problem lacked adequate information about what to do. Furthermore, the outcome was undetermined from the beginning because it depended on the cooperation of the children and the follow-through of the teachers and children's family. There were no routine procedures for teaching the children how to blow their noses; Louise developed procedures by drawing on her research at the day care center and her creativity. The custom-make solution was specifically designed for the children and teachers at the school.

You are correct also if you said that the primary problem was teaching the children how to blow their noses. There *is* no right answer for entry 3. Your response for entry 3 is based on your perception of creativity. Louise moved across uncharted territory as she generated a treatment strategy to meet the needs of the children and of their teachers. She didn't always know where she was going, yet she was willing to take the risk of trying new activities, to trust her intuition and be willing to take detours along the way. Louise's delight in learning, coupled with her personal belief "I can make a difference," stimulated her to set out courageously, like an explorer, to solve the problem.

Louise arrived at a successful solution without ever taking a course on the art of nose blowing! The expedition was a success for everyone involved. The children and the adults both gained from Louise's intervention with the students. The route that Louise took seemed so logical. How did she know how to teach nose blowing to the children in such a creative manner?

Louise executed a successful intervention program in her Nose Blowing Expedition because she spent time seeking to understand the problem. Initially, she met with the teacher to learn about the teacher's therapy needs for the students. After learning that the teacher's primary concern was that the children learn to blow their noses, Louise's first step was to turn to the literature. She was seeking answers to the question, "How do you teach nose blowing to children?" She searched the literature for information that would give her a developmental progression of how children learn to blow their noses. Her search was unsuccessful. This is when she courageously "took to the road."

Louise's travels took her to local day care centers. There she decided to conduct her own research on nose blowing. She wanted to observe how the children in the regular day care centers blew their noses. She would then use her observations of the way normal children blow their noses to develop an intervention for the children with special needs. Louise did a thorough job of understanding the problem in all its complexity. As a result of her time and effort to thoroughly understand the problem her intervention strategies were successful. They helped her successfully navigate through the occupational therapy process.

The "PACC"

The success of the Nose Blowing Expedition depended on Louise's ability to apply her CPS skills to the occupational therapy paradigm of occupational performance. To review, the three domains of occupational performance include Performance Areas, Performance Components, and Performance Contexts.

Use the **"PACC" Thinking Key** when you wish to examine a problem using an occupational therapy paradigm. The acronym PACC (pronounced "pack," as in "pack your bags") stands for Performance Areas, Components, and Contexts. Use the "PACC" Thinking

Key Field Organizer to extract the content from the story that corresponds to each of the three domains of occupational performance. In one sense, you use "PACC to pack your bag" with the necessary, specific information you need to help a client on a therapy expedition.

The "PACC" Thinking Key Field Organizer is divided into three parts. Each part represents one aspect of occupational performance.

- ◆ Part 1: Performance Areas
- ◆ Part 2: Performance Components
- ◆ Part 3: Performance Contexts

You will learn how to use the "PACC" Thinking Key by analyzing the Nose Blowing Expedition. The "PACC" Thinking Key will help to pack your travel bag with information from the story that relates to the three domains of occupational performance. Before you begin the activity, read through all the directions and the accompanying example. For this activity, you will need the yellow, green, and blue highlighter pens in your supply bag.

DIRECTIONS

1. Re-read the story "The Nose Blowing Expedition" and, using the color code below (this is the color code you used in Section 4), highlight the words or phrases in the story that correspond to the three domains of occupational performance. If you need to review the categories and subcategories of the three domains, refer to Figure 4.2.

   - ◆ Use a *yellow* highlighter to indicate parts of the story related to Performance Areas. (Recall that yellow symbolizes happiness and well-being. Occupational therapy practitioners help others achieve happiness within their daily occupational performance.)
   - ◆ Use a *green* highlighter to indicate parts of the story related to Performance Components. (Recall that green symbolizes growth and change.)
   - ◆ Use a *blue* highlighter to indicate parts of the story related to Performance Contexts. (Blue is associated with the sky and air; blue symbolizes context that is all-inclusive.)

   Study the first paragraph of "The Nose Blowing Expedition" quoted below. Each story element that corresponds to some area of occupational performance is italicized. Now turn to the "PACC" Field Organizer, Part 3 (p. 170) to see how the italicized story elements have been matched to the Performance Contexts portion of the "PACC." (Note that when you do the activity, these italicized words would be color highlighted. For the Performance Context domain, the words would be highlighted in blue.)

   Several years ago I was employed as a contract occupational therapist in a local *school for young deaf children*. In the *fall semester*, I received a *request from a teacher* concerning the possibility of providing a motor program designed to teach her *hearing impaired four to six-year-olds* to *blow their noses into a Kleenex*. I became intrigued by her request, put together some information on the subject, and developed and implemented the program.

2. Turn to the "PACC" Field Organizer. Begin with Part 1. Using your highlighted story as a point of reference, highlight in yellow all subcategories in the first column that correspond to the words and phrases you highlighted in yellow in the story. Turn to Part 2 and highlight in green all subcategories in the first column that correspond to the words and phrases you highlighted in green in the story. Do the same with the blue highlighter in Part 3.
3. Next, record the highlighted words or phrase as they appear in the story in the space to the right of the corresponding performance component. To clarify your response, if necessary, add your impression of how the story element relates to the performance. Use Part 3 to model your responses. See what else you might add to Part 3 in addition to the examples.

Note: When you analyze the story you may find that certain story elements can go into more than one part of the "PACC." For example, the story element from paragraph 1, children to learn how to blow their noses into a tissue, can be matched to any one or all of the areas of occupational performance, depending on how you view the situation. Before you begin the "PACC" Thinking Key Field Organizer, let's look at how the story element related to use of a tissue could be matched to more than one performance area.

Proper use and disposal of tissues promotes wellness by preventing the spread of germs. Thus the use of tissues fits into the Performance Area subcategory Health Maintenance. But if the person has difficulties interpreting light touch and is unaware of the need to use a tissue to wipe a runny nose, tissue usage may be classified under the Performance Components subcategory Tactile. One might also consider the fine motor coordination demands of tissue usage; hence a match with a second Performance Components subcategory, Fine Motor Coordination. Finally, if the person presents with developmental delays below age 12 months, you might classify tissue usage in the Performance Contexts category Developmental and decide that the child's use of tissue might not be a developmentally appropriate task to teach.

4. Next, record the paragraph number of each highlighted story element in the center column. Identifying the paragraph from which a particular story element was drawn will help organize your thinking when you go back and forth between the story and the three parts of the Field Organizer.

When you finish this activity, discuss your responses in the "PACC" Field Organizer with a traveling companion to see how differently the same situation is viewed by another person.

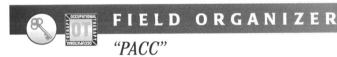

FIELD ORGANIZER

"PACC"

Part 1: Performance Areas

Performance Area	Story Paragraph #	Story Element from "The Nose Blowing Expedition"
A. Activities of daily living		
1. Grooming		
2. Oral hygiene		
3. Bathing/showering		
4. Toilet hygiene		
5. Personal device care		
6. Dressing		
7. Feeding and eating		
8. Medication routine		
9. Health maintenance	#1	*blow their noses into a Kleenex*
10. Socialization		
11. Functional communication		
12. Functional mobility		
13. Community mobility		
14. Emergency response		
15. Sexual expression		

Performance Area	Story Paragraph #	Story Element from "The Nose Blowing Expedition"
B. Work and productive activities		
1. Home management		
a. Clothing care		
b. Cleaning		
c. Meal preparation and cleanup		
d. Shopping		
e. Money management		
f. Household maintenance		
g. Safety procedures		
2. Care of others		
3. Educational activities		
4. Vocational activities		
a. Vocational exploration		
b. Job acquisition		
c. Work or job performance		
d. Retirement planning		
e. Volunteer participation		
C. Play and leisure		
1. Play and leisure exploration		
2. Play and leisure performance		

Part 2: Performance Components

Performance Component	Story Paragraph #	Story Element from "The Nose Blowing Expedition"
A. Sensorimotor component		
1. Sensory		
a. Sensory awareness		
b. Sensory processing		
(1) Tactile		*blow their noses into a Kleenex*
(2) Proprioceptive		
(3) Vestibular		
(4) Visual		
(5) Auditory		
(6) Gustatory		
(7) Olfactory		

(continued)

Performance Component	Story Paragraph #	Story Element from "The Nose Blowing Expedition"
c. Perceptual processing		
(1) Stereognosis		
(2) Kinesthesia		
(3) Pain response		
(4) Body scheme		
(5) Right-left discrimination		
(6) Form constancy		
(7) Position in space		
(8) Visual-closure		
(9) Figure ground		
(10) Depth perception		
(11) Spatial relations		
(12) Topographical orientation		
2. Neuromusculoskeletal		
a. Reflex		
b. Range of motion		
c. Muscle tone		
d. Strength		
e. Endurance		
f. Postural control		
g. Postural alignment		
h. Soft tissue integrity		
3. Motor		
a. Gross coordination		
b. Crossing midline		
c. Laterality		
d. Bilateral integration		
e. Motor control		
f. Praxis		
g. Fine coordination/dexterity		
h. Visual-motor integration		
i. Oral-motor control		

Performance Component	Story Paragraph #	Story Element from "The Nose Blowing Expedition"
B. Cognitive integration and cognitive components		
1. Level of arousal		
2. Orientation		
3. Recognition		
4. Attention span		
5. Initiation of activity		
6. Termination of activity		
7. Memory		
8. Sequencing		
9. Categorization		
10. Concept formation		
11. Spatial operations		
12. Problem solving		
13. Learning		
14. Generalization		
C. Psychosocial skills		
1. Psychological		
a. Values		
b. Interests		
c. Self-concept		
2. Social		
a. Role performance		
b. Social conduct		
c. Interpersonal skills		
d. Self-expression		
3. Self-management		
a. Coping skills		
b. Time management		
c. Self-control		

(continued)

Part 3: Performance Contexts

Performance Context	Story Paragraph #	Story Element from "The Nose Blowing Expedition"
A. Temporal aspects		
1. Chronological	#1	*four to six-year-olds*
2. Developmental	#1	*young . . . children*
3. Life cycle	#1	*preschoolers* (implied)
4. Disability status	#1	*hearing impaired children (developmental disability)*
B. Environment		
1. Physical	#1	*school for young deaf children*
2. Social	#1	*fall semester . . . request from a teacher . . . blow their noses into a Kleenex*
3. Cultural		

As you seek solutions to many of the problems encountered in practice, use the "PACC" Thinking Key to organize information about a client's occupational performance.

Create a Mind Map of Section

5

Mind Map Guidelines

1. Place the section's main concept in the center of the space using pictures or words or both.
2. Radiate ideas from the central thought.
   - Use images (be sure to use color).
   - Headline text—one or two words per line.
   - Print text (for easy reading).
3. Link the main concepts and generate more ideas from the linkages.
4. Have fun!

Section 5
SELF-ASSESSMENT

Now that I have completed the fifth part of my journey, I can:

○ distinguish among the seven Thinking Keys used to prepare for CPS.

○ describe how appreciating individual differences helps me understand a problem from the client's perspective.

○ explain the importance of establishing problem ownership when on a therapy expedition and identify the four criteria used to establish problem ownership.

○ explain why creating a shared vision enhances the client-therapist relationship.

○ distinguish between a well-structured and an ill-structured problem.

○ use the "PACC" to analyze data according to Performance Areas, Performance Components, and Performance Contexts.

NOTES

1. These seven Thinking Keys (mental strategies) are our adaptation of the Task Appraisal part of CPS used by Scott Isaksen, K. B. Dorval, and Donald Treffinger. See their *Creative Approaches to Problem Solving* (Dubuque, Iowa: Kendall/Hunt, 1994).

2. Sydney Parnes, *Visionizing* (Buffalo, N.Y.: Creative Education Foundation Press, 1992). Visionizing is a scientifically researched method of generating ideas. Parnes presents techniques to expand opportunity finding processes which are, for the most part, implicit in the general CPS method. The dreaming and visioning of what could be "are engineered into the best reality manageable" (p. ii) according to Parnes.

3. J. C. Moore, *Concepts from the Neurobehavioral Sciences* (Dubuque, Iowa: Kendall/Hunt, 1973), p. 44. Moore briefly describes twenty-two concepts related to rehabilitation. Although the monograph was published over twenty years ago, the concepts Moore addresses continue to hold true today.

4. Donald Treffinger, *Creative Problem Solving and School Improvement*, Idea Capsules Report No. 9002 (Sarasota, Florida: Center for Creative Learning, 1996), 15.

5. H. A. Simon, *The New Science of Management Decisions*, rev. ed. (Englewood Cliffs, N.J.: Prentice Hall, 1977), 35.

6. Stephen Covey, *The Seven Habits of Highly Effective People* (New York: Simon & Schuster, 1989).

7. Stephen Covey, *First Things First* (New York: Simon & Schuster, 1994).

8. A. VanGundy, *Techniques of Structured Problem Solving* (New York: Van Nostrand, 1988).

9. Ibid.

10. Published under the title "Occupational Therapy Teaches Nose Blowing." Reprinted from *Occupational Therapy Forum* 22, no. 2 (May 28, 1986): 17–18, by permission.

Get Ready to Understand the Problem: Opportunity Finding

6

Itinerary #6

At the end of the sixth part of your journey, you will be able to:

✓ explain how Opportunity Finding is related to the referral process

✓ describe how the invitational stem "WIBGI . . . ?" frames a problem in the Generating Phase

✓ use the "Head and Shoulders Test" to help a client select one option

✓ explain the purpose of clustering information during the Focusing Phase

✓ use "Highlighting" to help a client identify a "WIBGI . . . ?" statement that can serve as a starting point for solving his or her problem

Opportunity Finding Is Related to the Referral Process

Get Ready to understand the problem is one component in CPS. In Section 6 you will learn about one stage of this component. (Recall that the sequence in which we introduce the components and stages does not imply an explicit sequence for usage. The stages may be used in any order, according to the specific needs of the decision maker and the situation. Keep in mind that CPS is a flexible problem solving model.) To develop a comprehensive understanding of the problem, you will travel through three stages: Opportunity Finding, Data Finding, and Problem Finding. These three stages are half of the CPS process.

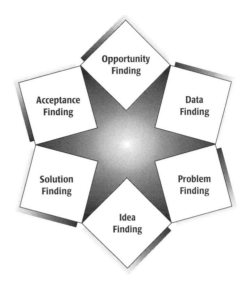

Opportunity Finding is an important stage of Get Ready to understand the problem, and depending on the situation, it can be the first stage. Opportunity Finding helps you to better understand the client's needs when you receive a referral for therapy services. The CPS literature refers to this stage as Objective Finding or Mess Finding. We renamed the stage Opportunity Finding because that name seems to better fit our role as health care providers. The name Objective Finding implies a search for the focus or objective of the problem. It is so named in the CPS literature because in this stage of Understanding the Problem, the scope of the problem is ill-defined and broad. This stage is also called Mess Finding because a problem solving situation that necessitates using this stage is so unclear that all you do know is that you have a mess. You need to organize the mess in order to identify the target area of the challenge before attempting to go forth to solve it.[1] Let's examine why the name for this stage is relevant to our discussion.

Consider the way a description or name has the power to instantaneously color the way you perceive an event.

"That was a *terrible* movie. Are your sure you want to see it?"

"He is a *horrible* mechanic. You may want to take your car somewhere else for repairs."

Chances are, you wouldn't choose to attend a "terrible" movie or to have your car fixed by a "horrible" mechanic. If a colleague or friend has ever given you friendly advice by using a one-word descriptor, you know the power that such words have in shaping your mindset.

By using the name Opportunity Finding (rather than Objective Finding or Mess Finding), you place a positive frame around the client's problem. Using the word *Opportunity* acknowledges the freedom that you have to view each challenge in a positive light.[2] Opportunity Finding is about improving a future state for the client. It is like making a wish for a better tomorrow for the client. Opportunity Finding is consistent with the occupational therapy process. Both are about helping others move toward a more productive future.

To help a client move toward a more productive future, a therapy guide begins by seeking to understand the scope of the client's problem. Sometimes the scope is very clear. At other times it is "fuzzy" and requires clarification. Use Opportunity Finding to identify the broad challenges, concerns, and opportunities within the problem.

In Opportunity Finding, you will ask yourself the following four questions:

1. What do I perceive as the **client's opportunities** to move forward in solving the problem?
2. What is the **global objective** of the problem that I am trying to help solve?
3. In what ways will the therapy program **increase** the client's (or the family's or the caregiver's) **independence** in the Performance Area category _____ (fill in as appropriate).
4. Will I be serving the client **directly** by working with him or her or **indirectly** by educating a family member or caregiver in ways to enhance his or her growth and development?

To better understand Opportunity Finding, let's look at a typical referral for occupational therapy services. Imagine that you receive a request for therapy service that states, "independence in self-care." The referral is a "well-stated problem." You have a definite place to begin your assessment and interview the parent or caregiver. "Enhancing independence in self-care" is the stated objective of the intervention program. The referral identifies the Performance Area to which you will direct your initial attention. (Of course, there may be additional areas you also wish to attend to in therapy after you complete the assessment process. The referral has the potential of providing a clear indication of where to begin in the therapy process.)

When the objective of therapy services has been clearly identified by the written referral, you can skip Opportunity Finding and move directly to another stage, such as Data Finding. If, however, you receive a referral for therapy services that states, "Evaluate and treat as needed," you must identify the challenge or opportunity involved in working with the client. "Evaluate and treat as needed" is a vague request for services. This is an "ill-stated problem" since it lacks adequate information that identifies the initial path to follow at the time of the assessment. Whenever the request for services is vague, a good rule of thumb to use is to begin CPS with Opportunity Finding.

Let's return to Louise Betteridge's Nose Blowing Expedition. In her story Louise tells us that she "received a request from a teacher concerning the possibility of providing a motor program designed to teach her hearing impaired four to six-year-olds to blow their noses into a [tissue]." The request for services from the classroom teacher had very clear parameters. Louise knew the objective because her mission had been identified by the teacher who requested therapy services. She could proceed to Data Finding. Had the referral been vague, Louise would have had to clarify the request for therapy services. To find out more about a referral for occupational therapy services use the Generating Phase of Opportunity Finding.

The Generating Phase of Opportunity Finding

"Wouldn't it be great if . . . ?" or simply, "WIBGI . . . ?" is an invitational stem. It is also a **Thinking Key**. The words "Wouldn't it be great if . . ." set the tone for creating a vision of a future state. When you begin thinking about a situation with the words "Wouldn't it be great if . . ." you start to imagine how the situation might be different. Using the invitational stem "WIBGI . . . ?" helps you expand your thinking about the situation. It creates a mind-set that shifts your thinking from the current problem to a positive future state.

When you think about a positive future state, you are doing what Sidney Parnes, an educator, writer, and leader in the CPS movement, calls "visionizing." "Visionizing" is a combination of "vision" and "actualizing." Parnes likens visionizing to the visual transformation that occurs when a therapy guide looks for opportunities, relationships, and implications surrounding a challenging situation.[3] The therapy guide is a "visionizer." And therapy goals are an expression of a vision of the client's future. Each goal reflects a vision of where you imagine the client to be within a designated time. As a visionizer, the therapy guide translates the vision into reality by implementing the therapy process.

Opportunity Finding allows the client to make explicit her wish to close the gap between where she is and where she wants to be. The gap between the current reality, the "now," and the time to come, the "future," is what creates a sense of tension. The tension is an emotional state expressed internally as a desire, motivation, or want.[4]

REFLECTIVE JOURNAL ENTRY 6.1

Complete the following thoughts:

1. I remember the time I had the following improbable wish: . . .

2. I worked hard to make it become a reality by . . .

3. During the time that I was working to make my wish become a reality, I remember feeling . . .

The experience you described in Reflective Journal Entry 6.1 illustrates the tension that is caused by a gap between your current reality and your wish for the distant future state. The tension created by the identified emotional state brings with it an emotional energy and excitement. This emotional energy gives momentum to your desire to solve what may initially appear to be an unsolvable problem. When the need to solve a seemingly unsolvable problem is strong, the amount of tension generated between your "now" and your desired "future" state motivates you to create a solution that would not otherwise have been possible.

A series of "Wouldn't it be great if . . . ?" questions offers you potential starting points from which to identify the client's problem. In the Generating Phase of Opportunity Finding you are looking for possible starting points rather than the definitive one. Therefore, when you complete the phrase "Wouldn't it be great if . . . ?" keep the question broad and brief. Your goal in Opportunity Finding is to capture the scope of the client's problem, not to define the problem. Express the "Wouldn't it be great if . . . ?" questions in headline format. Use short phrases to describe your wish.

To illustrate how wish statements are generated, let's return to the Nose Blowing Expedition and imagine that the initial request for occupational therapy services was stated in general (not specific) terms, which the therapist, Louise, clarified in the following manner:

> During an initial meeting with the teacher, Louise discovered that the teacher was dreading the "cold season." The children pass germs around the class, and as a result of the spread of germs, both students and the teacher miss school days. Maintaining an adequate attendance with minimal use of substitute teachers is an ongoing issue

for elementary school staff. The teacher would like to do something to improve the situation. The therapist developed ten wish statements from a discussion with the teacher.

Wouldn't it be great if . . .

◆ the children always threw their soiled tissues away?
◆ the children could blow their noses?
◆ the teachers didn't have to put on the children's boots?
◆ the children were healthy all winter long?
◆ the children could button up their own coats?
◆ the teacher's aide could teach the children how to keep their hands clean?
◆ the parents would not bring sick kids to school?
◆ the parents would recognize that sick children belong at home?
◆ the children learned how to put on their own snowsuits?
◆ the children could independently manage their hats and gloves?

Any one of the questions above could potentially offer a starting point to help the teacher deal with her problem. (Note that because these questions represent a wish for a future state, we call them wish statements. Because we are in Opportunity Finding, we also call them opportunity statements.) In contrast, stating the problem as "too bad the children spread germs all over during the cold season" is counterproductive to movement forward on the expedition. Focusing on the negatives obscures thoughts about potential opportunities for solving the problem. When you use the phrase "Wouldn't it be great if . . . ?" there is no place for thoughts such as, "It won't work," "That's a dumb idea," or "We don't have the resources." Opportunities for success thrive when stated in the affirmative. And when opportunities thrive, you can't help having a positive mindset.

The only mistake that you can possibly make when using the "WIBGI . . . ?" Thinking Key is to limit the number of wish statements that you generate. So remember to concentrate on broadening your thoughts in the Generating Phase. Stretch your mind to think out-of-the-box! And above all—defer judgment. Allow yourself time to express your wish statements without restraint. Headline your thoughts. Use only those words necessary to complete your opportunity statements. And always commit your thoughts to paper.

The more opportunity statements you generate, the greater your odds of producing a unique solution. So be wild; celebrate the impractical. You can always modify a wild idea later. Strive to generate a pre-set quota of opportunity statements. For example, decide to generate at least 10, 15, or 20 wish statements before entering the Focusing Phase. Continue *producing opportunity statements until you begin to duplicate previously stated ones.* When you begin repeating opportunity statements, you know you have completed the Generating Phase. It's time to move on.

In the words of the Nobel laureate Linus Pauling, "The best way to get a good idea is to get a lot of ideas."[6] His words reinforce the wisdom that the more opportunity statements you generate, the greater your potential of generating a "better" idea that will solve the problem.

Move forward on your journey now and practice your skill in writing wish, or Opportunity Finding, statements by completing the "WIBGI . . . ?"/"Highlighting" Thinking Keys Field Organizer. Choose a partner and decide who will role play Louise (the therapist) and who will be the teacher in the Nose Blowing Expedition. If you are performing the exercises alone, decide whether you will generate opportunity statements from the mindset of Louise or the therapist.

Note: In this Field Organizer, the "WIBGI . . . ?" Thinking Key is paired with the "Highlighting" Thinking Key (used in the Focusing Phase of Opportunity Finding). The "WIBGI . . . ?" Thinking Key is in the first column of the Field Organizer. The other five columns represent the "Highlighting" Thinking Key (i.e., Hits, A, B, C, and D). You will be directed to complete the Focusing Phase later.

---

1. Generate at least 10 wish statements to add to the 10 already listed. (There are more than 10 spaces on the Field Organizer, so don't limit yourself to 10 statements.) Begin each statement with the invitational stem "Wouldn't it be great if . . . ?"
2. Record your wish statements in the spaces in the first column, entitled "Generate." As you create opportunity statements, remember to hitchhike one idea to another.

 FIELD ORGANIZER

"WIBGI . . . ?"/"Highlighting"

Generate   **Focus**

WIBGI . . .	Part 1: Hits	Part 2: Clustering Hits into Hot Spots			
		A Performance Area	B Performance Area Subcategory	C Person	D
1. the children always threw their soiled Kleenexes away?	●	ADL*	Health maintenance	Child	
2. the children could blow their noses?	●	ADL	Health maintenance	Child	
3. the teachers didn't have to put on the children's boots?	●	ADL	Dressing	Teacher	
4. the children were healthy all winter long?	●	ADL	Health maintenance	Child	
5. the children could button up their own coats?	●	ADL	Dressing	Child	
6. the teacher's aide could teach the children how to keep their hands clean?	●	ADL	Health maintenance	Teacher's aide	
7. the parents would not bring sick kids to school?					
8. the parents would recognize that sick children belong at home?					
9. the children learned how to put on their own snowsuits?	●	ADL	Dressing	Child	
10. the children could independently manage their hats and gloves?	●	ADL	Dressing	Child	
11.					
12.					
13.					

*Activities of Daily Living

Generate		Focus			
WIBGI . . .		**Part 1: Hits**	**Part 2: Clustering Hits into Hot Spots**		
			A **Performance** **Area**	**B** **Performance Area** **Subcategory**	**C** **Person**	**D**
14.						
15.						
16.						
17.						
18.						
19.						
20.						
21.						
22.						

The Focusing Phase of Opportunity Finding

Now that you have generated additional Opportunity Finding statements, you are ready to move to the Focusing Phase. In the Focusing Phase, you will use Affirmative Judgment (introduced in Section 2). When you use Affirmative Judgment, your task is to consider what you like about the opportunity statements and which opportunity statements may not be the best fit to solve the problem. In Opportunity Finding you will work collaboratively with the client or the client's parents or caretakers to determine which "Wouldn't it be great if . . . ?" statement will set the course for solving the client's problem. Collaboration in this phase is important. The client's and the parents' or caregivers' opinions about the wish statements are essential to the development of the therapy expedition.

The "Head and Shoulders Test"

There are two Thinking Keys you can use to help a client judge all the options created in the Generating Phase of Opportunity Finding. The first is the **"Head and Shoulders Test."**[5] To use this **Thinking Key**, ask the client if there is one wish that stands head and shoulders above the rest. If the client is very interested in a single wish statement, move on to Data Finding to expand your understanding of that wish.

In the Nose Blowing Expedition the referral for occupational therapy services specified the need for a nose blowing program. The referral specifically indicated that the teacher had already decided that she wanted the children to learn how to blow their noses. That wish was "head and shoulders" above other wishes she might have had for therapy services in her classroom. Since you know that the teacher's wish in this story became a reality, for instructional purposes, you will use the "Head and Shoulders Test" Thinking Key to select a different wish to work on. Work with a partner for this activity.

DIRECTIONS

1. Turn back to the "WIBGI . . . ?"/"Highlighting" Thinking Keys Field Organizer and consider wishes in the list of "Wouldn't it be great if . . . ?" questions. Consider all the options on the list, including those both you and your partner recorded in the Generating Phase.
2. After the partner who is role playing the therapist reviews the list of wishes, he or she should use the "Head and Shoulders Test" (in the Field Organizer below) with the teacher to help him or her identify whether one option stands head and shoulders above the rest.
3. After the teacher selects a wish statement and records it in his or her "Head and Shoulders Test" Thinking Key Field Organizer, reverse roles. That is, the person who played the therapist in the first round will be the teacher in the second one (and vice versa). Repeat the "Head and Shoulders Test" in the new roles.

FIELD ORGANIZER

"Head and Shoulders Test"

Ask the client:

"Does any one option in the group stand **head and shoulders** above the rest?"

If the client is very interested in pursuing one of the options, confirm the option with the client and write it on the line below. (If not, return to the Generating Phase of Opportunity Finding and create more options.)

WIBGI _____ ?

Proceed to Data Finding using this wish statement.

When no one wish statement stands head and shoulders above the rest, use the **"Highlighting" Thinking Key** (it is the second Thinking Key you will use in the Focusing Phase of Opportunity Finding). This Thinking Key will help the client organize a large number of options through the process of clustering. Before you apply the "Highlighting" Thinking Key to the wish statements related to the Nose Blowing Expedition, let's discuss the process of clustering.

The Process of Clustering

When you cluster objects or opportunity statements, you place similar objects or statements into one category. Clustered information is easier to relate to than many individual pieces of information. Each cluster you identify is made up of a group of things that are related to one another in some way.

You probably cluster information each time you make a grocery list. You might create your grocery list throughout the week as you run out of household items or you might write one just before going to the store. When it's time to go to the supermarket, you review your list to see what else you need to purchase. Perhaps you cluster the items on your list into specific meal categories to help plan your food purchases for the coming week. Before leaving for the store, you check to see whether you have any of the items you need for the meals you plan to make in the coming week.

You will shop more efficiently and wisely when you organize the items on your list than when you compile the list without clustering the items. Even if you don't place the items on your shopping list into categories before you leave home, your shopping is made easier because grocery stores organize their food items in specific clusters. If stores did not cluster like items, you would be running from one side of the store to the other, as you searched for each item on the list.

REFLECTIVE JOURNAL ENTRY 6.2

Complete the following thoughts:

1. *I routinely cluster information when I . . .*

2. *When I cluster information in the situation above, I typically use the following categories . . .*

3. *The categories I list above are very different from those I use when I cluster . . .*

From Reflective Journal Entry 6.2 you can see that, depending on the situation, the categories you use to cluster things can vary widely and are often dependent on the context within which you are working. This is also true when clustering a list of wish statements. As the following list suggests, you can cluster a list of statements into broad categories and then organize them further into subcategories.

Sample Categories Used for Clustering

Sample Categories	*Sample Subcategories*
Performance Areas	Activities of Daily Living; Work and Productive Activities; Play and Leisure
Performance Components	Sensorimotor; Cognitive; Psychosocial
Level of difficulty in implementing	Simple vs. complex to solve
Time frames associated with pursuing	Need to be solved now vs. can be solved later
Degree of value for the client	High, medium, or low value
People involved in pursuing	Parents, siblings, teachers, ancillary school staff, administrators
Places where there might be an opportunity to pursue	Home, school, babysitter's home, grandparents' home, restaurant, stores

However you cluster the opportunity finding or wish statements, the clusters should help the client ultimately identify one statement that will move him closer to solving the problem.

"Highlighting"

"Highlighting" is a **Thinking Key** that is made up of three distinct but related parts.

- **Part 1** In Part 1 of "Highlighting," **Hits** are identified. Hits are promising options that the client is interested in pursuing. Some ways that an idea can *hit* the client is when the idea feels right, "sparkles," is realistic, understandable, workable, intriguing, or appropriate.
- **Part 2** In Part 2 of "Highlighting," Hits are clustered into groups called **Hot Spots** and given a label (e.g., dressing, grooming, play). The label reflects the focus of the cluster.
- **Part 3** In Part 3 of "Highlighting," the **Restatement** of Hot Spots occurs. The new "WIBGI . . . ?" statement that develops during the restatement process should reflect the essence of the Hits clustered in that Hot Spot.

Continuing in your roles as Louise (the therapist) and the teacher in the Nose Blowing Expedition, with a partner practice the three parts of the "Highlighting" Thinking Key one part at a time. You will need the orange dots in your supply bag to complete this task. Work together on all steps except in step 2 below, where the therapist directs the teacher.

DIRECTIONS

Part 1

1. Turn back to the "WIBGI . . . ?"/"Highlighting" Thinking Keys Field Organizer on p. 178 and review the list of wishes.
2. The person role playing the therapist should ask the person role playing the teacher to identify the Hits (promising options) by placing the orange dots in the Hits column in the "Highlighting" portion of the Field Organizer. In this context Hits are promising options that could support the teacher's desire to deal with the cold season. As the therapy guide, your role is to support the teacher in his or her selection of Hits. To get the teacher started, eight Hits have been identified from among the 10 opportunity statements provided.

Part 2

1. Look for relationships among the Hits (only those wish statements that have been identified with an orange dot) and cluster them into groups called Hot Spots (the last four columns in the Field Organizer, labeled A, B, C, and D).
2. Create a label that captures the theme of each Hot Spot. For your convenience, in this Field Organizer you will practice clustering the wish statements using preselected categories. The categories include:

   Column A, *Performance Areas:* Refers to the Performance Areas identified in Uniform Terminology: Activities of Daily Living (ADL), Work and Productive Activities (WPA), and Play and Leisure (PL). When you cluster the Hits using Performance Areas, analyze each Hit (a promising wish statement) and determine whether it falls under ADL, WPA, or PL, and record the appropriate label in column A opposite the wish statement.

   Column B, *Performance Areas Subcategories:* Refers to the specific activities listed under each category of the Performance Areas, such as grooming and oral hygiene. When you cluster the Hits using Performance Area subcategories, refer to the definitions of the subcategories located in the Uniform Terminology dictionary in Section 4. As you did in column A, place the appropriate label in column B opposite the wish statement. When you use subcategories to cluster the Hits you get a more detailed breakdown of the wish statements.

   Column C, *People:* Refers to the subject of the wish statement. Three groups of people are named in the first 10 wish statements: the children, the teacher, and the teacher's aide. In column C assign the label that corresponds to the subject of the wish statement. You might want to use "the parents" as a fourth group.

3. Complete the categorization process by recording the Performance Area, the Performance Area subcategory, and the people (columns A–C) only for those wish

statements you and your colleague generated. Categorize only those options identified as Hits by the person role playing the teacher. (Note: Steps 1–3 above often happen simultaneously when the relationship between a group of items is readily apparent. For example, if numerous options are generated that relate to developing play skills, you will cluster those items under the category label "play.")

4. Select another category for grouping the teacher's Hits in column D. To do so, look carefully at each of the Hits. Look for any themes or categories that might thread the Hits together. (You may want to refer to the list of sample categories on p. 181.) Write the name of the category at the top of column D in the Field Organizer. Complete the categorization process for your fourth category.

You may be asking yourself, "How many different ways are wish statements to be categorized?" You have been asked to group the teacher's Hits four different ways in order to see that there is more than one way to cluster wish statements, or options. When you are out in the field, use whatever system most efficiently helps the client consider all the options.

You have completed Parts 1 and 2 for the "Highlighting" Thinking Key: identifying Hits and clustering into Hot Spots. You will move on now to Part 3 for the Restatement of Hot Spots. Part 3 appears below as a new Field Organizer for the "Highlighting" Thinking Key.

First you will take the wish statements that the teacher identified as Hits in the Field Organizer for Parts 1 and 2 and transfer them to the appropriate Field Organizer for Part 3. In Part 3 you will record the wish statements (Area I) under the Hot Spots you identified in Part 2. Then you will restate the wish statements (Area II). Turn to the Field Organizer for Part 3 and familiarize yourself with how it is organized before you begin. Note that there are three versions of the Field Organizer for Part 3, one each for columns A, B, and C of Hot Spots.

DIRECTIONS

Part 3

1. Transfer all the Hits from column A, Performance Areas ("Highlighting" Part 2) to the "Highlighting" Part 3 Field Organizer on p. 184. Record each wish statement Hit under the appropriate Hot Spot cluster: ADL, Work and Productive Activities, or Play and Leisure. To get you started the eight Hits identified out of the first 10 wish statements provided have been transferred into one of the three Hot Spots listed above.

2. Analyze the Hits in each Hot Spot (cluster) and restate the label of the Hot Spot as an opportunity statement. The key to restating a Hot Spot is to avoid making the Restatement too broad or too narrow. The Restatement should reflect the main ideas stated in the cluster. For example, a Restatement of the label ADL for the Hot Spot Cluster One that reflects the Hits clustered under that label could be: "WIBGI the children could independently manage their noses and their outer garments?"

3. Record the new Hot Spot restatements in Area II at the bottom of the Field Organizer in the space provided. The restatement listed above has been recorded in Area II.

4. Repeat Steps 1–3, for columns B and C of the Field Organizer Part 2. Transfer Hits from column B to the "Highlighting" Part 3 Field Organizer on p. 185. Next, transfer Hits from column C to the "Highlighting" Part 3 Field Organizer on p. 186. Transfer all Hits into their respective Hot Spots according to their label. Space has been provided for an additional Performance Areas Subcategories Hot Spots (Cluster Three) that might emerge when you are clustering the Hits you generated. A sample Restatement has been provided in Area II.

5. Decide which Restatement (new opportunity statement) reflects your top priority for each of the clustering patterns (i.e., from columns A, B, and C): Performance Areas categories, Performance Areas subcategories, and People.

Hot Spots from Column A: Using Performance Areas to Cluster Hits

Area I: Wish Statements

Cluster One Labeled: *ADL*

WIBGI . . .

1. *the children always threw their soiled tissues away?*
2. *the children could blow their noses?*
3. *the teachers didn't have to put on the children's boots?*
4. *the children were healthy all winter long?*
5. *the children could button up their own coats?*
9. *the children learned how to put on their own snowsuits?*
10. *the children could independently manage their hats and gloves?*

_____

_____

_____

_____

Cluster Two Labeled: *Work and Productive Activities (Educational)*

WIBGI . . .

6. *the teacher's aide could teach the children how to keep their hands clean?*

_____

_____

_____

Cluster Three Labeled: *Play and Leisure*

WIBGI . . .

_____

_____

_____

Area II: Restatements

Hot Spot One: WIBGI *the children could independently manage their noses and their outer garments?*

Hot Spot Two: WIBGI

Hot Spot Three: WIBGI

Hot Spots from Column B: Using Performance Areas Subcategories to Cluster Hits

Area I: Wish Statements

Cluster One Labeled: *Health Maintenance*

WIBGI . . .

1. the children always threw their soiled tissues away?

2. the children could blow their noses?

4. the children were healthy all winter long?

6. the teacher's aide could teach the children how to keep their hands clean?

Cluster Two Labeled: *Dressing*

WIBGI . . .

3. the teachers didn't have to put on the children's boots?

5. the children could button up their own coats?

9. the children learned how to put on their own snowsuits?

10. the children could independently manage their hats and gloves?

Cluster Three Labeled:

WIBGI . . .

Area II: Restatements

Hot Spot One: WIBGI *the children took pride in having clean hands and a clean nose?*

Hot Spot Two: WIBGI

Hot Spot Three: WIBGI

FIELD ORGANIZER

"Highlighting" Part 3

Hot Spots from Column C: Using People to Cluster Hits

Area I: Wish Statements

Cluster One Labeled: *Children*

WIBGI . . .

1. *the children always threw their soiled tissues away?*

2. *the children could blow their noses?*

4. *the children were healthy all winter long?*

5. *the children could button up their own coats?*

9. *the children learned how to put on their own snowsuits?*

10. *the children could independently manage their hats and gloves?*

Cluster Two Labeled: *Teacher*

WIBGI . . .

3. *the teachers didn't have to put on the children's boots?*

Cluster Three Labeled: *Teacher's Aide*

WIBGI . . .

6. *if the teacher's aide could teach the children how to keep their hands clean?*

Area II: Restatements

Hot Spot One: WIBGI *the children loved to put on their outer garments and have proper nose etiquette?*

Hot Spot Two: WIBGI

Hot Spot Three: WIBGI

In actual practice you would work with only one "Highlighting" Thinking Key Field Organizer and select one Restatement (new opportunity statement) to explore in Data Finding. Time permitting, other opportunity statements can be worked through the CPS process.

If after using the "Highlighting" Thinking Key, the client still needs guidance in prioritizing the Hot Spots, use either the "Evaluation Matrix" or the "PCA" Thinking Key you will learn in Section 10.

The wish statement the client selects at the end of this stage will serve as the bridge to the next stage of CPS, Data Finding. Begin the Generating Phase of Data Finding with the client's wish statement. The purpose of Data Finding is to isolate the significant data that is needed to make the wish become a reality. This data then will help you and the client develop the Problem Statement in the Problem Finding stage. Opportunity Finding along with Data Finding and Problem Finding compose one component (half) of the CPS process, Get Ready to understand the problem.

Symbol for Opportunity Finding

Each stage of CPS is represented by an icon. When you complete your work with each CPS stage in the remaining sections of Unit I, you will see the icon for that stage. The icons will be used to trigger your thinking about using specific stages of CPS in Unit II.

The genie's lamp represents Opportunity Finding. The genie's lamp symbolizes the process of generating a wish in each Opportunity Finding statement. It represents the client's wish that will lead to defining the problem. Whenever you see the genie's lamp, you are being reminded to use Opportunity Finding.

Create a Mind Map of Section

6

Mind Map Guidelines

1. Place the section's main concept in the center of the space using pictures or words or both.
2. Radiate ideas from the central thought.
   - Use images (be sure to use color).
   - Headline text—one or two words per line.
   - Print text (for easy reading).
3. Link the main concepts and generate more ideas from the linkages.
4. Have fun!

Green dot: I understand the concept and can explain it to a traveling companion.

Red dot: I need to retrace my steps and review the material.

Section 6
SELF-ASSESSMENT

Now that I have completed the sixth part of my journey, I can:

○ explain how Opportunity Finding is related to the referral process.

○ describe how the invitational stem "WIBGI . . . ?" frames a problem in the Generating Phase.

○ use the "Head and Shoulders Test" to help a client select one option.

○ explain the purpose of clustering information during the Focusing Phase.

○ use "Highlighting" to help a client identify a "WIBGI . . . ?" statement that can serve as a starting point for solving his or her problem.

NOTES

1. Scott Isaksen and Donald Treffinger, *Creative Problem Solving: The Basic Course* (Buffalo, N.Y.: Bearly, 1985).
2. Victor Frankl, *Man's Search for Meaning*, 3d. ed. (New York: Simon & Schuster, 1984). Victor Frankl is the founder of logotherapy, the Third Viennese School of Psychotherapy (after Freud's psycho-analysis and Adler's individual psychology). Following his three-year imprisonment in Auschwitz and other Nazi concentration camps, Frankl attests to the tremendous and total capability one has to define one's attitude toward a situation. He states that the last of the human freedoms is the abil-ity to choose one's attitude in a given set of circumstances. Logotherapy helps people search for meaning in their lives in an effort to find happiness and the capability to cope with suffering. Frankl asserts, "Even the helpless victim of a hopeless situation, facing a fate he cannot change, may rise above himself, may grow beyond himself, and by so doing change himself, . . . [turning] a per-sonal tragedy into a triumph" (147). We drew on Frankl's thoughts to support our decision to change the original wording of CPS from Objective Finding to Opportunity Finding.
3. Sidney Parnes, *Visionizing* (Buffalo, N.Y.: Creative Education Foundation Press, 1992).
4. Frankl, *Man's Search for Meaning*. In a discussion about the psychological tension that builds as a result of the gap between what one has accomplished and what one desires to accomplish, Frankl takes issue with the idea that man needs equilibrium or "homeostasis" (i.e., a tensionless state). Instead, Frankl praises the healthy aspect of having an ongoing sense of tension within one's psyche. The tension should be appreciated as a robust indicator that one is "striving and struggling for a worthwhile goal, a freely chosen task" (110).
5. R. L. Firestein and Donald Treffinger, "Ownership and Converging: Essential Ingredients of Creative Problem Solving," *Journal of Creative Behavior* 17, no. 1 (1983): 32–38.
6. Parnes, *Visionizing*, 11. Parnes cites Linus Pauling to make the point that although Alex Osborn, an advertising man, originated CPS, scientists, psychologists, and people in other fields of endeavor also ascribed to similar ideas expressed in the CPS model.

Get Ready to Understand the Problem: Data Finding

Itinerary #7

At the end of the seventh part of your journey, you will be able to:

✓ explain how resource people help the therapy guide find data about the wish statement

✓ use the "5 Ws & an H" Thinking Key in the Generating Phase of Data Finding

✓ use the "5 Ws & an H else" Thinking Key

✓ use "Highlighting" Part 1 to identify Hits during the Focusing Phase of Data Finding

✓ use the "Storytelling" Thinking Key to find relationships among the Hits in the data list

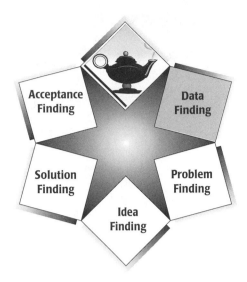

Resource People Help Find Data

Data Finding is the second of three stages dedicated to understanding the problem. In this stage, you will expand your understanding of the wish statement generated in Opportunity Finding. You will learn two Thinking Keys that will help expand your knowledge (which we refer to as data) about the context in which the problem lies and clarify the "burning" issues that need to be addressed in solving the problem. You will also be introduced to one new Thinking Key designed to help you identify relationships among data in the Focusing Phase.

For instructional purposes Data Finding follows Opportunity Finding. (Remember that in real practice, each of the six stages may be used at any time, in any order, depending on the demands of the situation.) In some situations Data Finding may be your first step in understanding the problem. When the objective of therapy services has been identified—through an external source such as the referral for services, your previous familiarity with the client, or the client's previous therapy history—you can skip Opportunity Finding and move directly to Data Finding.

Data Finding begins with the one "wish" (as in "WIBGI . . . ?") the client independently or with the therapy guide's assistance selected at the end of the Focusing Phase of Opportunity Finding. The wish is the opportunity statement that the client feels holds the most promise toward solving his problem.

In Data Finding your focus is on *finding* as much *data* as you can about the contents of the wish statement in order to help make it a reality. You will gather facts, feelings, observations, hunches, projections, and opinions about the wish statement from as many resources as possible. At this point you might be asking yourself, "From whom do I seek information?" or, "How do I know who can help me?" Every person who could be involved with making the client's dream come true is potentially a resource on your therapy expedition.[1] Your responsibility as a therapy guide is to seek out resources that will expand your understanding of the wish. The realization of the wish is what ultimately helps the client solve her problem. The following scenario is an example of expanding a wish statement with relevant data:

> Imagine that you receive a referral from a teacher about Jason, a new student in his classroom. Jason has a problem attending to any task for longer than two minutes at a time because he has a need to move constantly. When you sit down with the teacher and hold a "wishing session" he selects the wish, "Wouldn't it be great if Jason could move and study at the same time?"[2] To work on this wish the teacher, at your recom-

mendation, is willing to suspend a hanging swing in the classroom. To find data on the feasibility of accomplishing the teacher's wish, you consider what resources you have. The *maintenance staff* would be a central resource in determining how a hook might be installed in the ceiling. The *school principal* could help by providing the school policies that address installing equipment in the classroom. A *distributor of therapy equipment* could be a resource on the availability of ceiling support systems.

Each of the resource persons mentioned potentially can provide valuable insight about different aspects of the wish. Consider another scenario.

Imagine you are working with a special education resource teacher in a junior high school. The teacher has determined that her students have a problem with many life skills, such as money management, punctuality, and taking responsibility. From the "wishing session" you conducted with this teacher, her wish statement was, "Wouldn't it be great if the students could set up a midday sandwich shop at the school as part of their prevocational training?" As you explore the territory of this wish, you develop the following list of individuals who might serve as resources.

The *school principal* may know about other prevocational programs in the school district that could serve as models. *School board members* may know how to obtain funds for the initial start-up costs. *Parents* of the participating students may know about community resources that could support such a program. *Food service personnel* at the school might offer suggestions about menus and food preparation. The *graphic arts teacher* might offer to have an art class produce the advertising for the sandwich shop. The list goes on.

REFLECTIVE JOURNAL ENTRY 7.1

Complete the following thought:

Additional resource persons who might be interested in helping to make the midday sandwich shop become a reality are . . .

Every therapy expedition has a potentially wide range of resource people who could offer some type of information that will shed light on the journey. Receiving information from a resource person is like turning on a flashlight. Like the beam cast by the flashlight, a resource person helps you to see the area through which you are traveling. One resource person might offer technical advice. Another might offer ways to network a third person, who has the expertise you are seeking. Yet another resource person might offer advice about economic and time considerations. Each resource person offers a unique perspective on some aspect of the wish. *All those who share ownership of all or part of the problem are considered resources, but all resource persons do not necessarily share ownership of the problem.* A resource person might also have no greater role than simply to offer a piece of valuable information that helps you understand the problem or some aspect of the problem more clearly.

As you collect information from resource persons, bear in mind that data gathering involves more than collecting facts. It is also about people's feelings, observations, hunches, projections, and opinions about the wish statement. Understanding as many aspects of the client's wish as possible increases the probability of bringing the wish to reality.

Data Finding is the stage in the CPS process where you seek to find as much data as possible, as time allows and circumstances permit, from the respective resource persons. Since each therapy expedition is made up of a unique set of circumstances, each expedition will call for a unique combination of resource persons. In addition to the occupational therapist, the primary resource group on an expedition may include the child, the child's mother, a grandmother, and three aunts, and the school speech and language pathologist. In a different expedition, the primary resources may be the child, a grandmother, the classroom teacher, a tutor, a music therapist, and the occupational therapist. Each combination of resource persons creates a unique blend of talents from which the therapy guide can draw during the expedition. The more thoroughly a therapy guide understands the kind of help each resource person can offer, the greater the success of the therapy expedition. (Note: a successful therapy expedition is one in which the client's goals are met and, at the termination of the services, the client is satisfied.)

As you go about *finding data* while on a therapy expedition, write down all the information that you uncover. This is one process where it is important to record everyone's thoughts. So grab the paper and pen and be prepared to harvest every idea about the wish that crosses everyone's mind. The data you uncover during Data Finding will be a handy reference for the remainder of the CPS process.

The Generating Phase of Data Finding

The wish statement that emerged from Opportunity Finding is like the tip of the iceberg. Working with the client, you have identified a direction, a most likely place to begin the journey toward helping the client solve his problem. The client's wish statement at this point gives you a rough idea of where you are going on the expedition. However, you need to explore deeper for what lies below the surface. One **Thinking Key** that will help you identify data in the Generating Phase of Data Finding is the **"5 Ws & an H."**

The "5 Ws" are the basic questions reporters use to extract information for a news story. Reporters rely on who, what, where, when, and why questions to gain information about a situation. In Data Finding, these same "5 W" questions are asked. A further question, the "H" question, asks how or by what method the task will be accomplished.

Below is a brief description of what the 5 Ws and an H questions focus on.

"Who" questions ask about the people who are or possibly could be involved in helping make the wish a reality. Who has different perspectives about the wish? Who has strong feelings—positive or negative—about the wish? Who might have knowledge about some aspect of the wish?

"What" questions cover many aspects of the wish. What are the parts? What is the scope of the problem? What support systems exist to solve the problem? What objections, difficulties, limitations, or obstacles might there be in trying to solve the client's problem? What steps are necessary to help the client achieve his dream?

"Where" questions ask about all the places where the original problem occurred as well as where the opportunities exist for the wish to become a reality. Consider also, Where can you go to increase your knowledge about the opportunity? Where are possible obstacles? Where is the most harmony?

"When" questions address time frames. When did the original problem occur? When are there opportunities to make the client's wish come true? When is the best time to work on the client's wish? When is the worst time? When do we need to have our questions about the opportunity answered? When do strong feelings about the opportunity arise?

"Why" questions help to clarify the reason the problem has become an issue of concern. Why is this situation viewed as a problem? Why is a solution important?

"How" questions identify the steps, activities, or actions involved in the situation. When asking "how" questions, explore the emotional impact that the therapy expedition will have on the client. Ask how the client might be supported in the therapy plan.

When you pose who, what, where, when, why, and how questions to resource persons, you begin to gather information about the environmental context of the client's wish. You find out who might be able to help. Asking, "What is involved in turning the wish into a reality? Where and when might opportunities be found to act on the wish? Why are people interested in solving the problem? How might the problem be solved?" will help you zero in on the context of the situation and gather very specific information about the client's paradigm. The more familiar you are with the context within which a problem occurs, the more adept you will be at exploring the territory for opportunities to creatively help make the client's dream come true. (Recall the discussion in Section 4: the context is the frame of reference that brings meaning to the situation. Understanding the context of a problem is essential since the meaning of a problem can change as the context changes.)

As you become comfortable using the "5 Ws & an H" Thinking Key you will find many more questions for each W and the H than those listed above. Here's a quick reference guide.

Who	Identify people who are or could be involved (directly or indirectly) in creating opportunities to solve the client's problem.
Where	Name places and events to consider where opportunities could be found to help the client's wish come true.
What	Identify what is involved in creating opportunities to help the client's wish come true.
When	Explore time frames and duration related to when opportunities could be found to help the client's wish come true.
Why	Explore the reason the problem has to be solved.
How	Identify opportunities (such as methods or activities) that are possible and probable as well as those that may seem improbable in helping make the client's dream come true.

Now it's time to practice your skill at systematically collecting data into natural clusters using the "5 Ws & an H" Thinking Key. Note: The "5 Ws & an H" Thinking Key is joined together in one Field Organizer with the "Highlighting" (Part 1) Thinking Key, and the "5 Ws & an H else?" Thinking Key you will be introduced to later in this section. Turn to the Field Organizer that begins on p. 196 and familiarize yourself with how it is organized. The "5 Ws & an H" Thinking Key is located in column A. The "5 Ws & an H else" Thinking Key is located in column C. The two narrow columns (B and D) are reserved for "Highlighting" (Part 1). You will be directed to use the "Highlighting" Thinking Key in the Focusing Phase of Data Finding.

For this activity imagine that you are again a member of the Nose Blowing Expedition. As you imagine yourself on this expedition, you will need to think beyond what you read in the story.

When you use the "5 Ws & an H" Thinking Key, the more minds you involve the better (groups of four or more participants work well). For this Field Organizer, however, you may work with a partner or alone. If you are working in pairs or a small group, decide who will role play the therapist and who will role play the teacher. The therapist and the teacher share ownership of the problem and are two resource persons in the Nose Blowing Expedition. If you are working in a small group, have the members who are not playing the therapist or the teacher take on the roles of other possible resource persons within the context of the story (e.g., teacher's aide, parent, speech pathologist). The main point in structuring activities to include a resource group is to demonstrate the important role sharing ideas with others plays in the decision making process.

DIRECTIONS

1. Add at least five pieces of data to the information already listed in each of the six sections in column A, under the Thinking Key the "5 Ws & an H" on the left side of the Field Organizer. There is a section for each of the 5 Ws and an H questions. Use the question at the top of each section to trigger your thoughts. There are more than five spaces left in each section, so don't limit yourself. Collect data with the intention of thoroughly exploring the following wish statement:

   WIBGI the children could learn to blow their own noses?

   This statement is like the tip of the iceberg. To help make this wish a reality you will need to delve below the surface to uncover more information about this opportunity statement as well as the problem it is trying to solve. The "5 Ws and an H" Thinking Key will help you uncover these pieces of information.

2. Use the list on pp. 194–95 when responding to the questions posed in the "5 Ws & an H" Thinking Key as they relate to the Nose Blowing Expedition.

 FIELD ORGANIZER

"5 Ws & an H" / "5 Ws & an H else" / "Highlighting" Part 1

Wish Statement: *WIBGI the children could learn to blow their noses?*

The "5 Ws & an H"		The "5 Ws & an H else"	
A **Generate**	**B** **Hits**	**C** **Generate**	**D** **Hits**
Who might be involved in the opportunity?		**Who *else* might be involved in the opportunity?**	
1. *teacher of the children*	●	1. *siblings*	●
2. *four- to six-year-olds in the class*	●	2. *parents of the children*	●
3. *teacher's aide*	●	3. *babysitters of the children*	
4. *occupational therapist*		4. *grandparents of the children*	●

"5 Ws & an H" / "5 Ws & an H else" / "Highlighting" Part 1 (Continued)

The "5 Ws & an H"			The "5 Ws & an H else"	
A **Generate**	**B** **Hits**		**C** **Generate**	**D** **Hits**
5. the students' pediatricians			5. teachers in a regular day care center	
6.			6.	
7.			7.	
8.			8.	
9.			9.	
10.			10.	
What is involved in the opportunity?			**What *else* is involved in the opportunity?**	
1. nose-hand coordination	●		1. awareness of the need to blow without having to be told	●
2. knowing how to blow nose without snapping the neck forward	●		2. teach nose blowing through fun activities	
3. proper nose blowing etiquette	●		3. knowledge of how to dispose of tissues after use	●
4. learning how the nose works			4. no courses or books on how to teach nose blowing	
5. chronological age nose blowing develops			5. seems like an odd thing to teach	
6.			6.	
7.			7.	
8.			8.	
9.			9.	
10.			10.	

(continued)

"5 Ws & an H" / "5 Ws & an H else" / "Highlighting" Part 1 (Continued)

The "5 Ws & an H"		The "5 Ws & an H else"	
A **Generate**	**B** **Hits**	**C** **Generate**	**D** **Hits**
Where might opportunities occur to work on the wish?		**Where *else* might opportunities occur to work on the wish?**	
1. *local school for the deaf*	●	1. *at home with family*	
2. *near the coat rack*	●	2. *playing with friends at their home*	
3. *playground*		3. *when visiting relatives*	
4. *in the bathroom*		4. *at a restaurant*	
5. *in the hallway, outside the bathroom (while standing in line)*		5. *at the grocery store*	
6.		6.	
7.		7.	
8.		8.	
9.		9.	
10.		10.	
When might there be an opportunity to work on the wish?		**When *else* might there be an opportunity to work on the wish?**	
1. *upon arriving at school*	●	1. *upon rising in the morning*	
2. *after taking off coat*	●	2. *before going to bed at night*	
3. *after recess*	●	3. *before going to school*	
4. *after lunch*	●	4. *upon arriving home from school*	
5. *before going to the rug for reading time*		5. *in the morning before mealtime*	
6.		6.	

"5 Ws & an H" / "5 Ws & an H else" / "Highlighting" Part 1 (Continued)

The "5 Ws & an H"			The "5 Ws & an H else"	
A **Generate**	**B** **Hits**		**C** **Generate**	**D** **Hits**
When might there be an opportunity to work on the wish?			**When *else* might there be an opportunity to work on the wish?**	
7.			7.	
8.			8.	
9.			9.	
10.			10.	
Why is it important to look for opportunities in this area?			**Why *else* is it important to look for opportunities in this area?**	
1. *"cold season" approaching*			1. *stop the spread of cold germs*	●
2. *teachers will minimize exposure to cold germs if students blow own noses*	●		2. *decrease chafing from adults wiping students' noses*	
3. *children won't miss so much school because of colds*	●		3. *contribute to the children's general health by keeping others from becoming sick*	●
4. *children will feel good and be healthy*	●		4. *school won't have to pay substitutes to sub for sick teachers*	
5. *children will learn to use tissues to blow their noses rather than use their clothing to wipe their noses*			5. *children will do well at their schoolwork because they are healthy and able to focus*	●
6.			6.	
7.			7.	
8.			8.	
9.			9.	
10.			10.	

(continued)

"5 Ws & an H" / "5 Ws & an H else" / "Highlighting" Part 1 (Continued)

The "5 Ws & an H"		The "5 Ws & an H else"	
A **Generate**	**B** **Hits**	**C** **Generate**	**D** **Hits**
How will you make this wish a reality?		**How *else* will you make this wish a reality?**	
1. *nose blowing games*	●	1. *parent group*	
2. *mouth blowing games*	●	2. *videotape the children to show parents*	
3. *set up blowing games as an "Olympic" event*	●	3. *educate the students on health issues related to properly disposing of used tissues*	
4. *have children take turns being the master of ceremonies for the games*	●	4. *give each child his little pocket size tissues to carry during the day*	
5. *videotape segments of the children's Olympic blowing games*	●	5. *have children view segments of themselves in the Olympic blowing games and send funniest segment to <u>America's Funniest Home Videos</u> television program*	●
6.		6.	
7.		7.	
8.		8.	
9.		9.	
10.		10.	

The "5 Ws & an H Else"

To increase your depth of inquiry and further expand your thoughts after using the "5 Ws & an H" use the **"5 Ws & an H else" Thinking Key**. This Thinking Key adds the word *else*, as in: "Who . . . ? Who else . . . ?" "What . . . ? What else . . . ?" "Where . . . ? Where else . . . ?" "When . . . ? When else . . . ?" "Why . . . ? Why else . . . ?" and "How . . . ? How else . . . ?" to each of the 5 Ws and an H questions.

Adding *else* to each of the 5 Ws and an H questions will stretch your thinking even further beyond the information you know from Louise's story. Asking Who *else* . . . ? What *else* . . . ? Where *else* . . . ? When *else* . . . ? Why *else* . . . ? and How *else* . . . ?" about the Nose Blowing Expedition will expand your perception of issues that you systematically identified using the "5 Ws & an H" Thinking Key. The 5 Ws and an H else questions propel your thinking outward from the locus of the baseline information. Following is a description of how each of the 5 Ws and an H else questions can expand your thinking about the wish statement and the original problem in the Nose Blowing Expedition.

Who else? In the Nose Blowing Expedition, the "Who else?" questions can stimulate the resource group to think beyond the scope of the school personnel, beyond those persons who are immediately involved with the children in the classroom. By asking the "who else?" questions you begin to consider, for example, the family members of the students as part of the story.

What else? Asking "What else?" can stimulate the resource group to consider a wild idea like adding nose blowing to the students' curriculum basics. The "what else?" question can also prompt feelings about the oddity of categorizing nose blowing along with the rest of the academics in the class. Nose blowing does seem like a peculiar and at the same time, given its effect on the children's health, a necessary "subject" to teach in school. "What else" can also push you to explore the range of the skills and abilities involved in the completion of the task.

Where else? The "Where else?" question can transport the Nose Blowing Expedition from the school for the deaf to each child's respective home territory. The "Where else?" questions can stimulate thoughts about the need for students to be able to blow their noses when they are at their friends' houses, at the grocery store, or in a restaurant.

When else? Asking "When else?" can extend the value of the Nose Blowing Expedition beyond the time planned with the students in the classroom. The students' families would appreciate the lessons learned from the Nose Blowing Expedition whenever they are at home or out in their community. Exploring the "When else?" question has the capacity of deepening the resource group's perspective of the merit or relative worth of pursuing an issue.

Why else? The "Why else?" question can direct thoughts from the immediate issues related to nose blowing to concerns for the students' health. Asking "Why else?" can bring to mind how nose blowing skills can decrease the spread of cold germs and in turn can contribute to the improvement in the general quality of the children's health.

How else? Asking "How else?" questions can move the story from the obvious techniques associated with the nuts and bolts of teaching the children to blow their noses to the possible use of other strategies such as games, parent groups, and videotaping.

You are ready now to use the "5 Ws & an H else" Thinking Key to extend the data collection process you began with the "5 Ws & an H" Thinking Key. Turn back to the Field Organizer that begins on p. 196.

DIRECTIONS

Add at least five more pieces of data to the information already listed in each of the six sections in column C, under the "5 Ws & an H else" Thinking Key.

After completing the Field Organizer, turn to Appendix A (p. 463). You will see a completed Field Organizer to which you can compare your Data Finding lists. Note similarities and differences between the items in the two lists. Noting differences reminds you that no two therapy guides will approach any one problem exactly the same way. The more you celebrate your own originality, the more you will develop the confidence to take risks. Innovative solutions thrive in an environment where risk taking occurs. Push yourself as far as you can in identifying data before turning to Appendix A.

The Focusing Phase of Data Finding

When the therapy guide and the client analyze the data in the Focusing Phase of Data Finding, their thoughts should be anchored to the client's Opportunity Finding statement. Recall that the wish the client selects at the end of Opportunity Finding is that which she determines to be the most likely option that will lead to a solution to her problem. Recall also, that the family or caregiver will select the wish if the client is at a chronological or developmental age that precludes her making the decision independently.

In the Focusing Phase of Opportunity Finding, your aim was to select one wish statement. In Data Finding, your aim is on understanding how the pieces of data (gathered into sections according to the 5 Ws and an H questions) relate to each other. To consider the relationships among the data gathered, you will use the "Highlighting" and the "Storytelling" Thinking Keys.

"Highlighting" Part 1

In Data Finding, only Part 1 of the **"Highlighting" Thinking Key** is used. In place of Parts 2 and 3 of the "Highlighting" Thinking Key, the "Storytelling" Thinking Key is used in Data Finding. The aim of "Highlighting" in Data Finding is to identify all the Hits that might help make the therapy expedition a success. Return once again to the "5 Ws and an H else" Field Organizer and continue working with your partner or group.

DIRECTIONS

The person role playing the therapist should direct the person role playing the teacher or other resource person to place an orange dot in the Hits columns B and D next to any responses that might help make the teacher's wish statement a reality. (Recall that a Hit in Opportunity Finding is an *idea* that holds promise in helping solve a problem. In Data Finding, a Hit is any piece of *data* that you feel holds promise in helping you understand the client's wish and the problem it is attempting to solve.)

"Storytelling"

The **"Storytelling" Thinking Key** will help you look for relationships among Hits identified in Part 1 of the "Highlighting" process. With the "Storytelling" Thinking Key, you will connect selected Hits in such a way as to tell a story. When you create a story by linking information, you in turn construct a broader context within which to consider the individual pieces of data. Remember, in any problem solving situation, we need to acknowledge the relevance of the context in an effort to give meaning to the situation. The first question asked is not, "What's the problem?" but rather, "What's the story?"[3]

Practice using the "Storytelling" Thinking Key with the group you have been working with. Use the completed Field Organizer as an example. The blank one is for you to complete. To begin this activity, each group member should have a completed copy of the "5 Ws & an H"/"5 Ws & an H else"/"Highlighting" Part 1 Thinking Keys Field Organizer.

The storytelling process may be done in actual practice with a resource group of only two members, the client and the therapy guide, or it may involve several members of a resource group. In occupational therapy practice, often the therapy guide works alone and mentally constructs the story as she sees the relationship between all of the collected pieces of data.

DIRECTIONS

1. The person role playing the therapist should direct the person role playing the client (in this instance a group) to look for relationships among the Hits identified in the "5 Ws . . ." Field Organizer that could be joined into a story that will help you think about how to make the teacher's wish come true.
2. Turn to the blank "Storytelling" Thinking Key Field Organizer and begin the story by recording the wish statement selected from Opportunity Finding. First, drop the "WIBG" from the wish statement and start it with "If" (If the children . . .). Complete the statement by incorporating a Hit from the "5 Ws . . ." Field Organizer into the statement. For example, "If the children learned how to blow their noses *and properly discard the tissue, the children's teachers, classmates, family members, and babysitters will be less likely to be contaminated by cold germs.* See this sample recorded at the top of the completed "Storytelling" Field Organizer.

3. Develop the story, linking one Hit to the next, by creating sentences that incorporate Hits from the "5 Ws . . ." Field Organizer. Members of the resource group contribute ideas (linking one piece of data to the next) in a spontaneous manner. Develop the story in a logical progression (refer to the sample story provided in the completed "Storytelling" Field Organizer, where the Hits have been organized logically).

4. Write each story element on the lines provided and create a linking phrase between one story element box and the next, such as "For this to occur . . ." or "If this could occur . . ." The downward arrows between the write-on lines indicate the linkages between the story elements. As Hits are incorporated into the story, identify the source of the Hit (e.g., What #3–5, Why else #4) in parentheses. Recording where each Hit was drawn from will help you track the items as they are sequenced into the story and avoid duplication. One long story or multiple short stories can be created.

5. Next, direct the client to identify the themes that emerged from each story element and record the theme in the corresponding space at the bottom of the Field Organizer in Part B. Refer to the completed "Storytelling" Field Organizer to model your answers.

 FIELD ORGANIZER

"Storytelling" (Example)

Part A: Wish Statement

If the children could learn to blow their noses . . .

1. *and properly discard the tissue, the children's teachers, classmates, family members, and babysitters (Who #1–3, Who else #1–3) will be less likely to be contaminated by cold germs (Why #2, Why else #1). If the children's teachers, classmates, and family members remained healthy, the children's chances of remaining healthy all year would in turn increase (Why else #3).*

If this were to occur . . .

2. *the children will have a high attendance at school (Why #3). The more consistent the children's attendance at school, the more likely the children will do well in school because they are healthy and able to attend to their school work (Why else #5).*

For this to occur . . .

3. *the children need to learn proper nose blowing etiquette (What #3), which involves knowing how to blow through their noses without snapping their necks (What #2); obtaining a tissue to blow their nose rather than use their hand or their sleeve (Why #5); proper disposal of the tissue after use (What else #2); an awareness of when their nose is running so they can blow it as needed without being reminded to do so (What else #1); nose-hand coordination (What #1).*

In order to help the students develop proper nose blowing etiquette . . .

4. *the children could participate in a nose blowing program that includes routine times when the children know they would need to blow their noses, such as when coming in from the outside in the morning and after recess and lunch (When #1–4); games that included having the children blow through their mouth and their nose (How #1–3). The children could take turns being the master of ceremonies for the Olympic nose and mouth blowing games, which are videotaped (How #4–5).*

(continued)

Part A: Wish Statement

If this could occur . . .

5. the children could view themselves in their own Olympic blowing games and make a class project of selecting the funniest segment to send to the television show *America's Funniest Home Videos* in hopes of having their segment aired on national television (How else #5).

6. And to think it all started with the children learning how to blow their noses!

Part B: Themes from the Nose Blowing Story

1. health maintenance of the children, the teachers, and the children's families

2. the relationship between wellness and school performance

3. proper nose blowing etiquette

4. embedding nose blowing activities in: daily routines in order for the children to develop healthy habits, and special events that motivate the children to participate with a seemingly boring task.

5. technology can be used to promote the children's achievement of basic skills while simultaneously helping them maintain good health

6. extraordinary happenings can develop from simple beginnings when you start with an end in mind

FIELD ORGANIZER
"Storytelling"

Part A: Wish Statement

If the children could learn to blow their noses . . .

1. _____

    _____

    _____

↓

2. _____

    _____

    _____

↓

3. _____

    _____

    _____

↓

4. _____

    _____

    _____

↓

5. _____

    _____

    _____

↓

6. _____

    _____

    _____

"Storytelling" (Continued)

Part B: Themes from the Nose Blowing Story

1. _____

   _____

2. _____

   _____

3. _____

   _____

4. _____

   _____

5. _____

   _____

6. _____

   _____

Hits identified in the "5 Ws and an H else" Field Organizer that were not incorporated into a story element may trigger thoughts in another stage of CPS. (Keep this Field Organizer handy as a reference as you proceed through CPS.) You may choose to use the data recorded here in future sections.

Symbol for Data Finding

The computer, like the one to the left, represents Data Finding. The computer symbolizes the process of collecting data to understand the wish statement generated from the challenging situation. The heart on the icon's computer monitor is a reminder that in addition to facts, data includes feelings, impressions, observations, and questions. Whenever you see the computer icon with the heart, you are being reminded to use Data Finding.

Create a Mind Map of Section

7

Mind Map Guidelines

1. Place the section's main concept in the center of the space using pictures or words or both.
2. Radiate ideas from the central thought.
   - Use images (be sure to use color).
   - Headline text—one or two words per line.
   - Print text (for easy reading).
3. Link the main concepts and generate more ideas from the linkages.
4. Have fun!

Section 7
SELF-ASSESSMENT

Now that I have completed the seventh section of my journey, I can:

○ explain how resource people help the therapy guide find data about the wish statement.

○ use the "5 Ws & an H" Thinking Key in the Generating Phase of Data Finding.

○ use the "5 Ws & an H else" Thinking Key.

○ use "Highlighting" Part 1 to identify Hits during the Focusing Phase of Data Finding.

○ use the "Storytelling" Thinking Key to find relationships among the Hits in the data list.

NOTES

1. R. L. Firestein, and Donald Treffinger, "Ownership and Converging: Essential Ingredients of Creative Problem Solving," *Journal of Creative Behavior* 17, no. 1 (1983): 32–38.
2. G. Prince, "The Mindspring Theory: A New Development from Synectics Research," in J. P. Guilford and S. Parnes, *Source Book for Creative Problem Solving* (Buffalo, N.Y.: Creative Education Foundation Press, 1992).
3. R. Neustadt, and E. May. *Thinking in Time: The Uses of History for Decision-Makers* (New York: Free Press, 1986).

Get Ready to Understand the Problem: Problem Finding

Itinerary #8

At the end of the eighth part of your journey, you will be able to:

✓ explain how a problem statement reflects a client's and therapist's vision of the therapy route

✓ describe the value of reframing a problem using the invitational stem "In what ways might. . . ."

✓ use the "IWWM . . . Who–Does–What?" Thinking Key to generate problem statements

✓ create alternative wording in a problem statement using the "Substitution" Thinking Key

✓ use the "Ladder of Abstraction" Thinking Key to generate problem statements in response to "How" and "Why" questions

✓ use the "Head and Shoulders Test" and "Highlighting" Thinking Keys to select a problem statement in the Problem Finding stage

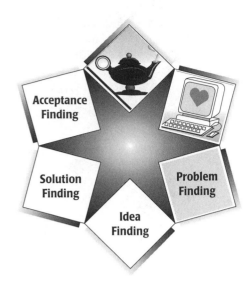

A Problem Statement Reflects a Vision of the Therapy Route

Problem Finding is the third stage of Get Ready to understand the problem. Problem Finding identifies the route you and the client will take for the remainder of the CPS process. Unlike Opportunity Finding, which seeks to describe the broad challenges within a situation, Problem Finding identifies the *specific* gap between what is and what should be. In this stage, you explicitly identify the link between the future opportunity you hope to achieve and the current reality you are trying to improve.

Identifying the problem is crucial to effective problem solving. As simplistic as it may sound, unless you accurately target the *right* problem, you may lose time and perhaps the opportunity to help the client solve the problem altogether. When you start out working on the wrong problem, you risk being off course for the rest of the journey.

We begin with an overview of Problem Finding to help organize your thoughts about where you will be going in this section. Like Opportunity Finding and Data Finding, Problem Finding begins with the Generating Phase. In the Generating Phase of Problem Finding you will create as many problem statements as possible. The following three Thinking Keys will help trigger your idea power:

"IWWM . . . Who–Does–What?"

"Substitution"

"Ladder of Abstraction"

The perspective from which you wish to view the problem will determine which of these three Thinking Keys to use.

When you have completed the Generating Phase, you will use Affirmative Judgment to evaluate the list of problem statements and the "Head and Shoulders Test" and "Highlighting" Thinking Keys to select one statement that best conceptualizes the future reality you both hope to create. This problem statement will define the route that you will take to help solve the client's problem. It will help you clearly envision what you and the client want to accomplish during the therapy process.[1] This vision will help guide you and the client throughout the therapy process. Once you have a clear vision of the journey ahead, developing appropriate and realistic therapy goals becomes a part of the therapy expedition. Therapy goals flow naturally from the problem statement identified in the Problem Finding stage.

One of the "seven habits of highly effective people," according to Stephen Covey, is to begin with an end in mind.[2] Creating a vision of what you want to accomplish in therapy is an example of beginning with an end in mind. To help create a vision, a therapy guide considers all the data collected in Data Finding: the facts, feelings, perceptions, and opinions that surround the wish statement within the context of the problem to be solved. When you and the client design a therapy expedition around a vision, the client has a clear destination to work toward. This is not to say that you won't encounter any detours along the way.

Detours are made when anything out of the ordinary occurs on the journey. When you know that detours are part of any journey, it's easier to manage them. Detours have many causes. Clients become ill; therapy appointments are canceled; therapy goals need to be restructured. Any disruption in the scheduled therapy routine can cause you to have to take a detour from the original trip plan. When the client has a clear vision of therapy outcomes, however, a detour need only prevent the client temporarily from arriving at her destination. The vision will help guide her back on course.

The Generating Phase of Problem Finding

In the Generating Phase of Problem Finding, your mission is to see a problem in as many different ways as possible and to come up with many problem statements. When you think about a problem, it's only natural to define it in terms of your personal paradigms. The Problem Finding step challenges you to restructure or *reframe* a problem in as many ways as possible. When you reframe a problem, it is necessary to shift your paradigm in order to look at a situation from a different perspective.

The Invitational Stem "IWWM . . ."

The wording that you select to frame a problem will affect your perceptions about the problem. Since keeping a positive mindset toward the client and his therapy-related challenge is an important function of CPS, you will learn to use the invitational stem "In what ways might . . ." (or "IWWM . . .") to frame a problem statement in positive terms. Stating a problem in positive terms will elicit a flow of ideas. Beginning a problem statement with the invitational stem "IWWM . . ." is a way to expand your thinking toward positive thoughts.

To complete a thought that you begin with "IWWM . . ." answer the question, "Who does what?" "Who" refers to the person who will carry out the action addressed in the problem statement. "Does" directs your thinking about what action may be done to help solve the client's problem. "What" refers to the object of the action in the problem statement.

In the problem statement "IWWM Louise teach the children how to blow their noses?" *Louise* represents "Who," *teach* represents "Does," and *how to blow their [the children's] noses* represents "What."

"IWWM . . . Who–Does–What?"

The invitational stem "IWWM . . ." combined with the question "Who does what?" becomes the **"IWWM . . . Who–Does–What?" Thinking Key.** To gain experience using this Thinking Key, let's look at five problem statements Louise and the teacher might have generated as they thought about how to help the children learn to blow their noses. Complete the "IWWM . . . Who–Does–What?" Worksheet.

DIRECTIONS

1. Read the Problem Statements in Part A and identify the "Who–Does–What" parts of each statement.
2. Record your answers in the appropriate columns in Part B. Refer to row 1 as a model.
3. Check your answers as you continue reading. Each statement will be analyzed in the following paragraphs.

"IWWM . . . Who–Does–What?" Worksheet

Part A: Problem Statements

1. IWWM Louise teach the children how to blow their noses?
2. IWWM the teacher help the children learn how to blow into a tissue?
3. IWWM the teacher's aide help the children blow through their mouths?
4. IWWM the children participate in blowing activities that are fun?
5. IWWM the children's parents reward their children for appropriate nose blowing behavior?

Part B: IWWM . . .

Who?	Does?	What?
1. *Louise*	*teach*	*the children how to blow their noses?*
2.		
3.		
4.		
5.		

Identifying "Who" shares ownership for the entire problem or any part of it is an important part of any problem solving task. Identifying all the people who could help to solve the problem gives you and the client a broader perspective. The problem statement that begins with "IWWM . . ." sets the stage for identifying all the people who could help solve the problem:

> IWWM **Louise** . . .
> IWWM **the teacher** . . .
> IWWM **the teacher's aide** . . .
> IWWM **the children** . . .
> IWWM **the children's parents** . . .

For each statement, once you identify the "Who," define the specific action to be taken by the person or people named under the "Does" in the "IWWM . . . Who–Does–What?" Thinking Key. Note that the problem statement uses an active verb. The verb targets the desired action you wish the person named in the problem statement to pursue. The choice of verb in the problem statement is very important because it describes exactly how the person named will move toward a solution:

> IWWM Louise **teach** . . .
> IWWM the teacher **help** . . .
> IWWM the teacher's aide **assist** . . .
> IWWM the children **participate** . . .
> IWWM the children's parents **reward** . . .

To complete the problem statement, identify the "What." The "What" portion of the problem statement clearly defines the object of the problem. The object in the problem statement should specify the issue that you plan to address. For example, if your therapy expedition focuses on enhancing the performance area of activities of daily living, the problem statement will reflect that performance area in the problem statement:

IWWM Louise teach **the children how to blow their noses**?

IWWM the teacher help **the children learn how to blow into a tissue**?

IWWM the teacher's aide help **the children to blow through their mouths**?

IWWM the children participate **in blowing activities that are fun**?

IWWM the children's parents reward **their children for appropriate nose blowing behavior**?

The choices you make for the "Who–Does–What?" portions of the problem statement will powerfully influence how you visualize helping the client solve his problem. Therefore, spend time formulating the wording of your problem statement. It will be time well spent.

Business theorists have written extensively about the strong influence visualizing has on goal achievement. Visualizing or imagining a future state is an integral part of CPS because it can dramatically enhance the quality of a client's long-term goals.[3]

When you are on a therapy expedition, you must first visualize your destination point in order to begin to move toward it. To do so you need to define two primary locations. First, you must define your starting point. This is your present reality. Second, you must define where you are headed. Therapy guides reach their therapy goals because they create a vision of the outcome of the therapy process. To generate the kind of thoughts that will help create that vision, formulate your problem statement using the "IWWM . . . Who–Does–What?" Thinking Key.

When you overlay your vision of the future state with a picture of the present state, you create what Peter Senge calls "creative tension."[4] Creative tension is what motivates all of us to pursue our goals. When speaking about motivation, some theorists refer to creative tension as the "just right" challenge;[5] others call it the "inner drive" to succeed.[6] Whatever term you prefer, Louise demonstrated it when she led the children on the Nose Blowing Expedition.

Louise knew how to blow her own nose. After all, she was an adult. She was an expert at nose blowing. Why then, didn't she begin a therapy program based on her personal knowledge and previous experience blowing her own nose? What did she do? She felt a need to learn more about the process of nose blowing. She was motivated first to go to the literature in search of information describing nose blowing from a developmental perspective. When her literature search on nose blowing proved to be nonproductive, her creative tension fueled her desire to do her own research—visit the local day care center to observe first hand how normal children blow their noses.

Move forward on your journey now and practice your skill in writing problem statements related to the Nose Blowing Expedition, using the "IWWM . . . Who–Does–What?" Field Organizer that follows. (Note that the Thinking Key "IWWM . . . Who–Does–What?" is paired with Part 1 of the "Highlighting" Thinking Key to reduce the amount of rewriting necessary in the "Highlighting" process. Part 1 of the "Highlighting" Thinking Key is located on the right side of the Field Organizer in the column labeled Focus. You will be directed to use the "Highlighting" portion of the Field Organizer in the Focusing Phase of Problem Finding.)

Pair up with a partner and assume the role of the therapist Louise or of the teacher in the Nose Blowing Expedition. (If working with a group of three or more assume the role of one of the resource persons.)

DIRECTIONS

1. Generate eight problem statements to add to the six already listed in the Field Organizer. Begin each statement with the invitational stem "IWWM . . . " and complete the statement by answering "Who–Does–What?"
2. Record the statement by writing the parts that answer Who? Does? and What? in the appropriate columns under Generate. Note: As you work, try to hitchhike one idea to another.

		Generate		**Focus**

IWWM . . .

	Who?	Does?	What?	Hits
1.	teacher	decrease	the absenteeism in the class during the "cold season"?	●
2.	teacher	involve	parents in rewarding proper nose blowing at home?	●
3.	Louise	request	parents to rule out nasal obstructions by the child's pediatrician?	
4.	Louise	convince	principal that all students could benefit from O.T. in order to learn how to blow their noses?	●
5.	team	help	the children learn proper nose blowing etiquette?	●
6.	children	learn	to dispose of their soiled tissues properly?	●
7.				
8.				
9.				
10.				
11.				
12.				
13.				
14.				

Use the "Substitution" Thinking Key to Create Alternative Wording

Stating a problem in different ways helps you see the problem in a new light and can help uncover surprising solutions. Use the **"Substitution" Thinking Key** to create alternative wording for your problem statement when you get "stuck" and need to see a problem with a fresh perspective. The "Substitution" Thinking Key has two parts, which you will practice using in the "Substitution" Thinking Key Field Organizer. Like the "IWWM . . . Who–Does–What" Field Organizer, this next Field Organizer includes Part 1 of the "Highlighting" Thinking Key.

DIRECTIONS

Part A

1. Select a problem statement that you wish to expand on and record the statement in the space provided at the top of the "Substitution" Thinking Key Field Organizer. For instructional purposes we have recorded the following statement for you: "IWWM Louise teach the children how to blow their noses?"
2. Circle the verb and the subject of the direct object in the problem statement. (In the sentence provided, the verb to circle is "teach" and the subject of the direct object is "the children.")
3. Take the verb that has been circled ("teach") and think up as many substitutions for that verb as you can. Record the words under "Does?" in rows 4–8. Use rows 1–3 to model your answers.
4. Take the direct object that has been circled ("children") and think up as many substitutions as you can. Record the words under "What" (in rows 4–8). Use rows 1–3 to model your answers.

Part B

1. Write the new problem statements that resulted from changing the wording in the original problem statement in the spaces provided in Part B. For example, when you substitute "show (the) teacher" for "teach (the) children" your new problem statement would look like this: "IWWM Louise show the teacher how to blow their noses?" Before this statement could become a usable problem statement, the wording in the direct object (". . . . how to blow their noses) would need to be adjusted to fit the new word substitutions ("show" and "teacher"). The updated version could be as follows: "IWWM Louise show the teacher *how to blow the noses of the students*?"

   Try this step again and substitute words from row 2 into the original statement. Write the new version of the problem statement on line 2, in Part B. Your new problem statement would look like this: "IWWM the therapist *encourage* the *principal* how to blow her students' noses?" Again, before you could use this statement you would need to tailor the wording of the original problem statement to fit the new word substitutions. The updated version could be: "IWWM the therapist *encourage* the *principal* to support an occupational therapy referral for the whole class?"

2. Complete the word substitutions in rows 3–8 and update the problem statements in Part B.
3. Indicate the statements that you reworded by recording the row number of the original statement to the left of the reworded statement. The new problem statement for row 1 has been recorded in Part B in the space provided.

FIELD ORGANIZER

"Substitution"/"Highlighting" Part 1

Part A

Problem Statement: IWWM *Louise teach the children how to blow their noses?*

IWWM . . .

Who?	Does?	What?
1. *Louise*	*show*	*teacher . . .*
2. *Louise*	*encourage*	*principal . . .*
3. *Louise*	*tell*	*parents . . .*
4. *Louise*		

(continued)

"Substitution"/"Highlighting" Part 1 (Continued)

Part A

Problem Statement: IWWM *Louise teach the children how to blow their noses?*

IWWM . . .

Who?	Does?	What?
5. *Louise*		
6. *Louise*		
7. *Louise*		
8. *Louise*		

Part B

	Hits
1. *IWWM Louise show the teacher how to blow the noses of the students?*	

Another version of the "Substitution" Thinking Key involves substituting words for the "Who" parts of the problem statement. For example, replace Louise with teacher, teacher's aide, or parents. You can also look for substitutions for part of the direct object. For example, replace "IWWM Louise teach the children *to blow their noses?*" with "IWWM Louise teach the children *to blow through their mouths?*" or "IWWM Louise teach the children *to breathe in and out through their noses?*"

Some substitutions in wording work better than others. Be prepared to discover surprises when you play with the wording of your problem statement. You may find that changing the wording opens you up to new thoughts and new directions related to the problem.

Remember, problem statements define the route that you *might* take to solve the problem. Your problem statement should reflect actions that the client and you feel have a probability of occurring. Your goal in creating the problem statement is to explicitly set up a future vision of what you want to accomplish.

Expanding the Problem Statement with the "Ladder of Abstraction"

To redefine the problem, or broaden it further, use the **"Ladder of Abstraction" Thinking Key**. To use this Thinking Key, take any problem statement and ask the question, "Why does the person want to do that?" For example, to the problem statement, "IWWM Louise teach the students how to blow their noses?" ask, "Why does Louise want to teach the students how to blow their noses?" You might answer that question with, "So the teacher does not have to wipe the children's noses." Your answer to the "Why" question can be converted into a new possible problem statement, such as, "IWWM the teacher avoid having to wipe the children's noses?" Turn to the next activity below, the "Ladder of Abstraction" Worksheet Using "Why" Questions. The worksheet shows you step-by-step how to use "Why" questions in the "Ladder of Abstraction" Thinking Key. The worksheet is divided into three columns.

- ◆ Column A directs you to begin the "Ladder of Abstraction" by recording a problem statement.
- ◆ Column B directs you to ask the question, "Why does the person want to carry out the action stated in the problem statement?"
- ◆ Column C directs you to record the answer to the question posed in column B. The answer recorded in column C can then be converted to a new problem statement, which begins the process all over again.

When you use the "Ladder of Abstraction" Thinking Key, keep abstracting the problem statement until you feel you have expanded the problem statement to your satisfaction. Now, resume your role as a member of the resource group working on the Nose Blowing Expedition and practice your skill with the "Ladder of Abstraction" Thinking Key using "Why?" questions.

DIRECTIONS

1. Read all questions and answers, beginning in row 1, column A, and proceed from left to right.
2. When you reach row 3, column C, convert that response into a problem statement and record it in row 4, column A.
3. Continue the process of abstraction in rows 4–7.

"Ladder of Abstraction" Worksheet Using "Why" Questions

A	B	C
Directions: Record problem statements.	*Directions*: Ask the question, "Why does the person want to carry out the action stated in the problem statement listed in column A?"	*Directions*: Record the answer to the question posed in column B. Convert this response into a new problem statement and record it in column A in the next row down in order to start the process of abstraction over again.
1. IWWM Louise teach the students how to blow their noses? IWWM the teacher avoid having to wipe the children's noses?	Why does Louise want to teach the students how to blow their noses? Why does the teacher want to avoid having to wipe the children's noses?	So the teacher does not have to wipe the children's noses. So she can decrease the risk of spreading cold germs to other children.

(continued)

A	B	C
Directions: Record problem statements.	*Directions*: Ask the question, "Why does the person want to carry out the action stated in the problem statement listed in column A?"	*Directions*: Record the answer to the question posed in column B. Convert this response into a new problem statement and record it in column A in the next row down in order to start the process of abstraction over again.
3. IWWM the teacher decrease the risk of spreading cold germs?	Why does the teacher want to decrease the risk of spreading cold germs?	So she can create a healthy environment where the children can grow and learn.
4. _____		
5. _____		
6. _____		
7. _____		

Asking "Why" questions broadens the problem statement. In the example above, in three steps the problem statement went from "IWWM Louise teach the students how to blow their noses?" to "IWWM the teacher create a healthy environment where the children can grow and learn?"

To make the problem statement more abstract, ask a "How" question. "How" questions reframe the question and direct your thinking to specific answers and methods. Let's see in what ways "How" transforms the problem statement, "IWWM Louise teach the students how to blow their noses?" This "IWWM" statement becomes, "How can Louise teach the children how to blow their noses?" In answer to this restated question, you might say, "Louise could engage the children in blowing activities that are fun." The answer is then turned into another problem statement to continue the process.

Resume your role as a member of the resource group working on the Nose Blowing Expedition and practice your skill with the "Ladder of Abstraction" Thinking Key, this time using "How" questions.

DIRECTIONS

1. Read all questions and answers, beginning in row 1, column A, and proceed from left to right.
2. Once you reach row 3, column C, convert that response into a problem statement and record it in row 4, column A.
3. Continue the process of abstraction in rows 4–7.

"Ladder of Abstraction" Worksheet Using "How" Questions

A	B	C
Directions: Record possible problem statements.	*Directions*: Ask the question, "How does the person want to carry out the action stated in the problem statement listed in column A?"	*Directions*: Record the answer to the question posed in column B. Convert this response into a new problem statement and record it in column A to start the process of abstraction again.
1. IWWM Louise teach the students how to blow their noses?	How can Louise teach the students how to blow their noses?	By engaging the children in fun blowing activities.
2. IWWM Louise set up fun blowing activities for the children?	How can Louise set up blowing activities for the children that are fun?	By having each child have his or her own plastic bag of blow toys.
3. IWWM Louise have each child have his or her own plastic bag of blow toys?	How can Louise have each child have his or her own plastic bag of blow toys?	By selecting blow toys that fit the skills and abilities of the children.
4. _____		
_____		
5. _____		
_____		
6. _____		
_____		
7. _____		
_____		

In just three "How" questions, the problem statements range from Louise's concern about how to teach the students how to blow their noses to how each child in the class might receive his or her own bag of plastic blow toys. In the examples above, asking "How" questions created three different perspectives on the problem of teaching nose blowing to the children.

To further stretch your thinking about a problem statement, add the questions "Why else?" and "How else?" to the ladder of abstraction process. See the sequence of questions below using the question "Why else?":

Initial statement: "Why does the teacher want the students to learn to blow their noses?"

Reply: "To relieve congestion."

Reply: "*Why else* does the teacher want the students to blow their own noses?"

Reply: "To become more independent with personal hygiene skills."

Reply: "*Why else* does the teacher want the students to blow their own noses?"

Reply: "To reduce the risk of spreading cold germs."

The "Ladder of Abstraction" Field Organizer includes the "Why?" "Why else?" "How?" and "How else?" questions in a ladder format.[7] When you go up the ladder you broaden the problem statement. When you move sideways on the ladder by asking "Why else?" and "How else?" you identify multiple responses at each level of abstraction. When you go down the ladder your answers become more concrete and specific.

Note that in the "Ladder of Abstraction" Thinking Key Field Organizer the upper right corner of each box is reserved for identifying Hits during the "Highlighting" process (see "Hit" dots in the middle column). You will be directed to use the "Highlighting" portion of the Field Organizers in the Focusing Phase of Problem Finding.

Resume your role as a member of the resource group working on the Nose Blowing Expedition and practice your skill with the "Ladder of Abstraction" Thinking Key by filling in the blank spaces in the Field Organizer. Complete Part A before moving on to Part B.

DIRECTIONS

1. Begin in the middle of the "Ladder of Abstraction" Field Organizer at "start here" and read the Initial Problem Statement.
2. Decide where you and your partner wish to go. You may move up in the ladder and make the initial statement more abstract or move down in the ladder and make the initial statement more concrete and specific.
3. Begin the process of abstraction by reading the "How?" and "Why?" questions and the answers to these questions, which have been provided in the middle column. Note: The arrows on the Field Organizer are used to demonstrate the direction of the question and answer process.

FIELD ORGANIZER

"Ladder of Abstraction"/"Highlighting" Part 1

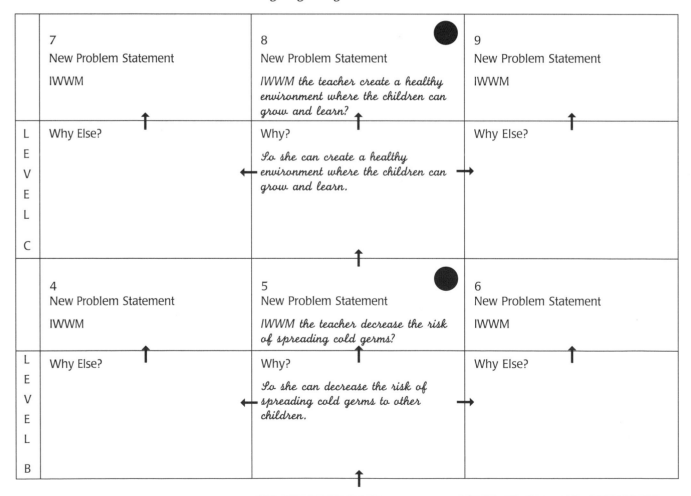

	7 New Problem Statement IWWM	8 New Problem Statement IWWM the teacher create a healthy environment where the children can grow and learn? ●	9 New Problem Statement IWWM
L E V E L C	Why Else? ↑	Why? So she can create a healthy ← environment where the children can → grow and learn.	Why Else? ↑
	4 New Problem Statement IWWM	5 New Problem Statement IWWM the teacher decrease the risk of spreading cold germs? ●	6 New Problem Statement IWWM
L E V E L B	Why Else? ↑	Why? So she can decrease the risk of ← spreading cold germs to other → children.	Why Else? ↑

"Ladder of Abstraction"/"Highlighting" Part 1 (Continued)

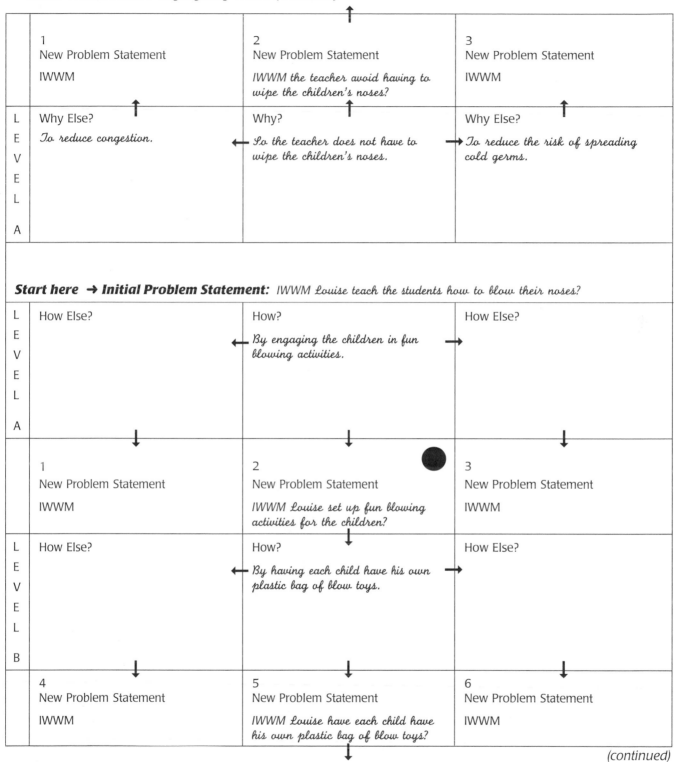

1 New Problem Statement IWWM	2 New Problem Statement IWWM the teacher avoid having to wipe the children's noses?	3 New Problem Statement IWWM
L E V E L A Why Else? *To reduce congestion.*	Why? *So the teacher does not have to wipe the children's noses.*	Why Else? *To reduce the risk of spreading cold germs.*

Start here → Initial Problem Statement: *IWWM Louise teach the students how to blow their noses?*

L E V E L A How Else?	How? *By engaging the children in fun blowing activities.*	How Else?
1 New Problem Statement IWWM	2 New Problem Statement *IWWM Louise set up fun blowing activities for the children?*	3 New Problem Statement IWWM
L E V E L B How Else?	How? *By having each child have his own plastic bag of blow toys.*	How Else?
4 New Problem Statement IWWM	5 New Problem Statement *IWWM Louise have each child have his own plastic bag of blow toys?*	6 New Problem Statement IWWM

(continued)

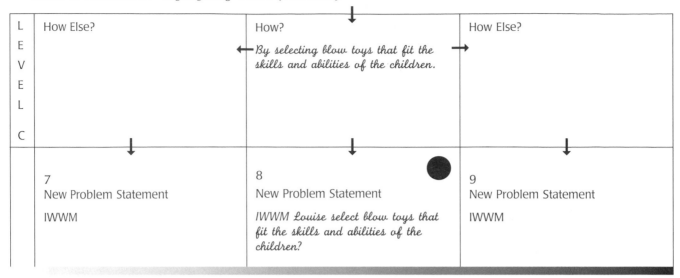

The "Ladder of Abstraction" is a Thinking Key that directs you to ask questions that can systematically develop a chain of abstract, yet related options. It is a useful strategy to use when you wish to expand your thinking about a subject. The "Ladder of Abstraction" explores the gaps within the problem situation. As you move from one statement to the next, you are systematically exploring pathways that might help close the gap between the present reality and the desired future state.

The Focusing Phase of Problem Finding

Now that you have generated many problem statements related to the Nose Blowing Expedition, you are ready to move to the Focusing Phase. In the Focusing Phase you work collaboratively with the client or the client's caretakers to determine which problem statement will set the course for solving the client's problem. To select one problem statement to be used for the remainder of the CPS process you will use either the "Head and Shoulders Test" Thinking Key or the "Highlighting" Thinking Key. You'll begin by completing the "Head and Shoulders Test" Field Organizer. Work with a partner for this activity.

DIRECTIONS

1. Turn back to the Field Organizers "IWWM . . . Who–Does–What?" (p. 214), "Substitution" (p. 215), and "Ladder of Abstraction" (p. 220) and consider all the problem statements you came up with in the Generating Phase. After the list of problem statements has been reviewed, the person role playing the therapist, Louise, should use the "Head and Shoulders Test" with the person role playing the teacher. Determine whether one option stands head and shoulders above the rest.
2. Record the problem statement in the "Head and Shoulders Test" Field Organizer. Next, reverse roles with your partner and repeat the "Head and Shoulders Test" in the new roles.

FIELD ORGANIZER

"Head and Shoulders Test"

Ask the client:

"Does one problem statement in the group stand **head and shoulders** above the rest?"

If the client is very interested in pursuing one of the statements or a combination of statements, confirm the problem statement with the client and write it on the line below.

IWWM _____ ?

Proceed to Idea Finding using this problem statement.

Even though you have already selected one option for the "Head and Shoulders Test," continue in your roles as Louise and the teacher and practice using the "Highlighting" Thinking Key with the next two Field Organizers, "Highlighting" Part 2 (p. 224) and "Highlighting" Part 3 (p. 226). Recall that "Highlighting" begins with the identification of all the Hits. In Problem Finding, Hits are the problem statements that show the most promise toward shining a light on the path to the solution. Take out the orange dots from your supply bag to complete this task. First you will identify the Hits. When the Hits have been identified, cluster the Hits into Hot Spots. Restate the Hot Spot labels into new problem statements that reflect the essence of the Hits clustered in each Hot Spot.

The person role playing Louise will direct the "Highlighting" process described below.

DIRECTIONS

Part 1

1. Review with the teacher the problem statements generated during the Generating Phase located in the Field Organizers "IWWM . . . Who–Does–What?" (p. 214), "Substitution" (p. 215), and "Ladder of Abstraction" (p. 220), which are all paired with "Highlighting" Part 1.
2. Direct the teacher to select the Hits from the list of problem statements by placing an orange dot in the space provided for Hits in each of the three Field Organizers (place the dot in the upper right corner of each space in the "Ladder of Abstraction" Field Organizer). To get you started, five Hits have been identified in the "IWWM . . ." Field Organizer and four Hits have been identified in the "Ladder of Abstraction" Field Organizer.

Part 2

1. Transfer the Hits from the "IWWM . . . ," "Substitution," and "Ladder of Abstraction" Field Organizers to the "Highlighting" Part 2 Field Organizer. Transfer the Hits from the Field Organizers in any order; there is no need to keep track of which Field Organizer each one came from. To get you started, the nine Hits that were identified in Part 1 of the "Highlighting" process have been transferred.
2. Look for relationships among the Hits by first identifying the central theme of each Hit. Record the central theme of each Hit in the right column of the Field Organizer titled Central Theme. The themes identified will serve as the label for the Hits when they get clustered into Hot Spots. Three themes emerged from the first nine problem statements: healthy environment, nose etiquette, and make nose blowing fun.
3. Move down to Part B of the Field Organizer and record all of the central themes that were identified in Part A (the first three have been recorded for you). These themes will be used to cluster the Hits into Hot Spots.

Part 3

1. Transfer all the Hits from "Highlighting" Part 2 into their respective Hot Spots (cluster) in "Highlighting" Part 3. To get you started, the three Hot Spots identified in "Highlighting" Part 2 have been transferred to a space designated for Hot Spots. They are: Hot Spot I:

Healthy environment; Hot Spot II: Nose blowing etiquette; and Hot Spot III: Make nose blowing fun. Space has been provided for you to add Hot Spots that emerge from the Hits you identified.

2. Analyze the Hits in each Hot Spot (cluster) and restate the label of the Hot Spot as a problem statement. The key to restating a Hot Spot is to avoid making the restatement too broad or too narrow. The restatement should reflect the main ideas stated in the cluster. For example, a restatement of the label *Healthy environment* (Hot Spot I) that reflects the Hits clustered under that label could be: "IWWM the teacher establish classroom routines that support a healthy learning environment?" Record the Hot Spot restatements in the lower portion of the field organizer in Part B.

3. Decide which restatement (new problem statement) reflects your top priority. Use that new problem statement for the remainder of the CPS process. As a rule of thumb, select a problem statement that is inclusive of the broadest number of challenges discussed without diluting the statement. The more inclusive the problem statement, the more comprehensive the solution will be. As need and time dictate, the remainder of the problem statements can be worked through.

FIELD ORGANIZER

"Highlighting" Part 2

Wish Statement: WIBGI *the children could learn to blow their noses?*

Part A

Hits		Central Theme
IWWM . . .		
1.	the teacher decrease the absenteeism in the class during the "cold season"?	healthy environment
2.	the teacher involve parents in rewarding proper nose blowing at home?	nose blowing etiquette
3.	Louise convince principal that all students could benefit from O.T. in order to learn how to blow their noses?	nose blowing etiquette
4.	the team help the children learn proper nose blowing etiquette?	nose blowing etiquette
5.	the children learn how to dispose of their soiled tissues properly?	nose blowing etiquette
6.	the teacher create a healthy environment where the children can grow and learn?	healthy environment
7.	the teacher decrease the risk of spreading cold germs?	healthy environment
8.	Louise set up fun blowing activities for the children?	make nose blowing fun
9.	Louise select blow toys that fit the skills and abilities of the children?	make nose blowing fun
10.		
11.		
12.		
13.		

Part B: Hot Spots Labels

1. _Healthy environment_   5. _____
2. _Nose blowing etiquette_   6. _____
3. _Make nose blowing fun_   7. _____
4. _____   8. _____

Wish Statement: WIBGI the children could learn to blow their noses?

Part A

Hot Spot I Labeled: *Healthy environment*

IWWM . . .

1. the teacher decrease the absenteeism in the class during the "cold season"?

3. Louise convince principal that all students could benefit from OT in order to learn how to blow their noses?

6. the teacher create a healthy environment where the children can grow and learn?

7. the teacher decrease the risk of spreading cold germs?

Hot Spot II Labeled: *Nose blowing etiquette*

IWWM . . .

2. the teacher involve parents in rewarding proper nose blowing at home?

4. the team help the children learn proper nose blowing etiquette?

5. children learn how to dispose of their soiled tissues properly?

Hot Spot III Labeled: *Make nose blowing fun*

IWWM . . .

8. Louise set up fun blowing activities for the children?

9. Louise select blow toys that fit the skills and abilities of the children?

Hot Spot IV Labeled:

IWWM . . .

"Highlighting" Part 3 (Continued)

Hot Spot V Labeled:

IWWM . . .

_____

_____

_____

_____

_____

Part B: Restatements of Hot Spot Labels

Hot Spot I: IWWM *the teacher establish classroom routines that support a healthy learning environment?* _____

Hot Spot II: IWWM _____

Hot Spot III: IWWM _____

Hot Spot IV: IWWM _____

Hot Spot V: IWWM _____

Once the client selects one problem statement, you are ready to move on to the next stage of CPS, Idea Finding. In Idea Finding you Get Set to find a solution by generating many ideas for carrying out the vision (problem statement) created for solving the original problem.

Following a path like the one Louise took on the Nose Blowing Expedition, we will begin the Idea Finding stage with the following problem statement: *IWWM a program be developed to teach the children how to blow their noses?*

Symbol for Problem Finding

The magnifying glass represents Problem Finding. It symbolizes the process of focusing in on the problem area that will be used to solve the client's problem. Whenever you see the magnifying glass icon, you are being reminded to use Problem Finding.

Create a Mind Map of Section

8

Mind Map Guidelines

1. Place the section's main concept in the center of the space using pictures or words or both.

2. Radiate ideas from the central thought.
   - Use images (be sure to use color).
   - Headline text—one or two words per line.
   - Print text (for easy reading).

3. Link the main concepts and generate more ideas from the linkages.

4. Have fun!

Remember, the more linkages that you generate between elements, the greater your ability to see how all the elements relate to one another.

Section 8
SELF-ASSESSMENT

Now that I have completed the eighth part of my journey, I can:

O explain how a problem statement reflects a client's and therapist's vision of the therapy route.

O describe the value of reframing the problem using the invitational stem "In what ways might. . . . "

O use the "IWWM . . . Who–Does–What?" Thinking Key to generate problem statements.

O create alternative wording in a problem statement using the "Substitution" Thinking Key.

O use the "Ladder of Abstraction" Thinking Key to generate problem statements in response to "How" and "Why" questions.

O use the "Head and Shoulders Test" and "Highlighting" Thinking Keys to select a problem statement in the Problem Finding stage.

NOTES

1. Sidney Parnes, *Visionizing* (Buffalo, N.Y.: Creative Education Foundation Press, 1992).
2. Stephen Covey, *The Seven Habits of Highly Effective People* (New York: Simon & Schuster, 1989).
3. Peter Senge, Sidney Parnes, and Joel Barker have written extensively on the powerful influence that creating a future vision of a situation has on the way you manage the decisions you make in the present. Peter Senge is the founder and director of the Center for Organizational Learning at MIT's Sloan School of Management. In his book *The Fifth Discipline: The Art and Practice of the Learning Organization* (New York: Currency Doubleday, 1990), Senge describes the dynamics that occur when groups work together. In his discussion of the "learning organizations," he eloquently describes how a leader needs to build a shared vision and hold that shared picture of the future when working with others. Sidney Parnes is professor emeritus of creative studies, State University College at Buffalo, and chairman of the board of the Creative Education Foundation. His book *Visionizing* is filled with outlines and exercises to enhance one's ability to develop skills at visionizing. The text is well referenced and recommended reading for anyone interested in learning about projecting thoughts into the future. Joel Barker calls himself a futurist. In his book *Paradigms: The Business of Discovering the Future* (New York: Harper Business, 1993) Barker presents a fascinating look at the life-span of a paradigm and how we can use our knowledge of defined paradigms within any given situation to strategically explore the future. Understanding paradigms of the present, according to Barker, will help us to envision the future.
4. Senge, *The Fifth Discipline*.
5. Mihaly Csikszentmihalyi, *Flow: The Psychology of Optimal Experience* (New York: Harper & Row, 1990).
6. A. J. Ayres, *Sensory Integration and the Child* (Los Angeles: Western Psychological Services, 1979).
7. "The Ladder of Abstraction" Field Organizer is derived from the Ladder of Abstraction Worksheet in Scott Isaksen, K. B. Dorval, and Donald Treffinger, *Creative Approaches to Problem Solving* (Dubuque, Iowa: Kendall/Hunt, 1994), 355.

Get Set to Find a Solution: Idea Finding

Itinerary #9

At the end of the ninth part of your journey, you will be able to:

✓ explain why it's important to generate lots of ideas during Idea Finding

✓ use "Brainstorming" to generate new ideas

✓ use the "CAMPERS" checklist to expand on ideas

✓ use "Force Fit" to generate novel ideas

✓ use "Attribute Listing" to analyze the components of a specific problem

✓ explain how to use the Reach for the Sky/Stick to the Basics Criteria Guide

✓ use "Highlighting" to identify ideas in the Focusing Phase of Idea Finding

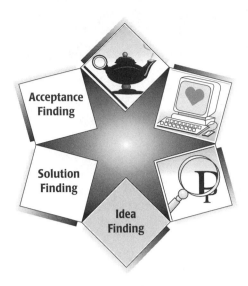

Generating Lots of Ideas

The component referred to as Get Set to find a solution is made up of one stage, Idea Finding. In Idea Finding you create the foundation for the solution. Like the previous stages to which you have been introduced—Opportunity Finding, Data Finding, and Problem Finding—Idea Finding has a Generating and a Focusing phase. There is a difference, however, in the emphasis on the two phases in Idea Finding. In the other stages there is equal accent on the two phases. In Idea Finding there is greater emphasis on the Generating Phase.

Idea Finding begins with the problem statement developed in the Focusing Phase of Problem Finding. The problem statement becomes a "springboard" from which to create more ideas. Sometimes the problem statement will have been clearly defined by another source. It may have come from the referral for therapy services or from a conversation with a client's parent, teacher, or other person who knows the client and is familiar with her functional performance needs.

Idea Finding is fun, challenging, and energizing because it relies on your creative potential. The Thinking Keys you will be introduced to in this section will show you how to build on your creative ability.[1] Creative ideas derive primarily from three sources:

- ◆ Your personal experiences
- ◆ Your ability to combine, adapt, and rearrange information from your personal experiences[2]
- ◆ Your imagination

Researchers who have studied the phenomenon of creativity have found that creative ability can be learned and honed through the use of specific thinking strategies.[3] In this section, five of these strategies will be presented as Thinking Keys. The Idea Finding Thinking Keys are designed to help you produce a large quantity of ideas.

There is a direct correlation between the number of ideas that you generate and the quality of the ideas. "The person who is capable of producing a large number of ideas per unit of time, other things being equal, has a greater chance of having significant ideas."[4] In the words of Alex Osborn, the originator of brainstorming, "quantity breeds quality."[5] The goal in Idea Finding is to stretch your imagination as far as you can to generate many ideas, options, paths, and approaches aimed at finding a solution. The guidelines associated with Deferred Judgment help create an environment for generating large quantities of ideas.

Some of the ideas you generate will be ready for use, while others will need refinement. Think of them as diamonds in the rough. That means you should look for value in every idea, however wild it may seem. To demonstrate this point, let's look for the merit in the three seemingly foolish ideas.

DIRECTIONS

1. Read the ideas listed in column A of the Look for Merit in Every Idea worksheet.
2. Record the *merit* of each idea in column B. If you have difficulty seeing the merit in any of the ideas, look at them from another person's perspective. For example, in the first idea below, imagine that you are the client rather than the therapist and describe the benefit of paying for therapy only after your goals are reached. Strive to see each situation from a fresh perspective.

Look for Merit in Every Idea Worksheet

A Idea	B The merit in this idea is . . .
1. Clients pay for therapy services only as each occupational therapy goal is met.	
2. Occupational therapy students go out on Field Work II at the beginning of their academic preparations rather than wait until the completion of the program.	
3. Write therapy goals for the child after one month of occupational therapy treatment.	

If you are used to making decisions analytically, that is, if you are used to processing information sequentially, as it is being presented, you will need to practice looking for merit in all ideas. Consider even those ideas that appear foolish at first. In analytical thinking, information is excluded immediately if it seems irrelevant. When you are looking for merit, nothing is irrelevant.

When you practice looking for merit in all ideas, you will increase your options for finding solutions. One way to practice is to look at an idea from another person's point of view. A fresh perspective will give you insights about an idea. New insights help you to shift your paradigm, to have what is also referred to as a *mindshift*. Mindshifts play an active role on therapy expeditions and can often lead to an "aha!" response. So, the greater your ability to shift among a variety of perspectives, the better your ability to make effective decisions. Or, as Albert Einstein is famous for saying, "No problem can be solved from the same perspective that created it."

The Generating Phase of Idea Finding

In this section you will learn about four qualities of creative performance and their associated Thinking Keys. These Thinking Keys will help you develop these qualities.

Qualities Associated with Creative Performance

Fluency: the ability to produce large quantities of ideas

Flexibility: the ability to shift from one method to another or combine methods

Originality: the ability to generate novel approaches

Elaboration: the ability to develop ideas by adding details that enrich the original thought

Depending on your need, you may choose to emphasize one quality of creative performance more than another. For example, if you need to generate a large number of ideas, use a Thinking Key that promotes fluency. If you need to expand your perspective on a situation by seeing it from another person's point of view, use a Thinking Key that emphasizes flexibility.[6] Each of the Thinking Keys in the Generating Phase of Idea Finding stimulates one of the qualities associated with creative performance. The list below pairs each quality with one of the Thinking Keys you will learn how to use in the Generating Phase of Fact Finding. This list will help you decide which Thinking Key is appropriate for a given situation.

Quality	Associated Thinking Key
Fluency	"Brainstorming"
Flexibility	"CAMPERS"
Originality	"Force Fit"
Elaboration	"Attribute Listing"

The "Brainstorming" Thinking Key Develops Fluency

Brainstorming is a popular group technique that adheres to the guidelines of Deferred Judgment. In this field book we introduce brainstorming as a Thinking Key. The **"Brainstorming" Thinking Key** helps to develop the creative quality of fluency. Fluency refers to the process of generating many ideas. The more rapidly you generate ideas, the more easily they seem to be accessed.

When a group brainstorms, all ideas are accepted. The voice of judgment remains silent. Alex Osborn feels that if you judge and evaluate ideas as they are thought up, the person whose idea is questioned will be more concerned with defending his or her questioned idea than with thinking up new and better ones.[7] An important aspect of brainstorming is the feeling of freedom to express whatever ideas come to mind, even wild and crazy ones. According to Osborn, if wild ideas are not forthcoming in a brainstorming session, internal evaluation is probably going on in the minds of the individual participants. For a brainstorming session to be successful, all participants must respect all ideas and be free from judgment of those ideas.

In a brainstorming session, all ideas must be recorded. Recording all ideas shows the participants that every one of their ideas is valued. The leader of a brainstorming session, referred to as a facilitator, sees to it that all contributions are acknowledged and that judgment is deferred, that is, that the group adheres to the "No Criticism Rule." When you, the therapist, use brainstorming in a therapy-related situation, you will most likely be the facilitator.

The facilitator has several choices for recording the ideas of the group. The size of the group and the set up of the room will determine what method is best in a given situation. In a group of three to five people, you can use a chalkboard or a large sheet of paper to record the ideas as the group generates them. This approach is a basic brainstorming method.

A modification to the basic method involves using Post-it notes (or another brand of self-sticking, removable notes). With this method, each member of the group is instructed to write one idea per self-sticking note. Ideas are to be printed and written with thoughts headlined. Conciseness is the key here. The facilitator then attaches the notes to a large piece of paper, which is placed where all can see. A benefit of this method is that as ideas are evaluated, the notes can easily be moved into clusters.

You are now ready to move forward and learn how to use the "Brainstorming" Thinking Key by applying it to the Nose Blowing Expedition. Note that the "Brainstorming" Field Organizer is divided into three main columns (A, C, E) with a narrow column (B, D, F) to the right of each larger column for later recording Hits in Part I of "Highlighting." The dots in the Hits column are discussed in the Focusing Phase of this section. Remember, when using the "Brainstorming" Thinking Key, the motto is, *The more minds the better.* For this activity, work with a group of four to five colleagues, with one chosen to be Louise, the therapist-facilitator.

DIRECTIONS

1. Generate ideas for the following problem statement: "In what ways might [IWWM] a program be developed to teach the children how to blow their noses?"
2. With Louise doing the writing, freely record ideas in the spaces provided. Remember to hitchhike one idea on another and record all ideas, even wild and crazy ones. Use the six brainstorming ideas recorded in the first two rows as models.

FIELD ORGANIZER
"Brainstorming"

Problem Statement: IWWM a program be developed to teach the children how to blow their noses?

A Idea	B Hit	C Idea	D Hit	E Idea	F Hit
1. Play Simon Says using some action with the nose for half of the commands.	●	2. Make up relay races that involve holding the nose while running.		3. Make up a relay race that involves rubbing the nose with a tissue before the next team mate begins.	●
4. Each day one child is named "Officer Nosey" and officiates at all nose blowing events for the day.	●	5. Incorporate the sound "ah-choo" into the children's songs (e.g., "If you're happy and you know it say, "ah-choo ...")	●	6. Make up a game that involves imitating sniffing like a rabbit.	●
7.		8.		9.	
10.		11.		12.	
13.		14.		15.	

Use the strategy of brainstorming anytime in CPS to trigger a free flow of ideas.

The "CAMPERS" Checklist Develops Flexibility

Flexibility is another quality associated with generating creative ideas. People who are flexible are able to view a problem from many different perspectives. Being flexible means being willing not to yield to old habits and routines. To avoid yielding to old habits you may need to move out of your "box" or comfort zone. You need to feel comfortable giving yourself permission to reject your previous ways of thinking, or old habits. Just because you have always thought about something a certain way doesn't mean that that's the only way to think about it. The unpredictable nature of a therapy expedition necessitates that you are comfortable working "outside the box." Dare yourself to generate many novel options for solving the problem at hand.

Use the **"CAMPERS" Thinking Key** to put flexibility into your thinking.[8] Campers are courageous, so be like a camper and take risks, explore unknown territories. When you are on a therapy expedition, refer to the words that make up the acronym CAMPERS to stimulate flexibility in your thinking.

Each letter of CAMPERS represents a word that completes the invitational stem "What can I . . .?" For instance, the C in CAMPERS stands for *combine*. Asking, "What can I combine?" stimulates you to think about how to solve the problem at hand by considering what objects, people, purposes, methods, or steps could be combined. The A in CAMPERS stands for *adapt*. Asking "What can I adapt?" stimulates you to think about how you can generate ideas for a solution by working with existing resources. Refer to the guide below for trigger questions related to the other letters of CAMPERS.

"CAMPERS" Reference Guide

Combine	How about a blend, or an assortment? Can I combine units, purposes, ideas, steps, or different kinds of people, disciplines, groups?
Adapt	Can I use existing materials, processes, or personnel to solve the problem? What else is like this? What other idea does this suggest? What can I apply to the new situation from a past experience? What or whom can I emulate?
Modify	What can be changed? What can be magnified or minimized? What can be added? What can be taken away? How can a new twist be added to an obvious situation? How can the meaning, color, motion, sound, order, shape, or form be changed? How can I increase or decrease the frequency? How can I make what I choose stronger, lighter, longer, shorter, thicker, thinner, higher, or lower? How can I duplicate, multiply, exaggerate, condense, streamline, omit, understate, or divide it?
Put to other uses	What are new ways to use what I choose as it is? What other uses would it have if it were to be modified? What are some absolutely outlandish uses? Does its form, weight, or structure suggest another use? Change the context?
Eliminate	What might be left out? Could fewer steps, materials, or people be involved? How can I make less be more?
Rearrange	Reverse roles? Interchange parts or people? Turn backward? What parts of the schedule or process can be transposed?
Substitute	Who else or what else instead? What other ingredients, materials, processes, places, or approaches could be used?

In the next activity, the "CAMPERS" Worksheet, try your skill at using the "CAMPERS" checklist to analyze five activities described in the Nose Blowing Expedition. You may want to refer to Louise's story in Section 5 to recall the details of the story.

1. Read each activity in column A and match it to the element of "CAMPERS" you feel it best fits. Use row 1 to model your responses. (Note: The activities in column A can be matched to more than one element of "CAMPERS." The answers you select depend on your perspective and the context of your previous experiences from which you draw your answers. There are no wrong answers in this activity, only differing viewpoints.)
2. In column B record the letter of the element that best matches the statement and briefly explain your choice. Use the sample questions listed in the "CAMPERS" Reference Guide to perform this activity.

"CAMPERS" Worksheet

A Activities from the Nose Blowing Expedition	B **C**ombine **A**dapt **M**odify **P**ut to other uses **E**liminate **R**earrange **S**ubstitute
1. Mouth blowing activities were incorporated into the treatment program before nose blowing was taught.	A—The idea of incorporating mouth blowing activities into the treatment program could match the element Adapt in "CAMPERS" by asking the Reference Guide question, "What other activity is nose blowing like?"
2. The children were first taught the concept of blowing by participating in mouth blowing activities.	
3. The children made a game of using tape to cover their mouths when nose blowing.	
4. Feathers, ping pong balls, and cotton balls were used in blowing games.	
5. Games that employed mouth blowing were changed to games that employed nose blowing.	
6. Activities using blowing skills were scaled down to table-top size using the blowing skills introduced in the first part of the program.	
7. The children progressed from blowing lightweight materials to blowing materials more difficult to move.	

Now practice using the "CAMPERS" Thinking Key to expand beyond the ideas listed in the Nose Blowing Expedition. Turn to the "CAMPERS" Field Organizer and note that it is divided vertically into three columns and horizontally into seven sections, one for each element in the acronym CAMPERS. Column A lists sample questions related to the elements. (You will use column C in the Contraction Phase of Idea Finding to identify the Hits.)

Pair with a partner and assume the roles of Louise and the teacher (or, if working in a larger group, take on the roles of the other members of the resource group). In this activity, you will generate ideas for the following problem statement: "IWWM a program be developed to teach the children how to blow their noses?"

DIRECTIONS

1. Respond to the questions in column A.
2. Record your responses in column B under the sample response to the first question. As you answer each question, reflect on the data gathered about the problem in Data Finding.

FIELD ORGANIZER
"CAMPERS"

Problem Statement: IWWM a program be developed to teach the children how to blow their noses?

A Sample Questions to Develop Flexibility in Your Thinking	B Responses to Questions in Column A	C Hits
What can I Combine? How might the children be grouped to teach them to blow their noses? How might the teaching staff be blended to teach the children to blow their noses? How might the steps of teaching nose blowing be combined? How might the nose blowing lessons be combined with the rest of the classroom instruction throughout the day?	Children could be placed in teams of four or five to play games.	
What can I Adapt? What other activities are similar to nose blowing? Which of the children's current repertoire of motor skills are similar to nose blowing? How could a child serve as a role model within the classroom?		
What can I Modify? What could be added to the motor program to motivate the children to blow their noses? How can the length of time spent on teaching nose blowing to the children be decreased? What strategies should I modify for those children whose immature mouthing behaviors preclude their use of tissues to blow their noses?		

"CAMPERS" (Continued)

A	B	C
Sample Questions to Develop Flexibility in Your Thinking	**Responses to Questions in Column A**	**Hits**
What can I Put to other uses? *In addition to the classroom, in what other contexts might the children learn to blow their noses?* ***What can I Eliminate?*** *What steps might be eliminated?* *What materials might be left out?* ***What can I Rearrange?*** *In what ways might the teacher's schedule be reversed to permit me to work on nose blowing the first thing when the children arrive at school for the day?* *In what ways might the classroom aide help me to implement the nose blowing program?* ***What can I Substitute?*** *Who else besides me might help the children to blow their noses?* *What else might be done in addition to my working directly with the children?* *What materials might be used to help the children learn to blow their noses?* *What approaches might I use to teach the children to blow their noses?* *What other place besides school might be used to teach the children to blow their noses?* *What other way might I communicate to the children the importance of learning to blow their noses?*		

Use the "CAMPERS" Reference Guide as a question "map" whenever you need to stimulate flexibility into your idea-generating session. You can organize the questions in any sequence or combination.

REFLECTIVE JOURNAL ENTRY 9.2

Complete the following thoughts:

1. *I feel I could use "CAMPERS" when . . .*

2. *The similarities I see between the "CAMPERS" Thinking Key and the "Brainstorming" Thinking Key are . . .*

The "Force Fit" Thinking Key Develops Originality

Ill-structured problems beg for novel ideas. **"Force Fit"** is a **Thinking Key** with which to generate novel ideas.[9] With this Thinking Key, you deliberately introduce into your situation something seemingly unconnected. You force a connection between the problem and a random object, idea, word, or sensation. Under normal circumstances, the connection would not be obvious and probably wouldn't even be considered.

The Force Fit Thinking Key uses random input to stretch your thinking in new and unusual directions. Identifying a random item and placing it within the same context as the problem you are trying to solve provokes ideas related to the problem situation. Use "Force Fit" when your goal is to generate a fresh novel idea for an ill-structured, challenging problem.

When you think about a problem it's easy to keep going back and forth over the same territory. Sometimes the harder you think about a problem the more stuck you seem to become. This happens because your concentration reinforces what you already know. To get unstuck, reroute the way the brain thinks about the problem and introduce a new stimulus to get the mind working in a new direction. Any random input—an object, a word from a dictionary, a geographical location—can serve as the new stimulus. For the random input to trigger new thoughts that will move you forward, the random stimulus needs to be something totally unrelated to your problem.

Now let's see how "Force Fit" can generate ideas related to the Nose Blowing Expedition. If we randomly select *book* and force fit it into the problem statement "IWWM a program be developed to teach the children how to blow their noses?" we might generate the following ideas:

> The teacher could look in a book of cartooning for simple ways to draw various types of noses, then select one or two of the simplest noses and draw them on a face to show the children.

> The children could look in their collection of children's books to see if any of the characters are shown blowing their noses.

> The children could participate in drawing noses for a little booklet about the nose blowing program that could be duplicated and sent home.

If we force fit *box* into the same problem statement, we might generate these ideas:

> Each child could have a small box of tissues with his or her name on it.

> The children could bring a box of new tissues to school and decorate it with various media. The children could then take the box home so that they have their own personalized box of tissues.

You are now ready to practice using the "Force Fit" Thinking Key on the Nose Blowing Expedition. For this activity, you will generate ideas that relate to the problem statement: "IWWM a program be developed to teach the children how to blow their noses?"

This problem statement is recorded at the top of the "Force Fit" Field Organizer. Refer back to this statement as you make associations that are triggered by the random input you select. Pair up with a partner and assume the roles of the therapist Louise and the teacher (or, if working in a larger group, take on the roles of other members of the resource group).

DIRECTIONS

1. Select three random inputs and record them in column A, rows 3, 4, and 5. (Refer to the examples in rows 1 and 2 to model your answers.) To select a random input, you might:

   ◆ look around the room for an object;
   ◆ open a dictionary and put your finger on a word;
   ◆ look in a catalogue, telephone book yellow pages, or newspaper advertisements;
   ◆ think of something from nature (e.g., mountain, sunset, river, tree); or
   ◆ think of an animal (e.g., fish, cat, bird, horse, cow, duck).

2. Consider in what ways each random input you selected could relate to setting up a program to teach the children how to blow their noses. Withhold any concern for the relevance of the input to the problem. "Force" at least five "fits" between each random stimulus you selected and the process of setting up a program for nose blowing.

When you finish using this Thinking Key you will have at least 15 fits that you have forced. Now try to go beyond 15. (The dots in the Hits column are discussed in the Focusing Phase.)

FIELD ORGANIZER
"Force Fit"

Problem Statement: IWWM a program be developed to teach the children how to blow their noses?

A Random Input	B Force a fit between the random input and the problem at hand	C Hits
1. Book	1. The children could make their own "nose" books. They could cut out pictures from magazines as well as draw noses. They could draw or cut out arms to show the people blowing their noses.	●
	2. The teacher could have an "official" book on her desk listing the names of all the children participating in the nose blowing program.	
	3. Each child could have a little nose blowing record book (made up of a few sheets of paper) in which the teacher places a star every time the child successfully blows his or her nose. The stars could be placed on noses drawn in the books.	●
	4.	
	5.	
	6.	
2. Box	1. The children could bring a box of new tissues to school to decorate with various media. The children could then take the box home so that they would have their own personalized box of tissues there.	●
	2. An official nose blowing box could be identified in the classroom for disposal of all soiled tissues.	●
	3.	
	4.	
	5.	
	6.	

(continued)

A Random Input	B Force a fit between the random input and the problem at hand	C Hits
3.	1. 2. 3. 4. 5. 6.	
4.	1. 2. 3. 4. 5. 6.	
5.	1. 2.	

A Random Input	B Force a fit between the random input and the problem at hand	C Hits
	3.	
	4.	
	5.	
	6.	

REFLECTIVE JOURNAL ENTRY 9.3

Complete the following thoughts:

1. *My thoughts about using the Thinking Key "Force Fit" to develop originality in my thinking are . . .*

2. *When I compare "Force Fit" with "Brainstorming" and "CAMPERS" I find that . . .*

The "Attribute Listing" Thinking Key Develops the Ability to Elaborate

The **"Attribute Listing" Thinking Key** helps you elaborate on your thinking about a problem by analyzing the parts (the attributes) of the problem.[10] "Attribute Listing" works best when you are trying to improve a process, technique, or object that has several parts.

To use this Thinking Key, first ask yourself, "What are the attributes of this problem or issue?" Consider the following scenario:

> You are working with Shelby, an elementary school–age student who has severely restricted range of motion in all joints secondary to juvenile rheumatoid arthritis. She wishes to be independent in dressing by the time she is in junior high school. Currently she cannot put on any of her shirts without the help of another person.
>
> You decide that the solution to Shelby's problem is in the design of her shirts and that you will look at ways to buy or make tops that she can put on by herself. First you consider the parts of the garment, beginning with the design of the shirt's neck, sleeves, and closures and then the material and the cut—narrow or full-bodied.
>
> Once you have identified each of the attributes, you look for ways to improve one or more of the parts. You consider whether the sleeves should be long, short, raglan, or puffy and whether the material should be nylon, wool, polyester or cotton. You also consider whether the material should be wrinkle-free and tug-resistant to tearing.

When you use "Attribute Listing" you assess each attribute one at a time, elaborating on that one part until you feel you have exhausted your ideas. In "Attribute Listing" it's more important to identify the significant elements than to focus on a specific number of factors.

Once you have looked at each attribute in detail by itself you can combine ideas you have generated. In the dressing example above, the outcome of combining ideas might be that Shelby and her parent go shopping for or make tops that are rayon, have a loose neck and raglan sleeves, and are free of closures.

Now let's apply the "Attribute Listing" Thinking Key to the Nose Blowing Expedition. For this activity, you will elaborate on four main elements of the problem statement: "IWWM a **program** be developed to **teach** the children how to **blow** their **noses**?" Four main elements drawn from this problem statement are:

◆ nose
◆ blow
◆ teach
◆ program

This problem statement has been recorded at the top of the "Attribute Listing" Field Organizer. Refer back to this statement as you expand your thinking about the attributes of the problem at hand.

Now turn to the "Attribute Listing" Field Organizer and note that it is divided into three columns. Column A identifies the main elements of the problem statement you will elaborate on, and column B allows space for recording your ideas. (You will use column C in the Focusing Phase of Idea Finding when you identify the Hits. The dots in the Hits column are discussed in the Focusing Phase.)

Pair up with a partner and assume the roles of the therapist Louise and the teacher (or, if working in a larger group, take on the roles of other members of the resource group).

DIRECTIONS

1. Review the Problem Statement and assess each attribute in column A, one at a time.
2. Record the ideas you generate in column B. Model your answers on the examples that have been supplied.

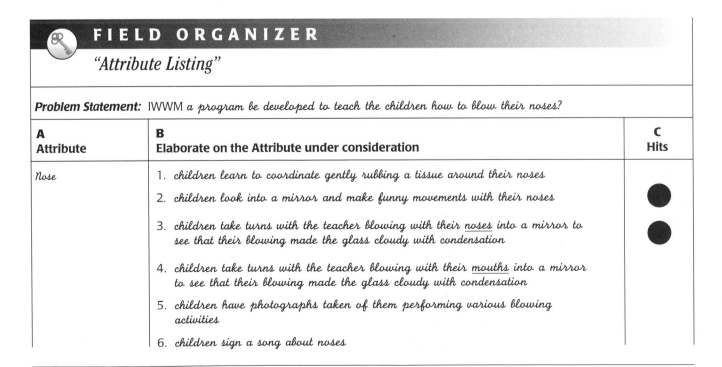

FIELD ORGANIZER
"Attribute Listing"

Problem Statement: IWWM a program be developed to teach the children how to blow their noses?

A Attribute	B Elaborate on the Attribute under consideration	C Hits
Nose	1. children learn to coordinate gently rubbing a tissue around their noses	
	2. children look into a mirror and make funny movements with their noses	●
	3. children take turns with the teacher blowing with their <u>noses</u> into a mirror to see that their blowing made the glass cloudy with condensation	●
	4. children take turns with the teacher blowing with their <u>mouths</u> into a mirror to see that their blowing made the glass cloudy with condensation	
	5. children have photographs taken of them performing various blowing activities	
	6. children sign a song about noses	

A Attribute	B Elaborate on the Attribute under consideration	C Hits
Nose	7. *Children imitate different animals sniffing (e.g., rabbit, puppy, kitten).* 8. 9. 10. 11. 12. 13. 14.	
Blow	1. *blowing out through the nose* 2. *blowing out through the mouth* 3. *breathing in through the nose* 4. *blowing out through the nose into a tissue* 5. *blowing out through the mouth into a tissue* 6. *blowing out through the nose with the mouth closed tight* 7. *blowing out through the mouth with the nose closed tight* 8. 9. 10. 11. 12. 13. 14.	● ●

(continued)

"Attribute Listing" (Continued)

A Attribute	B Elaborate on the Attribute under consideration	C Hits
Teach	1. *Louise teach the teacher* 2. *Louise teach the parents* 3. *Louise teach the teacher's aide* 4. *Louise teach the children* 5. *teacher teach the parents* 6. *teacher teach the teacher's aide* 7. *teacher teach the children* 8. 9. 10. 11. 12. 13. 14.	●
Program	1. *program integrates nose blowing into the daily routine* 2. *program includes the children instructing their stuffed animals in the classroom on how to blow their noses* 3. *program includes the children being videotaped as they teach their favorite stuffed animal how to blow her nose* 4. *home programs developed to have families reinforce proper nose blowing at home* 5. *certificate for children competing the nose blowing program* 6. *program includes a visit from a nurse who tells the children about germs* 7. *program includes a play in which the children take on the role of giant noses, germs, and tissues*	● ● ● ●

A Attribute	B Elaborate on the Attribute under consideration	C Hits
Program	8.	
	9.	
	10.	
	11.	
	12.	
	13.	
	14.	

Compare your Idea Finding list with the ideas in the "Attribute Listing" Field Organizer in Appendix A. Note the differences between your responses and the responses in Appendix A. Every item on your list that does not appear in the Appendix list is a reflection of your creative spirit. Celebrate your own originality and creativity for a moment before moving on.

REFLECTIVE JOURNAL ENTRY 9.4

Complete the following thoughts:

1. *When I was using the "Attribute Listing" Thinking Key to develop my skill at elaboration I felt . . .*

2. *When I compare "Attribute Listing" with "Force Fit," "Brainstorming," and "CAMPERS" I find that . . .*

Reach for the Sky or Stick to the Basics

What exactly are the outcome goals of your CPS efforts? Do you want to help the client solve his problem by reaching for the sky or by sticking to the basics? When you reach for the sky, you focus on generating "out-of-the-box," stimulating options that involve novel strategies. But when you stick to the basics, you design options that work within the paradigm or existing frame of reference.[11]

Three of the four Thinking Keys you have practiced in this section—"Brainstorming," "CAMPERS," and "Force Fit"—tend to stimulate expansive ideas. These Thinking Keys are all useful when you want to reach for the sky, to challenge existing paradigms and redefine the problem by looking at it from a totally new perspective. When you want to move in a new direction, use "Brainstorming," "CAMPERS," and "Force Fit."

But when you want to create a conservative solution, that is, a solution within the problem's existing structure or frame of reference, use "Attribute Listing." Conservative solutions bring gradual change that supports the current reality or context of the situation. Because there is less risk with conservative solutions, they may be the best route to take when you have limited time or a limited budget. To illustrate this point, imagine yourself as a therapist in the following situation.

> You see a high school student in his resource class. The student has a splint to use for computer keyboarding, but he is having trouble making it work because of an improper fit. You have two options. You can either make a new splint or modify the existing one. The first thing you do is consider the economics of the situation—your time to design and fabricate the splint and availability of splinting materials and necessary fabricating equipment. If there is no splinting equipment available in the school, you will need to order a low-temperature plastic especially for this student, incurring costs to the school. For all these reasons, you decide to try a conservative route first and modify the existing splint.

In some situations, reach-for-the-sky ideas work better than stick-to-the-basics ideas.[12] How do you decide which kind is more appropriate? Consult the following Criteria Guide.

Reach for the Sky/Stick to the Basics Criteria Guide

Criteria	Reach for the Sky	Stick to the Basics
Involvement of others		
◆ Those influenced by the decision are open-minded and willing to try anything.	×	
◆ Those influenced by the decision are deeply invested in the paradigm in which the problem occurs.		×
Resources		
◆ Resources are plentiful.	×	
◆ Limited time and/or limited budget		×
Nature of the problem		
◆ Chronic (recurring)	×	
◆ Acute (new)		×
Phase of therapy		
◆ Early: Client is beginning a therapy program.	×	
◆ Late: Client is close to discharge.		×
Therapist-client relationship		
◆ Trustful, mutually supportive	×	
◆ New, cautious, everything is questioned		×

The Focusing Phase of Idea Finding

Now that you have generated a quantity of ideas, you are ready to move on to the Focusing Phase of Idea Finding. You will now determine which ideas offer potential for finding a solution to the problem. In Idea Finding, use Part 1 of the Thinking Key "Highlighting" to identify the Hits. In Idea Finding, Hits are the ideas that show the most promise toward shining a light on the path to the solution.

Use your intuition to help you select Hits in Idea Finding. When you use your intuition rather than spending time analyzing each of your ideas, you avoid the risk of eliminating original ideas that are "diamonds in the rough." In the Focusing Phase of Idea Finding, concentrate on looking for options that hold promise rather than on looking for options to eliminate.

To perform Part 1 of "Highlighting," pair up with a partner and decide who will be Louise and who will be the teacher. In your role as Louise or the teacher imagine that your task in Idea Finding is to identify any ideas that will help you develop a program for teaching the children how to blow their noses. You will need the orange dots from your supply bag.

DIRECTIONS

1. Identify all the Hits listed in the Field Organizers for the following Thinking Keys: "Brainstorming," "CAMPERS," "Force Fit," and "Attribute Listing."
2. Place an orange dot in the Hits column located directly to the right of the options. To get you started, Hits have been identified in the "Brainstorming," "Force Fit," and "Attribute Listing" Field Organizers.
3. Transfer all the Hits you identified in step 1 to the "Highlighting" Part 1 (Idea Finding) Field Organizer. (Forty rows have been provided. The Hits we identified in step 1 have been transferred to the first 18 rows.)

 ## FIELD ORGANIZER

"Highlighting" Part 1 (Idea Finding)

Problem Statement: IWWM a program be developed to teach the children how to blow their noses?

"Hits" Transfer

1. Play Simon Says using some action with the nose for half of the commands.
2. Make up a relay race that involves rubbing the nose with a tissue before the next team mate begins.
3. Each day one child is named "Officer Nosey" and officiates at all nose blowing events for the day.
4. Incorporate the sound "ah-choo" into the children's songs (e.g., "If you're happy and you know it say, "ah-choo . . . ").
5. Make up a game that involves imitating sniffing like a rabbit.
6. The children make their own "nose" books. They could cut out pictures from magazines as well as draw noses. They could draw or cut out arms to show the people blowing their noses.
7. Each child could have a little nose blowing record book (made up of a few sheets of paper) in which the teacher places a star every time the child successfully blows his or her nose. The stars could be placed on noses drawn in the books.
8. The children could bring a box of new tissues to school to decorate with various media. The children could then take the box home so that they would have their own personalized box of tissues there.
9. An official nose blowing box could be identified in the classroom for disposal of all soiled tissues.
10. children look into a mirror and make funny movements with their noses

(continued)

"Hits" Transfer

11. children take turns with the teacher blowing with their noses into a mirror to see that their blowing made the glass cloudy with condensation

12. blowing out through the mouth into a tissue

13. blowing out through the nose with the mouth closed tight

14. Louise teach the parents

15. program integrates nose blowing into the daily routine

16. program includes the children instructing their stuffed animals in the classroom on how to blow their noses

17. certificate for children completing the nose blowing program

18. program includes a play in which the children take on the role of giant noses, germs, and tissues

19.

20.

21.

22.

23.

24.

25.

26.

27.

28.

29.

"Hits" Transfer

30.

31.

32.

33.

34.

35.

36.

37.

38.

39.

40.

Once you have a list of Hits from the Idea Finding stage, you are ready to evaluate those options that hold the most promise for moving you forward toward a solution. In Solution Finding, you will develop the criteria with which to evaluate Hits generated in Idea Finding.

Symbol for Idea Finding

The light bulb represents Idea Finding. The light bulb symbolizes the process of generating many ideas. Whenever you see the light bulb icon, you are being reminded to use Idea Finding.

Create a Mind Map of Section

9

Mind Map Guidelines

1. Place the section's main concept in the center of the space using pictures or words or both.
2. Radiate ideas from the central thought.
   - Use images (be sure to use color).
   - Headline text—one or two words per line.
   - Print text (for easy reading).
3. Link the main concepts and generate more ideas from the linkages.
4. Have fun!

Remember, the more linkages that you generate between elements, the greater your ability to see how all the elements relate to one another.

Green dot: I understand the concept and can explain it to a traveling companion.

Red dot: I need to retrace my steps and review the material.

Section 9
SELF-ASSESSMENT

Now that I have completed the ninth part of my journey, I can:

○ explain why it's important to generate lots of ideas during Idea Finding.

○ use "Brainstorming" to generate new ideas.

○ use the "CAMPERS" checklist to expand on ideas.

○ use "Force Fit" to generate novel ideas.

○ use "Attribute Listing" to analyze the parts of a specific problem.

○ explain how to use the Reach for the Sky/Stick to the Basics Criteria Guide.

○ use "Highlighting" to identify ideas in the Focusing Phase of Idea Finding.

NOTES

1. There are many publications that offer thinking tools to help structure your thinking. See R. Fobes, *The Creative Problem Solver's Toolbox* (Corvallis, Ore.: Solutions through Innovation, 1993); M. Michalko, *Thinkertoys* (Berkeley, Calif.: Ten Speed Press, 1991); and Roger von Oech, *A Whack on the Side of the Head* (New York: Warner Books, 1990), and *A Kick in the Seat of the Pants* (New York: Harper & Row, 1986). These four books present thinking strategies to apply to problem solving. Arthur VanGundy, *Techniques of Structured Problem Solving*, 2d ed. (New York: Van Nostrand, 1988), describes many thinking structures and provides a critique of the strengths and weaknesses of each one.

2. Some elementary and secondary school curriculums are now incorporating content on creative thinking. A structured handbook which if filled with graphic organizers or "thinking maps" for structuring one's thinking is written by Robert Swartz and Sandra Parks, *Infusing the Teaching of Critical and Creative Thinking into Elementary Instruction: A Lesson Design Handbook* (Pacific Grove, Calif.: Critical Thinking Press & Software, 1994).

3. Sidney Parnes, *Visionizing* (Buffalo, New York: Center for Creative Problem Solving, 1992), 10–11.

4. J. G. Guilford and Sidney Parnes, eds., *Source Book for Creative Problem Solving* (Buffalo, New York: Creative Education Foundation Press, 1992), 136.

5. Alex Osborn, *Applied Imagination*, 3d ed. rev. (New York: Charles Scribner's Sons, 1963), 124.

6. Scott Isaksen, K. B. Dorval, and Donald Treffinger, *Creative Approaches to Problem Solving* (Dubuque, Iowa: Kendall/Hunt, 1994).

7. Osborn, *Applied Imagination*. Alex Osborn, the originator of the term *brainstorming*, says that "pencils can serve as crowbars to move our minds. [Note-taking] empowers association, it stores rich fuel and otherwise would trickle out through our 'forgettery'; but above all, note-taking of itself induces a spirit of effort" (216). When you commit your thoughts to paper, you are practicing your ability to keep an open mind and defer judgment until all of your thoughts are revealed in writing about the situation under consideration.

8. Isaksen, Dorval, and Treffinger, *Creative Approaches to Problem Solving*.

9. In *Applied Imagination*, Osborn describes the technique of asking questions to spur ideas. Bob Eberle, in his book *SCAMPER* (New York: DOK, 1971), organizes the idea-sparking questions for easy recall under the acronym SCAMPER. To fit the travel theme in this field book, we adapted CAMPERS from Eberle's SCAMPER.

10. The "Attribute Listing" Thinking Key is based on the divergent thinking tool Attribute Listing described in Isaksen, Dorval, and Treffinger, *Creative Approaches to Problem Solving*, 250.

11. M. J. Kirton describes a system of viewing individuals as either "Adapters" or "Innovators." "Adapters are those individuals who prefer structure as they focus on key issues within the current reality. In contrast, Innovators focus on the future, the desired vision rather than the current reality. When making clinical decisions, sometimes having the mindset of an Adapter is most appropriate in generating ideas. Other times, thinking like an Innovator will support futuristic thinking and move onward from the current reality." M. J. Kirton, "Adapters, Innovators, and Paradigm

Consistency," *Psychological Reports* 57, no. 7 (1985): 487–90, and "Adapters and Innovators: Why New Initiatives Get Blocked," in J. Henry, ed., *Creative Management* (London: Sage, 1991), 209–21.

12. S. S. Gryskiewicz suggests several operational factors influence the category of ideas that would work best in ill-structured problem solving situations. See S. S. Gryskiewicz, "Predictable Creativity," in S. G. Isaksen, ed., *Frontiers in Creativity Research: Beyond the Basics* (Buffalo, N.Y.: Bearly, 1987), 305–13.

Go Forward with an Action Plan: Solution Finding

Itinerary #10

At the end of the tenth part of your journey, you will be able to:

✓ compare Solution Finding with Acceptance Finding

✓ explain how to use criteria to make a decision

✓ use the "Will It . . . ?" Thinking Key to create criteria

✓ show how "TRACS" will frame your thinking

✓ apply the "Making an Idea More Acceptable" Thinking Key

✓ unlock your intuition by using the "In-tuit" Thinking Key

✓ use the "AL-O" Thinking Key to join intuition with logic

✓ rate your ideas using the "Evaluation Matrix" Thinking Key

✓ use the "PCA" Thinking Key to prioritize ideas

✓ explain how rules of thumb and mindtraps relate to problem solving

✓ explain how rules of thumb can become mindtraps

✓ describe how a therapist might fall into a mindtrap

✓ use the "Mindtrap" Thinking Key to evaluate an action plan

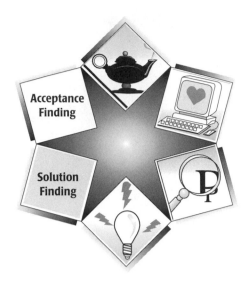

Solution Finding Transforms Ideas into an Action Plan

You have now arrived at the third component of CPS, Go Forward with an action plan. The third component consists of two stages: Solution Finding and Acceptance Finding (see Section 11). The action plan is created in Acceptance Finding; it is the actual travel route or itinerary of the therapy expedition. Before the action plan can be determined, however, possible solutions need to be considered.

In this section, you will learn how to (1) create a solution for a particular problem by recognizing conditions under which the ideas will have the greatest chance of succeeding; and (2) recognize and use criteria to isolate the "better" ideas that will lead to an action plan.

To insure acceptance of a tentative solution the therapy guide needs to perform a thorough and earnest evaluation of the options that emerged from Components I and II. Recall that in Component I, Get Ready to understand the problem, the therapy guide set a direction for the therapy expedition by establishing a vision or "destination point," gathering data, and identifying a specific route. In Component II, Get Set to find a solution, the therapy guide generated a large number of options from which to select a course of action. In Go Forward with an action plan, the therapy guide begins by considering various viewpoints, implications, potential consequences, and repercussions of pursuing a particular course of action.

In Solution Finding you will critically analyze and evaluate the relative worth of the options generated in Idea Finding. You will then select those options that seem to have the greatest potential for "solving" the problem. The evaluation process of Solution Finding begins with identifying the criteria by which to assess the *most promising* ideas. Identification of criteria is a mental yardstick to measure the options that hold the greatest promise for solving the problem. Establishing criteria will help you make objective decisions throughout the therapy expedition.

The Generating Phase of Solution Finding: Creating Criteria

Solution Finding, like the previous stages of CPS, has a Generating Phase and a Focusing Phase. In contrast to Idea Finding, however where the emphasis is on the Generating Phase, in Solution Finding, the emphasis is on the Focusing Phase.

Before we discuss ways to set criteria for a therapy expedition, think about the decisions you make every day. From the time you get up in the morning until you go to bed at night, you make one decision after another. All day long you are in a continuous cycle of deciding which actions to take and which to forgo. To make a decision means to make up one's mind, to come to a conclusion. Every one of the thousands of decisions you make each day is based on a set of criteria.

Reflect on a routine decision you made today—selecting what to wear. What criteria did you use to select each item that you now have on your body, including jewelry?

REFLECTIVE JOURNAL ENTRY 10.1

Complete the following thoughts:

1. This morning, my dressing choices consisted of . . .

2. The criteria I used to make the decisions I made about how to dress were . . .

3. The criteria that clinched my decision about how to dress were . . .

Most likely, your decision was influenced by one or more of the following criteria: the weather forecast, your plans for today, comfort, which clothes were clean and ready to wear, your mood, and the amount of time you had for dressing. Whatever criteria you selected, you probably mentally reviewed each one very quickly, made your decision, got dressed, and moved forward with your daily activities.

Most of the decisions you make throughout the day are made informally, spontaneously, and automatically. In these instances there is no need for a formal evaluation procedure to make a "better" decision. In fact, using a formal evaluation procedure for every daily decision would hinder the speed of your decision making. For certain decisions, however, you need to assess the criteria consciously and deliberately. Many of the decisions that therapy guides make during the therapy expedition require detailed attention to the criteria that lead to a decision.

A deliberate assessment of criteria begins with first identifying all the criteria you wish to consider. There are numerous strategies available for developing criteria. The three strategies that you will learn are presented in the following Thinking Keys:

"Will It . . . ?"

"TRACS"

"Making an Idea More Acceptable"

"Will It . . . ?"

The first Thinking Key for developing criteria involves the use of the invitational stem "Will it . . . ?" The "it" represents the idea or option under consideration. Completing the statement "Will it . . . ?" allows you to define concepts that identify specific domains of concern that can be turned into criteria. The context in which the proposed action will occur helps the therapy guide determine which domains to consider.

Let's explore the following Hit identified in the Nose Blowing Expedition: "The children could bring a box of new tissues to school to decorate with various media." To explore the value of pursuing "it," that is, the idea of having the children decorate their own tissue boxes, expand your thoughts about the option with the **"Will It . . . ?" Thinking Key** by pondering the four questions below.

1. Will it be *simple* to execute?
2. Will it be an *age appropriate* activity?

3. Will it hold the *children's interest*?
4. Will it be *fun*?

In each of the four questions above, a specific domain of concern is identified: ease of execution, age appropriateness, interest value, or entertainment value. Each of these domains can be turned into a criterion that explores the value of an idea.

Practice generating criteria with the "Will It . . . ?" Thinking Key Field Organizer. For this activity, imagine that you are deciding what kind of motor vehicle to purchase. Pair up with a partner or, if possible, work in a group of three or four (the more minds the better).

DIRECTIONS

1. To complete the question "Will it . . . ?" focus on possible considerations for purchasing a motor vehicle.
2. Now stretch your mind and, in column A, record as many questions as you can generate that have the potential of leading you to a decision about what kind of motor vehicle to buy. Use the examples in rows 1–3 to model your responses.
3. Determine the domain of concern that is embedded in each question in column A. Turn each domain of concern into a specific criterion against which you will evaluate the idea and record the criteria in column B. (Note, for example, when you ask in row 1, "Will it be small or large?" the *size of the vehicle* is the domain of concern and becomes a criterion influencing your decision to make the purchase.)

FIELD ORGANIZER
"Will It . . . ?"

Subject: Deciding to purchase a motor vehicle

A "Will it . . . ?"	B Criterion
1. be small or large?	size
2. be a car, truck, minivan, or jeep?	body style
3. be old or new?	age
4.	
5.	
6.	
7.	
8.	
9.	
10.	

The criteria you ultimately decide on should be tailored to match the context of the situation in which the decision will be made. Recall that, according to Uniform Terminology (Section 4), the Performance Contexts include the temporal aspects of the situation (client's age, stage of development, place in life phase, and disability status) and the environment (physical, social, and cultural).

"TRACS"

The **"TRACS" Thinking Key** keeps you on track during the therapy expedition. It's a useful tool for sorting your proposed actions into the five most common broad categories of criteria within the decision making process.[1] TRACS (pronounced "tracks") is an acronym for the following categories: **T**ime, **R**esources, **A**cceptance, **C**osts, and **S**pace. Study the list below and note that each criterion in the acronym is framed by questions that expand your thinking.

"TRACS" Reference Guide

Time	What are the temporal demands of the option? How long will it take to implement the option? How soon must it be implemented? What are the potential consequences of its being implemented earlier or later than planned?
Resources	What supplies, equipment, skills, or individuals are necessary to execute the option? What funding is available?
Acceptance	What level of acceptance or resistance might the option face from those who would be affected? Is the option feasible? Does it waste or conserve the energy of the people involved or materials used?
Costs	What expenses—in money and human effort—are associated with the option? Does the idea address the most efficient way to achieve the needed results? In what ways does the option increase or reduce the overall costs of the therapy expedition?
Space	What type and amount of space is needed to support the option? Is the space available?

The criteria that make up the acronym TRACS help a therapy guide select the "better" idea within a given situation. Do the next activity, the "TRACS" Field Organizer, using the "TRACS" Thinking Key to expand your thinking about the Nose Blowing Expedition's problem statement: "In what ways might a therapy program be developed to teach the children to blow their noses?" Expand your thinking by examining the five options listed below in terms of the criterion "time." These are examples of the kinds of options you might have generated in the Focusing Phase of Idea Finding in Section 9.

Work in pairs or small groups of three or four. As you go through the exercise, you will begin to see how a specific criterion influences the selection of certain options.

Hits from Idea Finding

1. The children are videotaped blowing their noses.
2. Louise and the teacher hold a nose blowing inservice in the evening for parents.
3. Louise works with each child individually when the child comes down with a cold.
4. Louise writes a step-by-step handbook on the art of nose blowing for the parents.
5. Louise and the teacher generate group activities that incorporate the movement components of nose blowing.

DIRECTIONS

1. Read each option in column A, rows 1–5, followed by the criterion phrase in column B to complete five questions.
2. In column C, record three responses to each question. Use the examples in row 1 to model your answers.

A Option	B Criterion	C Consideration
1. If the children were videotaped blowing their noses	what *time* would be involved?	1. Staff time to record the children 2. Time involved in obtaining photo releases 3. Time to edit tape for children's viewing
2. If Louise and the teacher hold a nose blowing inservice in the evening for parents	what *time* would be involved?	1. 2. 3.
3. If Louise works with each child individually when the child comes down with a cold	what *time* would be involved?	1. 2. 3.
4. If Louise wrote a step-by-step handbook on the art of nose blowing for the parents	what *time* would be involved?	1. 2. 3.
5. If Louise and the teacher generate group activities that incorporate the movement components of nose blowing	what *time* would be involved?	1. 2. 3.

Therapy guides keep on track with the "TRACS" Worksheet because it helps them examine the implications of their options before deciding which ones to include in their therapy expeditions. In the example above, a therapy guide might determine that organizing a videotaping session, which would include obtaining photo releases for each child, would too time-consuming to be cost-effective. After considering all of the options, the therapy guide would probably conclude that there is a more efficient way to achieve the same goal using less time and energy than would be involved with obtaining the photo releases for the video production.

Another therapy guide, with a paradigm that places a high value on the use of videotapes for educational purposes, might, in contrast, see a positive cost-benefit ratio in videotaping the children blowing their noses. To that therapy guide, becoming involved in activities that incorporate a video production would be a justified option.

Your paradigms play a significant role in influencing your decisions about the options that you select. Keep an open mind when deciding which options to use and which to filter out when you are involved in CPS. Use the "TRACS" Thinking Key to focus your thoughts.

"Making an Idea More Acceptable"

The **"Making an Idea More Acceptable" Thinking Key** improves an idea. This Thinking Key helps you to take the ideas that will eventually lead to the action plan and adapt them to the client's paradigm and value system. Therapy guides who prepare an idea for acceptance are sensitive to the need to make the solution acceptable to the people who share ownership of the problem.

Consider the following idea from the Nose Blowing Expedition: "Louise makes a home visit to each child who is absent from school with a cold." The cost-and-time–benefit ratio of this idea may make it seem impractical. Rather than abandoning the home visit option entirely, however, consider what part of the idea has value. Consider how the idea of making a home visit might be made more acceptable to those responsible for executing the therapy plan.

Inherent in the idea of Louise's making a home visit when a child is absent from school with a cold is the *essential criterion* that Louise individually contact each child's family. Once this criterion has been identified, it is possible to generate other options that might accomplish the same goal using different actions. To do this, unessential aspects of the idea are eliminated and the essential parts are retained and reworked into a new idea. In the example, an essential part is that Louise contact the families individually. Her effort to make home visits, then, might be changed to arranging a one-on-one conference with parents at the beginning of the school year, before or after school.

Louise might also communicate with the family about each child's progress on the Nose Blowing Expedition through a nose blowing booklet that travels back and forth between home and school. These examples are recorded in row 1 of the "Making an Idea More Acceptable" Thinking Key Field Organizer that follows. Practice reworking an idea with the intent of improving it by using the essential criteria of the idea. For this exercise, pair up with a partner.

DIRECTIONS

1. Read the idea in column A, row 2.
2. Next, read in column B the essential criterion embedded in the idea.
3. Record in column C at least two ideas that improve the original idea while retaining the essential criterion identified in the idea.

FIELD ORGANIZER

"Making an Idea More Acceptable"

A Idea to Be Improved	B Essential Criterion	C Possible Improvements
1. *Louise makes home visits when each child is absent from school with a cold.*	*Contact with family on an individual basis.*	a. *Invite each parent to schedule a meeting before or after school.* b. *Provide each child with a nose blowing booklet in which progress is reported. Send the booklet home throughout the Nose Blowing Expedition for the parents to read and record progress. Booklet would be returned when the child returns to school.*
2. *Louise will work with each child individually.*	*Each child has special attention.*	a. b.

When you prepare an idea for acceptance with the "Making an Idea More Acceptable" Thinking Key you increase the number of options to contemplate. Each of the three Thinking Keys therapy guides use in the Generating Phase of Solution Finding helps develop criteria by which to assess the most promising ideas. The primary strategy of each of the Thinking Keys is listed below.

Thinking Keys That Generate Criteria

"Will It . . . ?"	Generates questions that produce criteria
"TRACS"	Generates ideas framed by the five broad categories of criteria commonly used in decision making
"Making an Idea More Acceptable"	Generates criteria by identifying the essential element in an idea in need of improvement; the essential element then becomes the basis for improving the idea

The Focusing Phase of Solution Finding

In the Focusing Phase, you will use the criteria developed in the Generating Phase to identify solutions to the problem. These criteria systematically evaluate the Hits. The Hits are used to develop the plan of action—the "itinerary"—for the therapy expedition.

In this phase of Solution Finding you will use the following four Thinking Keys to evaluate ideas:

"In-tuit"

"AL-O"

"Evaluation Matrix"

"Paired Comparison Analysis"

The number of ideas coupled with the purpose of your evaluation will determine which Thinking Key to use.

"In-tuit"

The term *intuit* means to apprehend by intuition. When you use this Thinking Key you rely on your intuition to produce the criteria by which to evaluate the merit of an idea. When you rely on your intuition to assess information, the data categorized with logical rules and boundaries that previously seemed to envelop the information suddenly seems to dissipate. Intuition can act like an internal compass; it points us in the right direction, toward meaningful information, if we would only listen to it.[2]

In the three Thinking Keys you learned in the Generating Phase ("Will it . . . ?" "TRACS," and "Making an Idea More Acceptable") the development of criteria is based on external factors and involved asking questions such as, "How much will the idea cost?" or "What time is involved?" When you use the **"In-tuit" Thinking Key**, the criteria are based on internal, physiological factors that manifest psychologically. You might ask yourself, "What do I *sense* about this idea?" "Does this idea *feel* right?"

When you ask yourself, "What do I *sense* about this idea?" you are going deep "into" your inner way of knowing. You are tapping into that part of your inner self that defies rational knowledge. Thus the name "In-tuit" (pronounced "in to it").

When a therapy guide uses "In-tuit" to help make a decision he is sensitive to an internal voice that says, " 'Stop! Pay attention and take heed to what I am telling you!' Recognizing how you feel about something as it is happening is a keystone of emotional intelligence."[3] When you listen to your internal state you are attending to your emotional mind, as opposed to your rational mind. Ralph Waldo Emerson spoke of our inner way of knowing when he said, "What lies behind us and what lies before us are tiny matters, compared to what lies within us."[4]

Sensing what you feel can carry a deep kind of certainty about it. Feelings can be indispensable when we make rational decisions. The emotional mind "sends signals that streamline the decision by eliminating some options and highlighting others at the outset. The intellectual mind works best when it works hand in hand with the emotional mind."[5] Therapy guides need to develop an ability to harmonize the emotional with the rational mind.

Practice using the "In-tuit" Thinking Key by completing the "In-tuit" Field Organizer.

DIRECTIONS

1. Read each idea listed in column A and evaluate it by asking, "Do I *sense* that this idea will help solve the problem?"
2. Evaluate each idea with the criteria below according to your perception of the idea's potential for solving the problem.
   a. If you *feel positive that the idea has potential* for solving the problem, check "Yes" in column B.
   b. If you *sense that the idea will not help* to solve the problem, check "No" in column C.
   c. If you *feel that the idea has merit but needs to be reworked* using the Thinking Key "Making an Idea More Acceptable," check "Rework" in column D.

"In-tuit"

A Do I *sense* that this idea will help solve the problem?	B Yes	C No	D Rework
1. *Have children sit in a circle and practice blowing their noses on command.*			
2. *Teach each child how to blow his or her nose when he or she has a cold.*			
3. *Assign the teacher's aide the task of taking the children out in the hallway one at a time to practice nose blowing.*			
4. *Play Bingo using a nose blowing theme (e.g., in place of B-I-N-G-O, play for winning patterns of N-O-S-E or T-I-S-S-U-E).*			
5. *Play "Name the Softest Tissue" Game in which the children wear blindfolds to determine which tissue feels the softest on their noses.*			

Therapy guides continuously work on enhancing their sensitivity to how they feel about a decision. With the hundreds of decisions they must make every day, they realize the need to tap into their *internal* bank of knowledge. Their intuition allows them to arrive at a decision using their spontaneous understanding of a situation. Through practice, they build their confidence in using intuition and self-reflection to make decisions.

"AL-O"

"AL-O" teams your logic with your intuition. "AL-O" is an acronym for the words Advantages, Limitations, and Overcome (i.e., overcome the limitations). Using the **"AL-O" Thinking Key**, you view the advantages and limitations of an idea and determine how to overcome the limitations.

The decision making process can be enhanced when you develop a partnership between your logic and your intuition. Logical reasoning relies on readily available data that are part of your conscious awareness. Intuition is a product of your mind's capacity to act. It is not restricted by what is known. Much of what our intuition does cannot be done by logical reasoning. Intuition allows our thoughts to "leap chasms of missing information, make sideways detours, and bring together unusual, even illogical combinations [of information]."[6]

The literature on decision making documents that people naturally search out data that support an idea they favor. Conversely, they generally do not look for the advantages of an idea they dislike.[7] The natural human tendency to support decisions without thoroughly considering both sides makes "AL-O" an important Thinking Key.

Effective therapy guides acknowledge the element of uncertainty inherent in any decision making process. They also recognize that by examining both sides of an issue, they can minimize the number of surprise outcomes to their decisions. By looking at the limitations as well as the advantages of a decision, a therapy guide can prepare strategies to overcome the limitations.

To use the "AL-O" Thinking Key, begin with an idea that you sense will help solve a problem. Once you have an idea you would like to support, switch on your logical mind to examine the advantages and limitations, and consider strategies to overcome the limitations. Turn to the "AL-O" Thinking Key Field Organizer to see how this strategy is put into practice. Assume that you are examining the following idea from the "Nose Blowing" Expedition: "Develop group games that incorporate the components of nose blowing." (This idea appears at the top of the "AL-O" Field Organizer.)

Each column in the Field Organizer covers one aspect of "AL-O."

1. Use column A to record **advantages** of the idea under consideration. For example, one advantage of using group games to teach nose blowing is that group games are fun.
2. Use column B to record **limitations** of the idea under consideration. To identify limitations flip each advantage around and look at the other side. For example, the flip side of the advantage "group games are fun" is "group games can create excitement, causing children to become overstimulated, and unable to regulate their own behavior."

   When you flip advantages around to look at the other side, you practice "out-of-the-box" thinking, that is, you develop the necessary mindset to consider both sides of a situation. Call upon your "out-of-the-box" thinking when you want to challenge traditional concepts. Practice stretching your comfort zone by asking "What if . . ." questions.
3. Use column C to record ideas about how **to overcome** the limitation described in column B. Once a limitation is identified, you are ready to identify strategies to overcome that limitation. For example, to overcome the limitation that children become overstimulated while playing group games you might: keep the children calm by using variations in the quality of your voice, or stop the activity intermittently and help the children focus on the outcome.

After you identify several strategies for overcoming a potential limitation, you can go on to consider whether to include the option in your action plan.

Practice using the "AL-O" Thinking Key by completing the Field Organizer. For this exercise, imagine that you are part of the Nose Blowing Expedition. Pair up with a partner or work in a group of three or four. If you are working in pairs, assume the roles of the therapist Louise and the teacher; if you are working in small groups, assume the roles of Louise, the teacher, and other members of the resource team.

DIRECTIONS

1. Read the advantage in column A, row 2. Then read the limitation associated with this advantage in column B, row 2.
2. In column C, record three strategies for overcoming the limitation listed in column B, row 2. Use the examples provided to model your responses.
3. Repeat steps 1 and 2 using the advantage and limitation pair listed in row 3.

 FIELD ORGANIZER

"AL-O"

Idea: *Develop group games that incorporate the components of nose blowing.*

A Advantages	B Limitations	C How to Overcome Limitations
1. *Group games are fun.*	**Limitation:** *Group games can create excitement, causing children to become overstimulated and unable to self-regulate their own behavior.* *The issue becomes:* **How to** *keep the children from becoming overstimulated during a group game.*	a. *Keep the children calm by using variations in voice quality.* b. *Stop the activity intermittently and help the children focus on the outcome.* c. *Give a bear hug to any child who seems to be getting overly excited; require a deep breath before the child returns to the game.* d. *Provide structure to the game by making certain that the children know the rules.*

(continued)

A Advantages	B Limitations	C How to Overcome Limitations
2. *Group games can keep the motivation level high.*	**Limitation:** *Some children give up trying when they feel they are not doing as well as the other children.* *The issue becomes:* **How to** *avoid creating situations where the children become frustrated.*	a. *Reward all children for their efforts in the games.* b. c. d.
3. *Group games can create an exciting, lively environment that makes learning enjoyable.*	**Limitation:** *Some children prefer activities that they can perform on their own or in a one-to-one situation where there are fewer stimuli.* *The issue becomes:* **How to** *address the learning styles and preferences of all the children so they enjoy learning.*	a. *Respect individual differences and preferences for performing activities.* b. c. d.

A therapy guide avoids being blinded by a lack of foresight by regularly considering both sides of an issue. Using the "AL-O" Thinking Key will limit the probability that roadblocks will pop up on a therapy expedition. Use the "AL-O" Thinking Key when you have just one or two ideas that you wish to support; when you have many promising ideas to review, however, a grid or a matrix is more practical.

The "Evaluation Matrix"

The **"Evaluation Matrix" Thinking Key** helps to objectively compare Idea Finding options and rate them according to criteria you identified in the Generating Phase of Solution Finding.

To set up an "Evaluation Matrix," follow the steps below. (Refer to the "Evaluation Matrix" Field Organizer on p. 271.) Once you understand the general procedure, you will practice using the "Evaluation Matrix" by completing the Field Organizer.

Step 1: Select Options. Begin by transferring to the Evaluation Matrix the Hits you identified in the Focusing Phase of Idea Finding. Transfer only those Hits that you think offer the best opportunity for solving the problem. The number of options selected is not as critical as choice of the options.

As you transfer each idea to the vertical lines of the "Evaluation Matrix," rephrase each option using as few words as possible, as if you were writing a headline. For example, "Videotape children" is the headline version of "Videotape children blowing their noses and then have them view themselves."

Step 2: Select Criteria. Review the list of criteria that you generated using one or more of the Thinking Keys in the Generating Phase of Solution Finding (i.e., "Will it . . . ?" "TRACS," and "Making an Idea More Acceptable"). The criteria that you select will depend on the problem. Consider only those criteria that will best help define the "better" options that will eventually be part of the action plan. Remember, the action plan must be acceptable to all those who share ownership of the problem. Write the criteria under the column heading "Criteria" on the "Evaluation Matrix." (In the Field Organizer you are consulting as a sample the criteria Time, Resources, Acceptance, Costs, and Space are being considered.)

Step 3: Choose a Rating Scale. Choose a rating scale you feel will best grade the options you wish to consider. The rating scale can be made up of two or more numbers or symbols that represent levels of choice. For example, you might use a simple two-point scale to weigh the options, with 1 to represent a favorable feeling and 0 to represent an unfavorable feeling toward an option. Or you might use a scale with five or more numbers on it. Determine the complexity of the scale by looking at the number of options you have and deciding how discriminating you wish to be in the evaluation process and how much time you have. Be aware that the more numbers there are in a scale, the more time it takes to evaluate each item.

Another important consideration in the design of a scale is how easily it is understood by all who use it. For example, if you choose a five-point rating scale in which 3 is described as "good" and 4 is "very good," recognize the subjectivity of the word *good*, its meaning varies with each person who uses it.

REFLECTIVE JOURNAL ENTRY 10.2

Complete the following thoughts:

1. *When I hear the word* good *to describe an idea, I assume the following about the idea: . . .*

2. *When I hear the words* very good *to describe an idea, I assume the following about the idea: . . .*

"Good" is a difficult measure unless you define what "good" means. In general, avoid using one word descriptors to rate options unless you are able to define the word unambiguously. To minimize misinterpretation of the rating scale, establish clear descriptors for each number on the scale at the outset of the evaluation process. Symbols can be used in place of numbers to represent a value on an idea. Symbols conjure up emotions in ways that words do not.

Symbols have the power to tap into feelings and give an emotional perspective that is difficult to duplicate using numbers or words. In the two activities you will complete for the "Evaluation Matrix," you will find two symbols, which correspond with the following two-point scale:

◆ 1 (one) represents a favorable feeling

Favorable

◆ 0 (zero) represents an unfavorable feeling

Unfavorable

Step 4: Evaluate Each Option Against Each Criterion. To evaluate each option against each criterion, take the step you learned for the "TRACS" Thinking Key and complete the following sentence:

"If [the option], what [the criterion] would be involved?" For example, if you were to rate the option, "videotape children" against the criterion "cost," the question would be: "If *the children were videotaped* (option), what *cost* (criterion) would be involved?

If you think that showing a videotape to the children might involve high costs to the program, you would give the videotape option a low rating or unfavorable symbol.

Using videotapes might be an acceptable option if the following conditions are met:

◆ All video equipment is readily available
◆ You or someone involved in the therapy expedition is proficient with a video camera
◆ You know that all of the children in the class have signed photo releases on file
◆ You intend to videotape the children together in small groups to save time
◆ You feel that the children will benefit from watching the videotape

If all of these conditions were met, the videotape experience might receive a favorable rating.

Remember that costs can refer to money or to human effort. An option that will not cost much money relative to a budget might instead have high cost in terms of the expended effort and energy. Be specific when generating the criteria. To be a reliable tool, a criterion, like a ruler, must have clearly defined indicators.

As you continue with Step 4, individually rate each option against each criterion, beginning with row 1 and moving vertically from the top to the bottom of the list of options before moving over to the second criterion, then the third, and so on. When you consider each option against one criterion at a time, you will increase the objectivity with which you rate the options. The matrix also helps prevent you from becoming biased toward your favorite options.[8]

Look again at the "Evaluation Matrix" Field Organizer to see how the evaluation process works. The options listed in rows 1–5 are rated against the first criterion in the "Evaluation Matrix." The matrix uses a simple two-point rating scale with the smiley face symbol to show that the staff will support this idea and stand behind it, and the sad face symbol to show that the staff feels the idea is not a match for them at present but might be acceptable at a different time or under different circumstances. The criteria are drawn from the five broad categories represented by the "TRACS" Thinking Key.

To help you understand the ratings given to the five options in the "Evaluation Matrix" Field Organizer for the criterion "time," we have provided the following list of rationales for the ratings. The rationales are based on paradigms held by therapists and teachers we know out in the field.

"Evaluation Matrix" Ratings Rationale

A Option	B Rating	C Rationale for the Rating
1. Videotape children.		Resource persons are willing and able to videotape the children. Two people on the therapy expedition value video-taping as a regular instructional strategy in the classroom and frequently show funny video clips during class.

2. Hold an evening inservice for parents.

☹

The teacher, the teacher's aide, and the therapist all have young infants at home and find it difficult to attend evening meetings outside of their homes. Their preference is to meet with a group of three or four parents in the morning or to schedule a parent program during school time.

3. Write a handbook on nose blowing.

☺

The therapist feels capable of designing a simple four-page booklet with the help of a computer. She enjoys designing projects and since she's an "artist at heart," she feels competent to add simple sketches of children to the narrative.

4. Develop group games.

☺

The teacher, the teacher's aide, and the therapist enjoy games and routinely create simple games during the day. They have a large repertoire of games from which they quickly and easily adapt new games to suit a variety of educational themes.

5. Teach disposal management.

☺

The team feels that this is an important option to include on the therapy expedition. They agreed that if the adults and children (serving as monitors for each other) worked on the proper disposal of tissues, the goal could be reached within two weeks.

Step 5: Interpret the Scores. After the options are evaluated against each criterion, total the scores by adding the ratings for each option. Place the total in the far-right column. When the rating scale uses symbols, you can add the number of the symbols or convert the symbols into a numerical value (e.g., a smiley face is worth 1; a sad face is worth 0).

Whether you use numbers or symbols, a quick way to interpret the results on the matrix is to identify the strongest and the weakest options. The options that receive a high rating have greater potential for solving the problem than the options that receive a lower rating.

Practice using the "Evaluation Matrix" by completing the "Evaluation Matrix" Field Organizer. Pair up with a partner, assuming the roles of Louise and the teacher. Imagine that you are the resource team and need to evaluate options 1–5 using the following rating scale: a smiley face indicates that you will support pursuing the option; a sad face indicates that you cannot support the option at this time.

DIRECTIONS

1. Evaluate the options listed on the left side of the matrix for the criteria Time, Resources, Acceptance, Costs, and Space. Complete the evaluation for one criterion before moving on to the next.
2. Choose a value for each symbol and record the scores in the last column.

"Evaluation Matrix"

Options	Criteria					Rating
	T	**R**	**A**	**C**	**S**	Scale: ☺ **Favorable** ☹ **Unfavorable**
1. *Videotape children.*	☺					☺ =_____ ☹ =_____
2. *Hold evening inservice for parents.*	☹					☺ =_____ ☹ =_____
3. *Write handbook on nose blowing.*	☺					☺ =_____ ☹ =_____
4. *Develop group games.*	☺					☺ =_____ ☹ =_____
5. *Teach tissue disposal management.*	☺					☺ =_____ ☹ =_____
6.						☺ =_____ ☹ =_____
7.						☺ =_____ ☹ =_____
8.						☺ =_____ ☹ =_____
9.						☺ =_____ ☹ =_____
10.						☺ =_____ ☹ =_____

When using the "Evaluation Matrix," remember to ask yourself:

◆ Are the criteria clearly defined for all involved in the evaluation process?
◆ Is the rating scale clear and understandable to everyone who will be using it to make decisions?

The "Evaluation Matrix" is a decision making tool to use when you need to compare selected criteria against a limited set of possible options. But sometimes you are faced with a set of options that you perceive to have equal or near equal value.

"PCA": Paired Comparison Analysis

The **"PCA" Thinking Key** can be used to rate options that are close in value. In contrast to the "Evaluation Matrix," the "PCA" does not rely on a criteria-based rating system. Instead, it uses a ranking system to prioritize the options.

To use the "PCA" Thinking Key, follow the steps below. (Refer to the "PCA" Field Organizer on p. 273.) Once you understand the general procedure, you will practice using the "PCA" Thinking Key by completing the Field Organizer.

Step 1: Select Options. At the top of the Field Organizer, in Section I, list each Hit (option) you wish to prioritize. Begin each option with an action verb. For example, "Show the children videotapes of themselves playing fun nose blowing games during school hours." Note that this sentence can be broken down and worded in headline style:

- Action: show videotapes
- Object of the action: to children
- Headlined option: show videotapes to children

Be sure the options you select are mutually exclusive. That is, avoid having an overlap between options, and one option should not be a further elaboration of another one.

The option "Show the children videotapes during school hours" is closely related to the option "Give a copy of the videotape to the parents to show at home." Because both options include the act of showing videotapes to the children for the purpose of teaching them how to blow their noses, they are not mutually exclusive. The only difference between the options is where the videotapes will be shown. There may be a qualitative difference, however, because in the second option the parent would be seeing the video. If it is important to you that the parents view the videotape at home with the children, then the option might be worded like this: "Send the videotape home so that the parents and the children will view the videotape together." Or:

- Action: send videotape
- Object of action: home
- Headlined option: send videotape home

Step 2: Compare Options. After the options are listed in Section I of the "PCA" Field Organizer, begin the rating process by comparing option A to option B. In the Field Organizer that follows, that means comparing "Show videotapes to the children" with "Write a handbook for parents on the art of nose blowing."

Step 3: Record Choices. In Section II, locate the box that lists A and B as the two options being compared. In the box directly to the right, record which of the two options you prefer. In the example, we selected A over B. Continue comparing one option with the next by following the pairs of letters in each box until you have compared every option with every other option.

Step 4: Record Totals. After you finish rating the options, tally the letters. To tally the letters, count the number of times A was chosen. Record the number in Section III at the bottom of the Field Organizer. Next, count the number of times B was chosen and record that number in Section III. Continue on until you have a total score for each option.

Step 5: Rank Totals. Write the letter for the option with the highest total next to the number 1 in the Priority Order of Options box. Continue recording the letters in rank order. Rank ordering the options will help you to objectively determine which options you wish to pursue and in what order.

Practice using the "PCA" Thinking Key by completing the "PCA" Field Organizer. Pair up with a partner and assume the roles of Louise and the teacher. Perform steps 3, 4, and 5, above.

FIELD ORGANIZER
"PCA" (Paired Comparison Analysis)

Problem Statement: IWWM a program be developed that teaches the children how to blow their noses?

Section I: Options

A. Show videotapes to the children.

B. Write a handbook for parents on the art of nose blowing.

C. Develop group games that incorporate the components of nose blowing.

D. Show children how to dispose of soiled tissues.

E. Direct the children to individualize their tissue boxes by decorating them.

Section II: Option Comparison

Options	Choice	Options	Choice	Options	Choice	Options	Choice
A/B	A	A/C		A/D		A/E	
		B/C		B/D		B/E	
				C/D		C/E	
						D/E	

Section III: Totals

Total **A**	Total **B**	Total **C**	Total **D**	Total **E**	Priority Order of Options
					1.
					2.
					3.
					4.
					5.

The "PCA" Thinking Key is an effective tool to use when you are making a decision without the help of others or when you are working with a group who share ownership of a problem and need an objective measure.

A therapy guide who chooses to use the "PCA" with a group can develop a list of options before meeting with the others, or the group can generate the list of options. Therapy guides who lead the most successful therapy expeditions invite others to participate in the decision making process. They respect the needs of the client. That means, if the focus of the therapy intervention involves a young child, the family member most responsible for ensuring that the child's needs are met or the child's teacher who interacts with the child most of the day has the weighted opinion about which options will become part of the solution. A therapy guide never loses sight of the fact that those who share ownership of the problem will be most motivated to support the action plan when they have an active role in selecting the solution.

A Rule of Thumb Can Become a Mindtrap

As you make decisions on a therapy expedition, be mindful of the role that *rules of thumb* play in your decision making process. Rules of thumb are systematic thinking aids that influence judgment and simplify decision making.[9] Perhaps you have heard of one of the following rules of thumb: "Wait thirty minutes after eating before going into the water"; "Look both ways before crossing the street"; "The distance between fingertips with outstretched arms is equal to your height."[10]

Rules of thumb can be so automatic that you rely on them when you make decisions without being aware of their impact on your decision making process. They place a *perceptual frame* around your thoughts. A perceptual frame is an arbitrary boundary that one creates to contain the ideas that surround a particular notion about something or someone.

For example, you are in a position to recommend a software company to a colleague. Suppose you described their program as "always easy to install with clearly written manuals." By giving this description, you are placing a positive perceptual frame around the reason to purchase from this company. On the other hand, if you described their programs as "not user friendly," your perceptual frame or rule of thumb about this company's products might be perceived as negative. Consequently, your colleague would probably lean toward not purchasing a program from that company.

REFLECTIVE JOURNAL ENTRY 10.5

Complete the following thoughts:

1. *I once tried to convince my friend to change his [her] mind about . . .*

2. *To sway (bias) my friend's thinking, I placed the following perceptual frame around the subject of the discussion: . . .*

Rules of thumb are simplifying strategies that can be either helpful or constricting. They are constricting when you can use them to make a quick decision. They are destructive when they prevent you from considering all available information. When a rule of thumb becomes a "benchmark" or an assumed standard by which to make decisions, you fail to consider all of the factors needed to make a well-thought-out decision.

When rules of thumb are relied on to an extreme, they become *mindtraps*. Mindtraps sabotage your ability to make a "better" decision.[11] Mindtraps influence judgment in a variety of situations.[12] When these mindtraps operate, they create paradigms that are counterproductive to your producing rational and intuitive thoughts needed to find a solution.

When you are under the influence of a mindtrap, you no longer pay attention to or "mindfully" direct your thinking. You fail to consider all other information related to the situation. When you approach a problem with an automatic and sometimes overconfident mindset, you can make "mindless" decisions.[13] Efficient decision making requires "mindfulness." Effective therapy guides are aware that misusing a rule of thumb places one in danger of falling into a mindtrap.

When Therapy Guides Rely on Rules of Thumb

Therapy guides depend on many different rules of thumb when mapping out a therapy plan. Their rules of thumb are derived from theory and personal and professional life experiences. When therapy guides rely on one or two rules of thumb, however, they risk falling into a mindtrap that may misguide the therapy expedition and interfere with the making of better decisions along the way.

The following scenario illustrates how a rule of thumb that is derived from a therapy frame of reference can bias one's ability to make effective decisions.

> Donna and Dan are occupational therapists who provide therapy services to Brent. Brent is a seven-year-old who attends second grade at Community Elementary School. Donna works for a home health agency and sees Brent for therapy on Tuesdays and Thursdays, after school at home. Dan is employed by the Special Services Department of the local school system and works with Brent at school.
>
> Both therapists have Brent's best interest in mind. But neither therapist is willing to acknowledge the other's value in Brent's therapy program. Dan feels that what he does with Brent is more important than what Donna does. And Donna sees her sessions with Brent as more important to his future development than what Dan is able to achieve with him at school. As a result, the two therapists have difficulty communicating with each other.
>
> Donna's rule of thumb is grounded in a neurodevelopmental treatment (NDT) frame of reference. She is very concerned about how her client moves. When she implements a treatment program, she tries to avoid involving Brent in any activities that would cause abnormal movement patterns.[14]
>
> Dan, on the other hand, values functional outcomes when he develops a treatment plan. He is more concerned with whether Brent achieves success with functional tasks when he moves than he is with how Brent moves. Dan practices a motor learning theory when he creates a therapy expedition.[15] Hence, the construct of motor learning theory becomes his rule of thumb for guiding his treatment decisions.
>
> Because each therapist is structuring goals and treatment plans with different theoretical frames of reference, they both have difficulty seeing the value of the other's participation in managing Brent's ongoing developmental needs. They have fallen into mindtraps caused by their strong beliefs in one frame of reference or philosophy for managing Brent's developmental needs in therapy. Their respective frames of reference have such a powerful influence on what each feels is "best" for Brent that they are unable to communicate about Brent.

REFLECTIVE JOURNAL ENTRY 10.6

Complete the following thoughts:

1. *To free themselves from the influence of the mindtraps, I feel that Donna and Dan need to . . .*

2. *One way they might have avoided falling into the mindtraps is to . . .*

Whenever therapy guides use one rule of thumb as a "filter" through which to view a client's needs, they risk falling into a mindtrap. Mindtraps can be averted if you make up your mind to look at a situation from a broad perspective. For Dan and Donna, taking a broad perspective would have meant seeking more than one frame of reference when making decisions related to Brent's therapy needs.

Had either Dan or Donna been open to other viewpoints, that one might have initiated dialogue with the other. An open exchange of information might have led them to a mutual understanding of the decisions each one made about Brent's therapy program.

Therapy guides who are aware of the rules of thumb of decision making are less likely to fall into a mindtrap. The rules of thumb used in decision making fall into a variety of categories. Three of the common categories are listed below. After you have learned the rules of thumb in this section you will be asked to consider the mindtraps Louise avoided by being mindful of common rules of thumb during the Nose Blowing Expedition.

Categories of Rules of Thumb Used in Decision Making

Availability

1. Ease of Recall
2. Retrievability
3. Presumed Associations

Anchoring and Adjustment Phenomenon

Representativeness Bias

The Availability Rule of Thumb

The Availability Rule of Thumb biases your thinking toward repeatedly selecting the same path that led you to successful decisions on previous occasions. Each subcategory is discussed below.

In the following scenario, see how the Availability Rule of Thumb can influence the choice you make based on previous experiences.

Imagine that you always use your mother's chocolate chip recipe when baking cookies. Because of your vivid memories of the mouth-watering aroma emanating from the oven as you walked into your mother's kitchen and the soft, succulent texture and wonderful taste of her chocolate chip cookies, you have never considered using another recipe. Under the Availability Rule of Thumb, your culinary creativity is limited by your choosing to rely exclusively on strategies for which you hold vivid memories and whose memories are readily available to you.

REFLECTIVE JOURNAL ENTRY 10.7

Think about a task that you perform every day. Then, keeping in mind the Availability Rule of Thumb, recall a decision you once made that involved choosing one action over another because "that's the way I have always done it in the past." Now, complete the following thought:

Whenever I . . .

Note that the Availability Rule of Thumb has three subcategories or mindtraps: Ease of Recall, Retrievability, and Presumed Associations. As you read about the subcategories, think about the decision you described in Reflective Journal Entry 10.7.

Ease of Recall. The decision maker judges events that are vivid or recent as occurring with a higher frequency than they actually do. For an illustration of the Ease of Recall mindtrap, read the following scenario.

Sandra, a recent graduate in her first two months of employment, works in an early intervention program. She took over a twelve-client caseload from her predecessor. One of Sandra's clients is Tommy, a toddler who had been attending the program with his mother and aunt for the past two and a half years. During the past year, the family has missed more than half of the scheduled sessions, attending only one to two sessions a month. Within the past month, however, the family has attended every scheduled appointment.

One day while Sandra was waiting for Tommy's father to arrive, the center director called Sandra into her office and recommended that Sandra speak to the father about reducing the number of therapy appointments scheduled each month. The family had a history of canceling half of the scheduled sessions each month, she informed Sandra. She went on to explain that the center had a waiting list and that it was the therapist's responsibility to reduce the number of sessions scheduled each month if the family frequently canceled appointments.

Sandra felt that the center director was being unfair to Tommy's parents. She challenged the director's request to reduce the number of therapy sessions for Tommy. During her experience with Tommy's parents, they had never missed a session.

What was the flaw in Sandra's thinking? She was relying on the parents' attendance record as she knew it from her brief period of employment. She had neglected to consider the parents' cancellation rate within the past year. As a result, Sandra had fallen into the Ease of Recall mindtrap. She was biased by the attendance record in the recent past. Had Sandra asked herself the following two questions, she might have understood the center director's perspective on the situation.

1. How am I determining the frequency of these events?
2. What is the actual frequency of these events?[16]

REFLECTIVE JOURNAL ENTRY 10.8

Complete the following thought:

In Sandra's position, I would have thought about . . .

Retrievability. Relying on the way events are stored in memory, the decision maker tends to over- or underestimate the number of times an event occurs. The following scenario illustrates the Retrievability mindtrap.

Leonardo is a staff therapist on the children's unit in a large rehabilitation hospital. The hospital's therapy department has a supply room that the department director expects all occupational therapy staff to use when obtaining small adaptive equipment for clients.

On four different occasions in two weeks Leonardo went to the supply room in search of equipment for one of his young clients. Each time he found that the supply room was out of small spoons and scoop bowls. Leonardo assumed that the supply room inventory was no longer carrying adaptive feeding equipment for children because the majority of the patients were adults. Consequently, Leonardo began ordering equipment for his clients from an outside vendor.

When Leonardo had been ordering outside the hospital for about a month, the director learned about her employee's ordering practices. She immediately summoned Leonardo into her office and asked him to explain why he had been ordering supplies from outside vendors. She told him that by using outside vendors, he was adding additional expenses to the department, since supply room equipment was purchased at a special low cost. It was only during the meeting with the director that Leonardo learned that many items in the department's supply room had been on back order and had just arrived.

Where was the flaw in Leonardo's thinking? What biased his thoughts so that he assumed that the supply room no longer was stocked with equipment for children? Except for the last two weeks, Leonardo had been able to obtain small spoons and scoop bowls from the supply room when he needed them. But because of the way he organized information about the supply room's inventory in the recent past, Leonardo perceived that the supply room was no longer an option for purchasing equipment for his young clients. To arrive at this decision, he focused on the times that he was *unable* to get the equipment that he needed rather than viewing these times as exceptions.

Leonardo had fallen into a Retrievability mindtrap. He overestimated the number of times that the supply room was able to fill his order. He assumed (incorrectly) that it no longer stocked child-sized equipment. Had Leonardo asked himself the following questions, he might have saved himself the trouble of looking for outside vendors and saved the department some money.

1. Am I over- or underestimating the number of occurrences of the event?
2. Am I organizing information in my mind in a way that might lead to a misperception of the situation?

REFLECTIVE JOURNAL ENTRY 10.9

Complete the following thought:

In Leonardo's position, before ordering equipment from an outside vendor, I would have thought about . . .

Presumed Associations. The decision maker mentally links two separate events that occur at the same time. Because of the co-occurrence of events, the decision maker assigns an inappropriately high probability to the possibility that the events will occur at the same time again. The decision maker is often very resistant to considering the possibility that the two events do not always occur together.[17] For example, some people believe that all children with a medical diagnosis of cerebral palsy have cognitive deficits. If you were to ask these individuals why they believe cerebral palsy and intelligence are related, most likely they would describe their experience with a child who had cerebral palsy and attended a special school program for children with learning deficits. Despite their limited experience with children with special needs, their perception of all children with cerebral palsy is that they have learning disabilities in addition to the movement disorder. Now consider another scenario, which illustrates the Presumed Associations mindtrap.

Claire is an occupational therapist who was working on a research grant to gain financial support for a program for children with autism. During her investigation she called the Research Department Head at the American Occupational Therapy Association (AOTA).[18]

Midway through the telephone conversation with Claire, the department head asked her, "Do you think I'm an occupational therapist?" That's when Claire realized that she had wrongly assumed that all department heads at AOTA were occupational therapists.

Based on her acquaintance with several occupational therapists who work at the national headquarters, Claire assumed that all of the departments within AOTA are headed by occupational therapists. Claire had not considered the possibility that someone other than an occupational therapist would head a department at AOTA, because she had failed to properly analyze the situation. She fell into the Presumed Associations mindtrap.

Claire might have avoided the Presumed Associations mindtrap if she had only realized that there are always four separate combinations by which to evaluate the association between two unrelated groups of information or events. A four-square matrix illustrates this association.

To better understand how the four-square matrix works, let's analyze the common assumption that people who are wealthy are also happy. In this assumption there are two essential conditions: happiness and wealth. For each of these essential conditions (happiness and wealth) there is an opposite condition: not happy and not wealthy. When you look at both sides of two different situations you come up with four conditions:

Group 1: Happy people

Group 2: Unhappy people

Group 3: Wealthy people

Group 4: Not wealthy people

To assess the relationship between the groups, this information can be plotted on a matrix. In the Four-Square Matrix that follows, note that Groups 1 and 2 are recorded along the left side of the matrix and Groups 3 and 4 are recorded across the top of the matrix. The groups are then merged into the following four different combinations, as shown in Figure 10.1:

Combination 1: Happy people who are wealthy

Combination 2: Happy people who are NOT wealthy

Combination 3: UNhappy people who are wealthy

Combination 4: UNhappy people who are NOT wealthy

Figure 10.1. *Four-Square Matrix to Expand Your Perspective*

	Group 3 Wealthy people	Group 4 NOT wealthy people
Group 1 Happy people	Combination 1 Happy people who are wealthy	Combination 2 Happy people who are NOT wealthy
Group 2 UNhappy people	Combination 3 UNhappy people who are wealthy	Combination 4 UNhappy people who are NOT wealthy

Now let's return to Claire's scenario with her call to AOTA and see how the matrix might have helped her avoid falling into the mindtrap. She was dealing with two separate groups of information: AOTA staff members who head departments and AOTA staff members who are occupational therapists. When you look at the opposite side of AOTA staff members who head departments (Group 1) you see that there are AOTA staff members who do not head departments (Group 2). And when you look at the opposite side (Group 3) you recognize that there likely exist AOTA staff members who are not occupational therapists (Group 4).

When Groups 1–4 are merged on the four-square matrix, they yield four different combinations. Combination 1 represents the assumption that Claire made: All staff members who head departments at AOTA are occupational therapists. Had Claire considered the other three combinations, or options, she might not have assumed that the department head was an occupational therapist.

Complete the Four-Square Matrix Worksheet.

Record the three other options Claire might have considered to avoid falling into a Presumed Associations mindtrap.

Four-Square Matrix Worksheet

	Group 3 AOTA staff members who are occupational therapists	*Group 4* AOTA staff members who are NOT occupational therapists
Group 1 AOTA staff members who head departments	*Combination 1* *AOTA staff members who head departments who are occupational therapists*	*Combination 2*
Group 2 AOTA staff members who do NOT head departments	*Combination 3*	*Combination 4*

Compare your combinations in four-square matrix exercise with the following:

Combination 2: AOTA staff members who head departments and who are NOT occupational therapists.

Combination 3: AOTA staff members who do NOT head departments and who are occupational therapists.

Combination 4: AOTA staff members who do NOT head departments and who are NOT occupational therapists.

When you are considering whether two events or situations are necessarily linked, use the four-square matrix to evaluate whether they are mutually exclusive. Checking for four possible combinations will lessen the probability of your falling into a Presumed Associations mindtrap. Ask yourself the following two questions to decide whether there is a relationship between two events.

1. Have I considered the four possible outcomes of the two events?
2. How will the knowledge that the events are mutually exclusive alter my decision?

REFLECTIVE JOURNAL ENTRY 10.10

Complete the following thoughts:

1. *The last time I made a false assumption because I failed to carefully analyze all aspects of a situation was when . . .*

2. *When I discovered that my assumption was inaccurate, I . . .*

The Anchoring and Adjustment Phenomenon Rule of Thumb

The second rule of thumb category we discuss is the Anchoring and Adjustment Phenomenon. A decision maker who is operating under the influence of this rule of thumb is influenced by first impressions. The first information presented is perceived to have a greater value than what follows even though it's not of greater importance. The first information carries such a special significance that it is anchored in the decision maker's mind as the best information. The decision maker frequently develops a perception that nothing can measure up to the first information. There is an emotional attachment to the information, even when it is *inaccurate* and often despite attempts to correct the inaccuracies. The first impression may be so strongly anchored that adjustments cannot be made and subsequent information continues to be biased in the direction of the initial "first" information. The "first" information becomes the golden standard against which all other information is measured. Hence, the rule of thumb is referred to as the Anchoring and Adjustment Phenomenon.[19]

The following scenario illustrates the Anchoring and Adjustment Phenomenon.

Dierdra is a ten-year-old child with spastic diplegia cerebral palsy. She has just been discharged from the hospital after undergoing surgery to lengthen her hip flexor muscles. One of the reasons for the surgery was to increase her independence in self-care activities. Dierdra will be receiving four weeks of home based therapy before returning to school.

Three days before discharge, the hospital occupational therapist chose to teach Dierdra how to put on her pants, socks, and shoes using a long-handled dressing stick. The therapist had considered teaching dressing without any adaptive equipment. She felt, however, that Dierdra would be more independent if she learned the proper use of the dressing aid. So Dierdra's mother agreed to purchase the recommended piece of equipment for home use.

On the second day that Dierdra was home, she met her home health occupational therapist, Shelly. Unlike the therapist at the hospital, Shelly thought that Dierdra did not need any special equipment to dress herself. In contrast, Dierdra and her mother insisted that they wanted to continue using the dressing aid. Their insistence on using the dressing aid was based on the first impression created by the hospital therapist who taught Dierdra how to dress using the dressing aid. At that point Shelly recognized that Dierdra and her mother were influenced by how they were first taught to dress. They had anchored their understanding of how to dress using the piece of adaptive equipment.

Shelly was sensitive to the fact that whatever dressing methods she recommended to Dierdra and her mother would not be given full consideration. She understood that she was introducing a technique that was different from the one they had previously learned.

Shelly realized that Dierdra and her mother were not ready to consider ways to dress without a long-handled reacher. Her new clients were not ready to adjust their thinking or neutralize the anchoring effects of the dressing aid. Because Shelly was aware of the Anchoring Adjustment Phenomenon, she also thought that it was better for Dierdra to use the long-handled reacher until Dierdra was proficient with the dressing aid and was interested in a new technique.

Shelly recognized the Anchoring and Adjustment Phenomenon by asking herself the following two questions:

1. Is the client's thinking anchored by a first impression, first offer, first experience?
2. Have I investigated the legitimacy of making adjustments to neutralize the effect of the anchor? Or can I adapt to the anchor and allow it to become part of the action plan?

> **REFLECTIVE JOURNAL ENTRY 10.11**
>
> *Imagine yourself in Shelly's position. Consider your response to Dierdra and her mother's insistence on using the dressing aid even though you feel it is unnecessary. Then complete the following thoughts:*
>
> *I explain to Dierdra and her mother that . . .*

The Representativeness Bias Rule of Thumb

A third category of rules of thumb is the Representativeness Bias. A decision maker who makes predictions about a situation based on the way it is like another situation of similar quality and magnitude is influenced by the Representativeness Bias. The decision maker influenced by the Representativeness Bias applies a strategy that has worked in the past under a similar set of circumstances. The bias reflects a tendency to base decisions on "templates" of mentally stored information. A mental template is a pre-set pattern of thinking that developed gradually and is the outcome of a series of similar experiences. The decision maker who uses these templates to perceptually frame a similar situation and fails to think beyond the frame falls victim to the Representativeness Bias mindtrap.

The Representativeness Bias can be helpful to the decision maker when it approximates the success of an earlier decision based on similar occurrences. However, more often it can contribute to making a poor decision. If you rely on the Representativeness Bias when there is insufficient information or when the information you have is faulty, you risk falling into the Representativeness Bias mindtrap. Researchers have demonstrated that when decision makers misuse the Representativeness Bias Rule of Thumb they are being insensitive to baseline information and sample sizes.[20] These concepts are described below.

Baseline data is the starting point of information; it is a base to which future information is compared. When a change occurs within a situation, the change is measured against the baseline information. Consider, for example, the experience of starting a physical training program. If you want to increase your running endurance, the first thing you do is to identify your baseline endurance level for time and distance. From that baseline endurance level you measure the changes that can be attributed to the physical training program. Sensitivity to the baseline information is critical to evaluating the success of all therapy expeditions. Unless you know where you began, you will have difficulty determining whether positive (or negative) movement was made away from the point of entry.

A sample size is a small number of people, things, or events that are representative of a larger group. Since it is impractical to interview every person, observe every event, or consider every thing within a group before making a decision, polling a segment of the larger group is an efficient method to gather information on which to make a decision. Generally speaking, the larger the sample size the more accurately the information represents the whole group.

When you make any kind of decision you are dealing with data. Statistics is a way of dealing with data. A therapy guide needs a cursory understanding of statistics to support CPS and improve the ability to predict outcomes—positive and negative—of a decision.

Examine this scenario about Jason to see how a therapy guide uses statistics to make decisions.

Jason is a bright four-year-old, described as "high strung" by his mother. He has many problems performing all tasks related to the activities of daily living performance area. Performing self-care tasks are especially stressful for Jason and his mother.

Jason's mother complains that Jason eats only bland, soft, and semi-solid foods that are at room temperature. His diet consists of macaroni and cheese at almost every meal. Bath time, especially shampooing, is traumatic for both Jason and his mother. Jason doesn't like to "get wet," his mother reports. But once he is wet, he seems to enjoy the bath.

He also has difficulty sequencing words into cohesive sentences. Jason has been receiving speech therapy since he was two years old because of the atypical speech and language pattern that he demonstrates. His pediatrician recently referred Jason to occupational therapy. The referral stated, "Evaluate and treat as needed to increase Jason's tolerance for daily life skill."

Imagine that you are Jason's occupational therapist and are about to evaluate him. Asking yourself the following questions before beginning the evaluation will prevent you from falling into the Representativeness Bias mindtrap.

1. In what ways can I seek accurate baseline information about the situation?
2. How can I interview the family about the child so that my questions are direct and not skewed by my perception of the situation?
3. Am I judging the occurrence of events or behaviors on a large enough sample size? In other words, is the magnitude of the child's problems reported by the family so great that the family member perceives the problems to occur more frequently than they actually do occur?

To better understand the issues around Jason's feeding behaviors, begin collecting data on what he eats at each meal, including type, texture, and quantity of food. A knowledge of the daily menu will be valuable information when you begin to develop the action plan. To gather accurate baseline information, ask Jason's mother to keep a meal diary for five days; ask her to record what food she serves and what food Jason actually eats. To make Jason's mother's job of reporting the information as easy as possible, give her a calendar with large spaces on which to record Jason's meals. The calendar will help organize the data that you are asking her to report back to you. The completed calendar will allow you to objectively evaluate Jason's feeding behavior and help you to understand Jason's "eating problem."

After analyzing Jason's week of eating, you will need to ask yourself the following two questions:

1. Is Jason's eating behavior different from that of other four-year-olds?
2. In what ways is Jason's eating behavior out of the ordinary?

To determine how Jason's behavior varies from the norm it is important to understand the range of eating patterns preschoolers demonstrate. If you don't have this knowledge, you may need to seek it. One way to gather the data is to conduct a mini-research project; visit a local day care center and observe four-year-olds during snack and lunch time.

Ask Questions to Avoid Falling into a Mindtrap

Rules of thumb, when used appropriately and mindfully, can unlock doors to your thinking. Conversely, rules of thumb used mindlessly can become mindtraps and sabotage your thinking. Asking questions is the best way to avoid falling into a mindtrap. Never assume anything.

The Mindtrap Question Checklist lists a series of questions that are designed to help you avoid the pitfalls of a mindtrap. Ask yourself these questions before making a decision to expand your thinking beyond the immediate details and scope of the situation. The Mindtrap Question Checklist is also a useful tool for helping to understand the results of the decision making of others. To use the Mindtrap Question Checklist for other people, substitute the person's name in place of "I" when asking the questions.

Mindtrap Question Checklist

Rule of Thumb Category	Questions to Ask to Avoid Falling into a Rule of Thumb Mindtrap
Availability ◆ **Ease of Recall:** perceiving events that are vivid or recent as occurring with a higher frequency than they actually do.	☐ How am I [is _____] determining the frequency of these events? ☐ What is the actual number or frequency of these events?
◆ **Retrievability:** over- or underestimating the number of times an event occurs based on the way the events are stored in memory.	☐ Am I [is _____] over- or underestimating the number of occurrences of the event? ☐ Am I [is _____] organizing information in my mind in a way that might lead to a misperception of the situation?
◆ **Presumed Associations:** mentally linking two separate events in such a way that the events are perceived as co-occurring.	☐ Before making a decision have I [has _____] considered the possible existence of all four combinations of two separate events? ☐ Am I [is _____] ready to change my [his/her] opinion about the relationship between these two events even though I [he/she] previously thought the two events were linked?
The Anchoring and Adjustment Phenomenon: being influenced by the first information presented, assuming that this information has more value than subsequent information.	☐ On what previous experience or information is my [_____ 's] thinking anchored? ☐ Is my [_____ 's] anchor for this information so strong that an adjustment away from the anchor is not likely?
Representativeness Bias: making predictions about a situation based on the way it is like just one other situation of similar quality and magnitude.	☐ Am I [is _____] seeking accurate baseline information about the situation, or are my questions skewed by my perception of the situation? ☐ Am I [is _____] judging the occurrence of events or behaviors based on a large enough sample size?

Potential Mindtraps Along the Nose Blowing Expedition

Let's return to the Nose Blowing Expedition. Consider which mindtraps Louise might have fallen into had she not been mindful of the routes she took. Louise begins her Nose Blowing Expedition with information about the teacher and the teacher's aide's need to teach the children how to blow their noses. Louise was aware that she didn't have all of the information necessary to develop a therapy program.

Although she was not exactly sure where to start the task of teaching nose blowing to young children, she first explored the published literature for information. She looked for developmental scales on nose blowing. Finding no published information on the development sequence of nose blowing, she ventured out into the community to do her own field research on nose blowing. Her "field" consisted of the local day care centers. She had no guarantees of what she would find, but she listened to her intuition. Her inner sense "told" her that taking a side trip on her Nose Blowing Expedition might provide insights about the development of nose blowing skills in young children.

While visiting the day care centers, Louise used her skill at asking questions to interact with the parents and teachers of children between the ages of two and five. And alas! Louise acquired important data about the art of nose blowing in preschoolers. She learned that approximately 95 percent of normal children acquire the skill of nose blowing by age four.

REFLECTIVE JOURNAL ENTRY 10.12

Complete the following thought:

If Louise had spoken to only one parent and one teacher [HINT: sample size] about when children learn to blow their noses, I believe she would have been at risk for falling into the _____ mindtrap because . . .

Imagine what would have happened to the Nose Blowing Expedition if Louise had chosen not to visit the day care centers? After all, taking the time to explore nose blowing among normal children might seem to be a waste of time—especially when she wasn't exactly sure what she was going to find and more than likely was not financially compensated for her time observing the children in the day care.

Did Louise really need to take the side trip to the day care centers? She was proficient at blowing her own nose. She had done it for years and was very successful at it. She could easily have based her therapy program on the way her parents taught her to blow her nose when she was a child. Yet something sparked Louise's interest in gathering more information about how young children develop the skill of nose blowing.

REFLECTIVE JOURNAL ENTRY 10.13

Complete the following thought:

If Louise had relied on her personal experiences blowing her own nose [Hint: based on how Louise's parents taught her to blow her nose], I believe she would have fallen into the _____ mindtrap because . . .

If Louise had not taken the side trip to the child care centers, she would have risked developing an intervention plan supported by erroneous judgments. To effectively work with the children at the school for the deaf, she needed information about when children typically learn to blow their own noses. What she knew about nose blowing from her own experience would have been inadequate for developing a treatment plan. Louise's side trip to the local child care centers helped her avoid falling into an Availability mindtrap.

Symbol for Solution Finding

The almost completed puzzle with the last piece about to be placed represents Solution Finding. The puzzle symbolizes the process of looking for the "better" solution that fits the context in which the client's problem occurs. Whenever you see the puzzle icon, you are being reminded to use Solution Finding.

Create a Mind Map of Section

10

Mind Map Guidelines

1. Place the section's main concept in the center of the space using pictures or words or both.
2. Radiate ideas from the central thought.
   - Use images (be sure to use color).
   - Headline text—one or two words per line.
   - Print text (for easy reading).
3. Link the main concepts and generate more ideas from the linkages.
4. Have fun!

Remember, the more linkages that you generate between elements, the greater your ability to see how all the elements relate to one another.

Section 10
SELF-ASSESSMENT

Now that I have completed the tenth part of my journey, I can:

○ compare Solution Finding with Acceptance Finding.

○ explain how to use criteria to make a decision.

○ use the "Will It . . . ?" Thinking Key to create criteria.

○ show how "TRACS" will frame my thinking.

○ apply the "Making an Idea More Acceptable" Thinking Key.

○ unlock my intuition with the "In-tuit" Thinking Key.

○ use the "AL-O" Thinking Key to join intuition with logic.

○ rate my ideas using the "Evaluation Matrix" Thinking Key.

○ use the "PCA" Thinking Key to prioritize ideas.

○ explain how rules of thumb and mindtraps relate to problem solving.

○ explain how rules of thumb can become mindtraps.

○ describe how a therapist might fall into a mindtrap.

○ use the "Mindtrap" Thinking Key to evaluate an action plan.

NOTES

1. Scott Isaksen, K. B. Dorval, and Donald Treffinger, *Creative Approaches to Problem Solving* (Dubuque, Iowa: Kendall/Hunt, 1994). Isaksen et al. use the acronym CARTS to identify five commonly used criteria. To fit the travel theme of this field book, we adapted TRACS from CARTS.
2. Philip Goldberg, *The Intuitive Edge* (New York: Jeremy P. Tarcher, 1983).
3. Daniel Goleman, *Emotional Intelligence* (New York: Bantam Books, 1995), 43.
4. Quoted in Julia Cameron and Mark Bryan, *The Artist's Way: A Spiritual Path to Higher Creativity* (New York: G. P. Putnam's Sons, 1992), 6.
5. Goleman, *Emotional Intelligence*, 28.
6. Goldberg, *Intuitive Edge*, 36.
7. M. Bazerman, *Judgment in Managerial Decision Making*, 3d ed. (New York: John Wiley & Sons, 1994); E. de Bono, *CoRT Thinking: Teacher's Notes* (Des Moines, Iowa: Advanced Practical Thinking, 1986); R. M. Dawes, *Rational Choice in an Uncertain World* (New York: Harcourt Brace Jovanovich, 1988).
8. Isaksen, Dorval, and Treffinger, *Creative Approaches to Problem Solving*.
9. Max Bazerman, in his *Judgment in Managerial Decision Making*, 3d ed. (New York: Wiley & Sons, 1994), presents well-researched information in support of the mental-processing demands of decision making. His book is filled with examples from the behavioral decision-research literature and provides a valuable resource to decision makers who wish to improve their judgment skills.
10. Tom Parker, *Rules of Thumb* (Boston: Houghton Mifflin, 1983).
11. Anthony LeStorti, executive consultant of Ideatects in Philadelphia, Pennsylvania, coined the term *mindtraps* to refer to the way that a heuristic has the power of becoming counterproductive to optimal decision making.
12. Bazerman, *Judgment in Managerial Decision Making*, cites research on cognitive bias. Bazerman identifies 13 biases that result from overreliance on judgmental heuristics. The biases include ease of recall, retrievability, presumed associations, insensitivity to base rates, insensitivity to sample size, misconceptions of chance, regression to the mean, the conjunction fallacy, insufficient anchor adjustment, conjunctive and disjunctive events bias, overconfidence, the confir-

mation trap and hindsight, and the curse of knowledge. For a complete explanation of these biases, see his chapter 2, "Biases," 12–47. Much of the research Bazerman cites is by A. Tversky and D. Kahnemann. (See n. 20.)

13. Ellen Langer, *Mindfulness* (New York: Addison-Wesley, 1989). Langer, a professor of psychology at Harvard University, has studied the psychological and physical costs that people pay when they fail to pay attention to why they do what they do. According to Langer, people who act without full consciousness of the current situation act mindlessly. When presented with a new situation, people who act mindlessly rely on old frames of reference to categorize information. They use the old frames of reference as a template for planning their actions. In contrast, people who act mindfully continually reconfigure the categories that lead to new frames of reference tailor-made to fit each new situation. The process of creating new categories forces people to pay attention to the situation and its context—to be mindful of what they do as they are doing it.

14. K. Bobath, *A Neurophysiological Basis for the Treatment of Cerebral Palsy* (Suffolk, Eng.: The Lavenham Press, 1980).

15. M. Lister, ed., *A Contemporary Management of Motor Control Problems: Proceedings of the 11 Step Conference.* Alexandria, Va.: Foundation for Physical Therapy, 1991.

16. Anthony LeStorti, of Ideatects, developed a checklist of questions to help identify and guard against cognitive biases. LeStorti recommends using the checklist to lessen the potential of falling into mindtraps.

17. L. J. Chapman and J. P. Chapman, "Genesis of Popular but Erroneous Diagnostic Observations," *Journal of Abnormal Psychology* 72 (1967): 197–204.

18. AOTA is the national organization that oversees the profession of occupational therapy. It provides services to its members and information related to occupational therapy to others outside of the profession.

19. Bazerman, *Judgment in Managerial Decision Making*.

20. Tversky and Kahnemann have published many studies about the influence of the representativeness bias on decision making. See A. Tversky, and D. Kahnemann, "The Belief in the 'Law of Numbers,' " *Psychological Bulletin* 76 (1971): 105–10; "Judgment Under Uncertainty: Heuristics and Biases," *Science* 185 (1974): 1124–31, "The Framing of Decisions and the Psychology of Choice," *Science* 211 (1981): 453–64; "Extensional Versus Intuitive Reasoning: The Conjunction Fallacy in Probability Judgment," *Psychological Review* 90 (1983): 293–315; "Rational Choice and the Framing of Decisions," *Journal of Business* 59 (1986): 251–94.

Go Forward with an Action Plan: Acceptance Finding

Itinerary #11

At the end of the eleventh part of your journey, you will be able to:

✓ explain the purpose of identifying forms of "support" and "resistance" when planning a therapy expedition

✓ use the "Potential Sources of Support and Resistance" Thinking Key to identify the supporters and resisters of the action plan

✓ identify the factors that influence how people deal with change

✓ identify the two kinds of change that influence therapy outcomes

✓ describe mindsets that support change and those that are barriers to change

✓ identify three context-related factors that support change

✓ develop an action plan with the "Generating Potential Actions" Thinking Key

✓ use the "LIST" Thinking Key to organize actions into long-term, intermediate, and short-term plans

✓ develop an action plan using the "Planning for Action" Thinking Key

✓ develop an action plan with the "What's Next? Question Series," "If–Then," "What If . . . ? Question Series," and "Think Positive" Thinking Keys

✓ finalize a plan with the "Action Plan Adoption Checklist" Thinking Key

✓ explain how to gather feedback about an action plan using the "Preparing to Seek Feedback" Thinking Key

✓ use the "Flow Checklist" Thinking Key to evaluate a treatment plan

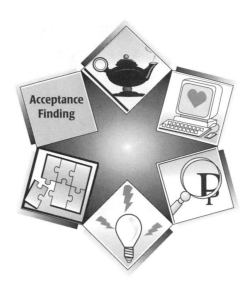

The Generating Phase: Sources of Support and Resistance

Acceptance Finding is the sixth stage of CPS and the second part of Component III, Go Forward with an action plan. In the Acceptance Finding stage you will learn that in order for a therapy expedition to be successful, it must gain the acceptance of its participants.

In the first part of Component III, Solution Finding, you learned how to use criteria to transform ideas into solutions. In Acceptance Finding you will learn how to lead the client from the present to a desired future state by creating a therapy expedition plan of action. To insure the success of the action plan, the therapy guide must look at the proposed plan from many perspectives. Analyzing the plan from several different points of view helps her think about ways to make the plan acceptable to all who will be influenced by the plan (e.g., the child, family members, caregivers, teacher, babysitters). Gathering support for the plan is one of the first steps in creating an action plan; a well-conceived plan may fail if there is insufficient support from the people whose lives will be most influenced by it.

The Generating Phase of Acceptance Finding begins with an examination of the plan from different perspectives. The therapy guide considers the forces that will either help move the plan forward or block its progress. The two forces that either help or hinder the plan fall into the following two general categories:

1. potential *sources of support* for the plan of action; and
2. potential *sources of resistance* to the plan of action.

Sources of support are the persons, places, times, or things that support an environment or climate conducive to moving the plan forward. The sources of support are called "supporters." Supporters move an action plan forward but can also help to deal creatively with sources of resistance, or "resisters." Resisters are persons, places, times, or things that block or inhibit the quality of the therapy process. By identifying and then seeking to understand all the potential sources of resistance to the therapy plan a therapy guide increases the probability of leading a successful therapy expedition.

A therapy guide recognizes the importance of identifying early on all individuals and situations that might challenge the plan. Therapy guides anticipate trouble spots and proactively respond to and control for potential problems. To identify supporters and resistors, consider everyone who is expected to interact with the client during the therapy expedition. Ask yourself the following question: "Who will, in any way, have an influence on the client's ability to achieve the goals set forth in the action plan?"

If the client is an infant or a child who is not yet enrolled in a school program, the people who most influence the action plan are the child's parents, other family members, babysitters, and caregivers. Therapists whose clients attend school programs have an additional sphere of individuals to consider—teachers, classroom aides, and possibly volunteers. Identify all individuals who will be influenced by the therapy expedition. Next identify those who will most likely support the expedition and those who may resist the plan or any part of it.

Imagine, for example, that you are working with four-year-old Timothy. His therapy expedition involves developing independence in self-care skills. One of his goals addresses toilet self-management. The goal states, "Timothy will pull his pants down past his knees." For the therapy expedition to be a success, Timothy's caregivers and early childhood classroom staff need to help him develop self-help skills in clothing management each time he goes to the bathroom.

Timothy's mother and father want Timothy to learn to manage his clothing during toileting. Consequently, both parents diligently use verbal cues to coax their son to pull his own pants down every time he goes to the bathroom. Timothy's parents are supporters in the therapy expedition. Ms. Jones, the classroom aide in Timothy's preschool classroom, on the other hand, physically assists Timothy each time he goes to the bathroom. Currently, she is a source of resistance to the therapy expedition. She is blocking Timothy's ability to take responsibility for himself during toileting. If Timothy is to eventually gain independence in self-help toileting skills, your role as a therapy guide and a supporter of Timothy's therapy expedition is to seek to understand why Ms. Jones helps Timothy and your challenge is to bring Ms. Jones "on board" as a source of support to the expedition.

REFLECTIVE JOURNAL ENTRY 11.1

Jot down your thoughts about why Ms. Jones might be resisting the therapist's efforts for Timothy to help himself during toileting.

1. *Three reasons I could give for Ms. Jones's helping Timothy are . . .*

   a.

   b.

   c.

2. *Ms. Jones might better understand Timothy's needs if I explained that . . .*

The following are possible explanations for why Ms. Jones helps Timothy in the bathroom:

- Ms. Jones is not clear about the goal of independent dressing.
- According to how Ms. Jones views Timothy's abilities, asking him to pull his pants down is an unrealistic goal.
- Ms. Jones does not know how to manage Timothy's behaviors and pulls down his pants to avoid a confrontation.
- Ms. Jones regularly helps the children pull down their pants and therefore forgets that Timothy requires a special kind of assistance.

Hypothesizing about why Ms. Jones helps Timothy will expand your thinking about the dilemma. Once you have thought of various reasons why Ms. Jones is not supporting Timothy's goals, speak directly to her. Speaking to Ms. Jones face-to-face will help you understand why she helps Timothy. When you know why Ms. Jones helps Timothy, you are better prepared to work with her and gain her assistance in supporting Timothy's action plan.

Individuals are not the only sources of resistance that can block the success of a therapy expedition. Time, location, and things are also sources of resistance. The location of the therapy expedition can be a source of resistance if the environment (e.g., at home; in the classroom; or outside, in the community) does not support the goals of the action plan. Consider, for example, how time influences an action plan involving dressing skills when the therapy guide provides services in the classroom. Furthermore, the best times to work on dressing skills would be in the morning when the student arrives and at the end of the day when he prepares to leave school, because at those times he is most likely taking off or putting on outerwear. Another time to work on dressing is during bathroom breaks or physical education class. If, however, the therapy guide is unable to schedule the student during times of routine clothing management, the physical environment and time would be considered sources of resistance to the therapy expedition.

The funding source that covers therapy services for the client could also be a source of resistance. If, for example, a client's insurance coverage defines the number of occupational therapy visits to be less than what the client needs, the client's insurance plan could be considered a resister to the therapy expedition.

After the therapy guide identifies the sources of resistance, he seeks to understand the reason behind the resistance. The sooner a therapy guide examines the possible sources of resistance and thoroughly explores reasons for the resistance, the sooner he can either work toward converting a resister into a supporter or creating a strategy to deal with the source of resistance.

"Potential Sources of Support and Resistance"

The **"Potential Sources of Support and Resistance" Thinking Key** will help you to systematically identify the potential sources of support and resistance on the therapy expedition. In Acceptance Finding, this Thinking Key once again uses the 5 Ws & an H question set (who, what, where, when, why, and how) that was introduced in Data Finding (Section 7).

Turn now to the Field Organizer for the "Potential Sources of Support and Resistance" Thinking Key and note that it is divided into columns A, B, and C. Column A lists phrases that introduce questions beginning with one of the 5 Ws & an H questions. Columns B and C list phrases that can complete the questions started in column A. The questions completed in column B are about sources of support; the questions completed in column C are about sources of resistance. Pair up with a partner and practice using the "Potential Sources of Support and Resistance" Field Organizer from the point of view of the therapist Louise on the Nose Blowing Expedition (To review the story, turn to p. 162.).

DIRECTIONS

1. Read the proposed idea at the top of the Field Organizer.
2. Create the first question by combining the phrase "WHO might . . ." in column A, row 1, with the phrase "contribute time and resources to move the plan forward?" in column B, row 1.
3. Answer the question "Who might contribute time and resources to move the plan forward?" by identifying those individuals who could contribute time, talent, or resources to support the plan. Record your responses in column B.
4. Combine the phrases in columns A and C, row 1, to create the question "WHO might limit or restrict forward movement of the plan?" Identify the people who will potentially inhibit the plan from moving forward and record your responses in column C.
5. Continue creating questions in rows 3 through 6 by combining the phrase in column A with the phrase in column B and then with the phrase in column C, row by row, to trigger thoughts about potential sources of support and resistance for the proposed plan.
6. Record the answers to the questions created in rows 3 through 6. Use the examples in rows 1 and 2 to model your responses.

To respond to some of the questions using the Nose Blowing Expedition you will need to extend your thinking beyond the printed words of the story. Not all potential sources of support and resistance are explicitly stated. For this exercise, think outside of the box to expand the list of sources of support and resistance that you think might affect the therapy expedition.

"Potential Sources of Support and Resistance"

Proposed idea: *Teach the children the skill of nose blowing using games and relay races.*

A 5 Ws & an H	B Potential Sources of Support	C Potential Sources of Resistance
1. **WHO** might . . .	*contribute time and resources to move the plan forward?* *The teacher and the teacher's aide, if they believe that play is the vehicle through which children learn best.* *Parents who reinforce recommended nose blowing techniques at home.*	*limit or restrict the forward movement of the plan?* *The teacher and teacher's aide, if they believe that in order to learn how to blow a nose, children need to practice holding a tissue and blow into it until they get it correct; if they don't reinforce the nose blowing program on the days that the therapist is not present.* *Parents who don't reinforce recommended nose blowing techniques at home.*
2. **WHAT** things, objects, or activities might be . . .	*helpful?* *Visits to the children's doctors to rule out nasal obstructions.* *Supplies to carry out games and relay races.* *Availability of local child care centers that allow visitors.*	*an impediment?* *Lack of documentation about nose blowing behaviors in the literature.* *Time to communicate with parents about the details of the nose blowing program.* *Local day care centers who do not allow visitors to observe the children.*
3. **WHERE** are . . .	*locations where the plan can be accomplished?*	*locations that block progress of the plan?*
4. **WHEN** might there be . . .	*an appropriate time to work on the plan [specify hours, day, week, month]?*	*an inappropriate time to work on the plan?*
5. **WHY** might the plan be . . .	*supported?*	*resisted?*
6. **HOW** might I anticipate . . .	*strengths in the plan?*	*weaknesses in the plan?*

As you generate sources of support and resistance you may find one variable acting as both a supporter and a resister. For example, a student's teacher can support the therapy expedition by implementing a special positioning program on days when the therapy guide is present in the classroom. However, if the same teacher ignores the child's special seating and positioning needs the rest of the week when the therapy guide is not present, the teacher is also a source of resistance to the therapy expedition. When an individual appears to be both a source of support and a source of resistance to a therapy expedition, the therapy guide needs to address the resistance issue in the course of developing the action plan.

Factors That Influence How People Deal with Change

Since the focus of a therapy plan is to help a client move from a current reality to a desired future state, change plays a major role on a therapy expedition. The therapy guide is a "change agent" who manages the change. Therapy guides actively seek to understand why members of the expedition respond with varying levels of support and resistance to the change that is brought about by the therapy plan. The extent to which individuals are able to accept change within an expedition is influenced by the following factors:

◆ *kind* of change
◆ *mindset* of the individuals impacted by the change
◆ *context* in which the change will occur

Kind of Change. On a therapy expedition there are two broad categories of change. One change involves creating a new paradigm for the client. The second relates to improving the client's performance within a familiar, recognized paradigm.

A client's paradigm is like a map of a designated territory, not the territory itself. A client's paradigm is a map that influences his behavior and perception of a situation. Since a therapy expedition will create a change for anyone involved with the action plan, therapy guides need to understand the paradigm of those persons on the expedition.[1] The scenarios of Philip and Jeffrey, below, demonstrate how the type of change on an expedition influences the therapy process.

First, meet Philip. See how change involves creating a new paradigm for Philip and his caregivers.

Philip, who is 18 months old, was recently diagnosed as having cerebral palsy. Philip's pediatrician referred Philip to an early intervention program "for developmental growth and development." Philip's parents' reason for seeking therapy services was "to teach Philip to walk."

You meet Philip's family during the multidisciplinary initial evaluation meeting. Based on your assessment of Philip, you question whether walking is a realistic goal for him now or in the future.

Your evaluation shows that Philip rolls from his back to his stomach. Based on the movement patterns he displays in his upper body and trunk, you speculate that he is possibly showing an interest in trying to sit. In deference to the parents' reason for bringing Philip to therapy, focusing on walking does not appear to be a realistic goal for the next six months.

Since Philip's parents' expectations (paradigm) for the immediate future differ from yours, your immediate goal is to build a bridge of understanding. Without such a bridge, Philip's parents will have difficulty shifting the expectations they now hold for their son's future. A shift in their thinking can come about through effective communication, nurturing, and support by you, the therapy guide. For in order to have a successful therapy expedition you and Philip's parents must agree on the destination point.

Before you can define a realistic destination point for a therapy expedition, you need to connect, early on in the journey, with the client's or the client's caregivers' perception of the potential benefits of therapy. Making this connection will require your compassion, coupled with skillful inquiry. When you value the expressed needs of the clients you serve, you increase the probability of a successful therapy expedition.

Next, meet Jeffrey. In Jeffrey's story, change involves working with parents whose future vision for their son is shared by you.

> Jeffrey is now 24 months old. When he was referred for therapy services, he was beginning to walk. He demonstrated difficulties maneuvering between closely spaced objects and was still unsteady on his feet. Although he was walking by himself, his parents were aware of his need to refine the way he moved through space. They understood that the therapy program would involve creating situations to challenge his motor performance through a variety of play activities. From your point of view, Jeffrey's parents came to therapy with a realistic perception of the treatment process.

The therapy goals in Jeffrey's case involved enhancing Jeffrey's performance within a paradigm familiar to Jeffrey's parents. In contrast to Jeffrey's situation, the plan of action for Philip was to help the parents understand Philip's developmental needs while at the same time supporting their emotional needs to see Philip advance developmentally.

Therapy expeditions that involve a shift in the client's, the family's, or the therapist's paradigm are more difficult to execute than therapy expeditions that occur within a paradigm familiar to all "traveling companions." When the success of a therapy expedition depends on working within a new paradigm for the client, the therapy guide expends a great amount of effort, energy, and compassion at the outset of the therapy expedition helping the client (or the client's family if the client is a young child) reframe his or her thinking about the forthcoming therapy experience.

In the Nose Blowing Expedition, Louise created a new paradigm for teaching nose blowing. She might have tackled the problem head on by teaching the children how to hold the tissue and blow into it. But instead she chose a new set of rules for teaching nose blowing. She developed a treatment program around games and relay races. The story tells you that her strategy motivated the children to develop the movements necessary for blowing their noses. It is likely, however, that at the outset of the plan the teacher needed to understand Louise's reasons (paradigm) for using games and relay races with the children, rather than taking a more direct approach to the problem.

REFLECTIVE JOURNAL ENTRY 11.2

Imagine that you are Louise and you wish to explain to the teacher your reasons (paradigm) for wanting to use games and relay races to teach nose blowing skills to the children, then complete the following thought:

I think nose blowing skills can be taught through games and relay races because . . .

When a therapy expedition calls for a paradigm shift, you need to explain the need for such a change. Taking the time to prepare the way for a paradigm shift will increase the probability of gaining support for the proposed therapy plan.

Mindset of the Individuals Impacted by the Change. Mindset is the manner in which a person responds to events; a person's mindset flows out of his or her paradigm.[2] (Mindset is presented in Section 3 in relation to the qualities associated with a therapy guide.) In the present discussion, we are concerned with the mindset of persons with whom the therapy guide will be working. Awareness of the mindset of everyone else on the therapy expedition helps the guide determine whether she is working with resisters to, or supporters of, the action plan.

REFLECTIVE JOURNAL ENTRY 11.3

Complete the following thoughts:

1. *The last time I can remember that someone strongly supported a major change was when . . .*

2. *The last time I can remember that someone strongly resisted a major change was when . . .*

"Check the Mindset"

There are many mindsets that indicate a person's readiness for or resistance to change. The **"Check the Mindset" Thinking Key** will help you identify mindsets or ways of thinking by looking at the behaviors of the people on an expedition. For example, if the teacher on the Nose Blowing Expedition accepts the idea of using games to teach nose blowing, she might suggest some children's games that could be adapted to teaching nose blowing. Such a response would indicate that the teacher is *a risk-taker*. If, however, the teacher is resistant to new ideas (e.g., she refuses to use games to teach nose blowing), she might suggest that Louise teach the children to blow their noses only by practicing blowing into a tissue. Such a response would indicate that the teacher is a *conformer*.

Turn to the "Check the Mindset" Field Organizer, below, and read the list of five pairs of mindsets. Each pair represents a continuum from resistance to change (on the left side) to readiness for change (on the right). The five pairs of mindsets are as follows:

1. Conforming–Willing to take risks
2. Rigid–Flexible
3. Narrow-minded–Open-minded
4. Needing to know–Tolerant of ambiguity
5. Self-centered–Empathetic

Note that the mindsets indicative of a readiness for change are the same ones used to describe the qualities associated with a therapy guide (see Section 3). In the "Check the Mindset" Field Organizer each mindset is accompanied by a description that will trigger your thoughts about the actions of a person with that particular mindset.

Imagine that you are Louise, the therapy guide of the Nose Blowing Expedition. Practice using the "Check the Mindset" Thinking Key Field Organizer. You will be recording actions that the teacher in the Nose-Blowing Expedition might have demonstrated.

DIRECTIONS

1. Read the behaviors in rows 1 and 2 that reflect the mindset of the teacher as *Willing to take risks* (right side of the continuum) and as *Flexible* (right side of the continuum).
2. Read the mindsets on both sides of the continuum in rows 3–5. Select one mindset on each continuum and fill in the circle next to the mindset. (Note that since you are evaluating the teacher on the Nose Blowing Expedition, you will choose mindsets indicative of a readiness for change, on the right side of the Field Organizer.)
3. Think of a behavior the teacher could demonstrate that reflects each of the mindsets on the right side.

4. Record the behaviors on the lines below each mindset in rows 3–5. Use the examples in rows 1–2 to model your responses.

FIELD ORGANIZER

"Check the Mindset"

Resistance to Change	Readiness for Change
1. ○ **Conforming**	**Willing to take risks** ●
Prefers to act according to the standard or norm.	*Willing to expose self to chance; seeks out opportunities that may move the action plan forward.*
_____	*The teacher suggested adapting children's games to teach*
_____	*nose-blowing skills.*
2. ○ **Rigid**	**Flexible** ●
Unyielding and consequently unable to change the course of action or switch gears readily.	*Able to change the course of action (switch gears) whenever it is necessary to meet the demands of the situation.*
_____	*The Teacher was willing to work individually with the*
_____	*student who had a cold and congestion during the Nose*
_____	*Blowing Expedition.*
3. ○ **Narrow-minded**	**Open-minded** ○
Unreceptive to new ideas or strategies. Prefers to use routine ideas and activities that are familiar.	*Acknowledges that there are few absolutes in therapy. Receptive to new ideas or strategies. Open to new possibilities.*
_____	_____
_____	_____
4. ○ **Needing to know**	**Tolerant of ambiguity** ○
Needs to have discrete answers.	*Feels comfortable waiting for the "better" answer to emerge.*
_____	_____
_____	_____
5. ○ **Self-centered**	**Empathetic** ○
Values personal needs and perspectives over the needs of others.	*Identifies with the feelings or thoughts of others.*
_____	_____
_____	_____

When looking for cues that indicate levels of support or resistance to the therapy plan, use the "Check the Mindset" Thinking Key to sharpen your observation and listening skills.

Context in Which the Change Will Occur. A person's resistance to, or support of, an action plan can be influenced by human and nonhuman factors in the environment (context). The following three context-related factors can support or work against change:[3]

- ◆ Time
- ◆ People
- ◆ Resources

Time. For a therapy expedition to be successful, there must be adequate time to develop the treatment plan and communicate the details of the plan to the client (depending on his age) and caregivers as well as anyone else who shares ownership in the problem. The therapy guide must also have adequate time to implement the treatment plan and to follow up after the scheduled therapy sessions have terminated. The more carefully the therapy guide fine tunes time schedules to coordinate the needs of the various people on an expedition, the more likely that everyone on the therapy expedition will accept change in a positive light.

Continuity of people. The greater the continuity of people involved in an expedition, the greater the chance of making progress on the action plan. Whenever essential personnel within the therapy expedition (e.g., therapist, physician, social worker, teacher) change, the challenges within the therapy process increase. Each new member who joins an expedition must spend a significant amount of time "learning the ropes." She must acquire knowledge in:

1. the particulars related to the expedition (i.e., what activities the client likes and dislikes, the best time to schedule appointments, the client's medical history and diagnosis; who shares ownership of the problem), and
2. the interpersonal communication styles, verbal as well as nonverbal, of all team members.

Any interruptions in the makeup of the team can interfere with the flow of the action plan. Consistency among members of an expedition helps to build a cohesive team that can learn together how to best meet the needs of a client.

Stability of resources. Therapy expeditions require resources to support the therapy process. Such resources include funding for the therapist's services as well as for the space, equipment, and supplies required to provide high quality therapy intervention. Resources also include the expertise and talents team members contribute to the therapy process. Resources can make the difference between whether an expedition is a well-run operation or one that struggles to reach its destination point. A steady flow of resources gives everyone involved in the expedition a sense of stability.

Stability of time, people, and resources supports an environment where change can be cultivated. Each of these three factors relates to the context within which the therapy expedition occurs, and together they can have a profound influence on the mindset of individuals on the therapy expedition.

A therapy expedition must have adequate support and commitment from those involved if it is to be a success. Capitalizing on the sources of support for a therapy plan while creatively dealing with the sources of resistance will help you gain acceptance for the therapy expedition. By imagining the way others will respond to the therapy plan, you will increase your ability to structure a plan of action to which people will feel committed. That commitment is important. After all, the real agents of change in any therapy situation are the people who are dedicated to seeing the change happen. A therapy guide knows that he is with the client only a small percentage of the client's life. The lasting changes that the client makes as a result of the therapy intervention are due to the ongoing efforts of the client's daily support system (of family, caregivers, babysitter, day care center personnel, classroom teacher, and teacher's aide). When the client's support system is stable over time, the flow of resources remains strong, and the goals are appropriate, there is a high probability that the client will attain his goals.

"Generating Potential Actions"

The last exercise you will engage in during the Generating Phase of Acceptance Finding involves identifying actions that can lead to developing an action plan. Recall the guidelines of the Generating Phase: think up as many ideas as you can so that you will have a variety from which to select. Look for strategies that are beyond the obvious.

Use the **"Generating Potential Actions" Thinking Key** to frame your thinking with a "forward mode" toward an action plan. When you use this Thinking Key you answer the following two questions:

1. What possible actions can be taken to move the plan forward?
2. What are possible sources of resistance to the proposed plan?

You will practice using the "Generating Potential Actions" Thinking Key by completing the "Generating Potential Actions" Field Organizer with reference to the actions taken in the Nose Blowing Expedition. First, turn to the Field Organizer and note that the two questions above are restated at the top of columns A and B. To begin, we noted what possible actions Louise on the Nose Blowing Expedition took to move the action plan forward. One action was to check whether she could locate any published information about the developmental progression of nose blowing. This action is recorded in column A, row 1.

The ten actions recorded in column A were either specifically stated or implied in the Nose Blowing Expedition story. An example of an implied action is that Louise needed to make an appointment with the day care centers before visiting them. This action is recorded in column A, row 2.

For each one of the potential actions recorded in column A, rows 1 through 10, one possible source of resistance is recorded in column B. For example, in row 1, a possible source of resistance to making an appointment to visit the local child care centers might be the time Louise will take to speak with the child care center directors. Recognizing sources of resistance ahead of time can help a therapy guide plan for ways to deal with them. Now complete the "Generating Potential Actions" Thinking Key Field Organizer with a partner.

DIRECTIONS

1. Read the actions and sources of resistance in columns A and B, rows 1–10.
2. In column A, rows 11–15, record five more actions that Louise might have taken based on information stated or implied in the story.
3. In column B, rows 11–15, record one possible source of resistance to each of the actions recorded in column A.

FIELD ORGANIZER

"Generating Potential Actions"

Proposed plan: *Teach the children how to blow their noses through games and relay races.*

A Actions That Move the Plan Forward	B Sources of Resistance That Block the Plan
1. *Check references for developmental information about nose blowing.*	*Limited or no written information on nose blowing.*
2. *Make appointments to visit local child care centers.*	*May take many calls to speak with the child care center directors who must approve visitation.*
3. *Observe children at child care centers and speak with teachers and parents about their impressions about nose blowing behaviors.*	*No therapy service reimbursement for visiting the child care center.*
4. *Seek school principal's permission to send a letter to parents about having their children checked for nasal obstructions.*	*Principal may not have time to review letter right away.*

(continued)

Proposed idea: *Teach the children how to blow their noses through games and relay races.*

A Actions That Move the Plan Forward	B Sources of Resistance That Block the Plan
5. *Send a letter home with a slip to be returned to the school indicating the parents' willingness to follow up on the request to have their children checked for nasal obstructions.*	*Parents may object to what they perceive to be an unnecessary visit to the doctor's office.*
6. *Develop a computerized matrix form to record children's baseline nose blowing performance.*	*Therapist may not have computer skills to create a matrix on the computer; creating a handwritten (or a computerized) form will take time.*
7. *Gather baseline data on the children's nose blowing skills.*	*Gathering baseline data could be time consuming.*
8. *Develop a plan for how to sequence the nose blowing activities based on the analysis of the baseline data.*	*A wide range of nose blowing skills within the class could make developing a program to meet the needs of all the children in the program difficult.*
9. *Meet with the teacher to discuss proposed activities to get additional ideas and feedback.*	*Teacher may be more interested in having the children practice blowing into a tissue than in teaching nose blowing through games.*
10. *Schedule nose blowing activities.*	*Finding time to schedule nose blowing activities in with the rest of the curriculum may be difficult.*
11.	
12.	
13.	
14.	
15.	

Now that you have examined potential sources of support and resistance to the therapy plan, you are ready to move to the Focusing Phase. This is the final step of developing an action plan.

The Focusing Phase: Traveling from the Present to the Future State

In the Focusing Phase of Acceptance Finding, you will generate a specific plan of action. The plan will move you from the current reality of the initial assessment to a desired future state based on the goals of the action plan. The plan includes actions to be taken and the time line within which they will occur. The time line is an arbitrary projection based on your best knowledge of all of the factors related to the expedition.

The context of the situation will influence the occupational performance scenario that is scripted by the action plan. The context includes

- the service delivery system (i.e., home health, school system, acute care),
- the payer source (i.e., health maintenance organization, private insurance, state funding sources, self-pay),
- the time frame of the service delivery (e.g., a complete school year, a six-week hospital admission), and
- the individuals who will be supporting the therapy goals.

If the therapy expedition occurs within the context of the school system, for example, the time line is measured by the school calendar. Because of the administrative structure within most school programs, therapists record the students' annual progress on Individual Educational Plans at the completion of the school year. In contrast to the school system, the time line of an action plan for a child receiving services in a rehabilitation center might be only six weeks. The rehabilitation center's time line is based on the anticipated discharge date established by the members of the rehabilitation team.

The task of the therapy guide is to organize actions for the therapy plan into the following three categories: long-term, intermediate, and short-term actions. The categories are based on the projected duration of the therapy expedition. Plotting the route of the therapy expedition is both a skill and an art. The following guidelines will help you structure the plan:

1. *Establish long-term actions first.* Begin each therapy expedition with an end in mind. Establish the long-term actions first in order to avoid taking detours that may consume time and delay progress and to ensure that all the members of the therapy expedition have a clear vision of the destination point. Long-term actions are like a beacon of light. They establish the reference point by which all shorter-term actions will be measured.[4]
2. *Establish the intermediate point of progress.* Once the long-term actions are in place, establish what progress you anticipate the child will make at the halfway point, that is, at a point halfway between completion of the long-term actions and the client's point of entry to the therapy expedition.
3. Next, use the intermediate actions as a reference point and move backward again to determine the progress that the child needs to make by the quarter point. (See Figure 11.1.)

Plotting out a therapy expedition action plan is like plotting out a trip.

Figure 11.1. *Therapy Expedition Plot Map*

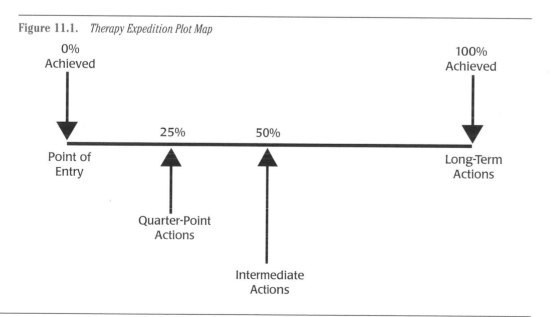

A therapy guide uses the same kind of thinking you described in the journal entry above. A therapy guide first gets the lay of the land by hypothesizing what goals the client could potentially achieve within a designated amount of time. And because a therapy guide has a tolerance for ambiguity, she accepts that she may need to revise the long-term action plan depending on the progress made along the way. With experience, she develops skill at adjusting the short-term actions that lead to the projected long-term actions that conclude the therapy expedition.

Imagine that you are working in a rehabilitation hospital. Your newest client is Rose, an eight-year-old child who suffered a complete severance of the spinal cord at the level of the sixth thoracic vertebrae; her anticipated in-patient admission is eight weeks. One of her long-term goals is that she will be independent in functional mobility skills using a wheelchair at the time of discharge.

When you first meet Rose, she is weak and requires maximum physical assistance with all transfers in and out of the wheelchair. She has difficulty maneuvering the wheelchair around small spaces in the bedroom and dining area. In other words, Rose demonstrates 0 percent independence in functional mobility skills. Based on the rehabilitation team's long-term action plan, her therapy expedition will focus on taking her from 0 percent independence to 100 percent independence in eight weeks.

For Rose, an intermediate step toward independence in functional mobility is to develop sufficient strength and endurance to transfer in and out of the wheelchair and maneuver the wheelchair through space. Therefore, by four weeks, Rose needs to be able to display an increase in upper body strength to a point that allows her to move her lower body. Working backward from the intermediate point, you envision that Rose at the intermediate point must have a minimum strength capability to perform all her upper extremity dressing independently.

The long-term actions set the tone for all the intermediate steps. The intermediate steps provide the halfway point, and the short-term goals are those steps that will be first on the action plan on the therapy expedition. Use the following strategy to organize a therapy plan. Start with an end point in mind.

Point of referral	0%	independence in functional mobility skills
Point of discharge	100%	independence in functional mobility skills (long-term goal)
Halfway point	50%	independence in functional mobility skills (intermediate goal)
One-quarter of the way	25%	independence in functional mobility skills (short-term goal)

The long-term actions for a plan will be influenced by a variety of factors, including the client's

◆ abilities,
◆ awareness of the need to actively participate during the therapy experience,
◆ funding source that dictates the duration of the therapy expedition,
◆ expectations, and
◆ support system (i.e., family, caregivers, teachers, babysitters).

"LIST"

The **"LIST" Thinking Key** helps organize the therapy plan actions into long-term, intermediate-point, and short-term actions (shown in the Field Organizer on p. 306). The "LIST" represents all the actions you foresee at the outset of the therapy expedition. "LIST" is an acronym whose letters sequentially represent the first letters of the words Long, Intermediate, Short, and Term. The more thorough the "LIST" the better your ability to plan for successful outcomes and minimize the number of unexpected detours. The "LIST" Thinking Key works with two other Thinking Keys: "Generating Potential Actions" and "Plan for Action." ("Plan for Action" is introduced later in this section.)

You will use the "LIST" Thinking Key to put into three categories the actions for the Nose Blowing Expedition that you recorded in the "Generating Potential Actions" Field Organizer. The categories are long-term, intermediate, and short-term actions. (Note: The numbers on the "LIST" are for discussion purposes only; they do not imply a rank order or value to the items under each section.)

Select a partner. Decide who will role play Louise and who will role play the teacher as you work on the "LIST" Field Organizer.

DIRECTIONS

1. Turn back to the "Generating Potential Actions" Field Organizer (p. 301). "Louise" will review the actions with "the teacher" in the following way:
   a. "Louise" reads the actions listed in column A of the Field Organizer, and
   b. with "the teacher," "Louise" sorts the actions into long-term, intermediate, and short-term goals.
   (For this activity, "long-term" refers to actions to be taken between the first and second months, "intermediate" refers to actions to be taken between the second and the fourth weeks, and "short-term" refers to actions to be taken within the first two weeks. Actions 1 through 10 from the "Generating Potential Actions" Field Organizer have already been recorded on the "LIST" Field Organizer. Your task is to sort the actions that you recorded in the "Generating Potential Actions" Field Organizer into one of the three categories on the "LIST" Field Organizer.)
2. Record the actions that you have sorted under the appropriate category on the "LIST" Field Organizer.
3. Add to the "LIST" any additional actions that you consider important but that were not included in the original list in the "Generating Potential Actions" Field Organizer.

The three actions in the Long-Term Actions section of the "LIST" Field Organizer, "Prepare a list of materials needed for teaching nose blowing," "Gather materials needed for teaching nose blowing," and "Teach nose blowing activities," were not on the original list of actions in the "Generating Potential Actions" Field Organizer. They were added because they are important actions that support Louise's need to have the necessary materials available when she is ready to execute the action plan. Whenever you think of additional steps along the way be sure to add them to your list.

FIELD ORGANIZER

"LIST"

Long-Term Actions to Take <u>*between the first and second months*</u>

1. Prepare a list of materials needed for teaching nose blowing.
2. Gather materials needed for teaching nose blowing.
3. Teach nose blowing activities.
4.
5.
6.
7.
8.

Intermediate Actions to Take <u>*between the second and fourth weeks*</u>

1. Develop a computerized matrix form to record children's baseline nose blowing performance.
2. Gather baseline data on the children's nose blowing skills.
3. Develop a plan for how to sequence the nose blowing activities based on the analysis of the baseline data.
4. Meet with the teacher to discuss proposed activities to get additional ideas and feedback.
5. Schedule nose blowing activities.
6.
7.
8.

Short-Term Actions to Take <u>*within the first two weeks*</u>

1. Check references for developmental information about nose blowing.
2. Make appointments to visit local child care centers.
3. Observe children at child care centers.
4. Seek school principal's permission to send a letter to parents about having their children checked for nasal obstructions.
5. Ask parents to have their pediatrician rule out nasal obstructions.
6.
7.
8.

The "LIST" Field Organizer is a useful tool for detailing the needs of the therapy expedition and prioritizing the actions within the time constraints of the expedition.

"Plan for Action"

Use the **"Plan for Action" Thinking Key** to develop the specific steps that will be part of the therapy expedition's itinerary, that is, to plan for implementation of the ideas. "Plan for Action" uses the 5 Ws & an H question set. Each section of the "Plan for Action" Field Organizer (see below) poses a series of questions for each action. The questions are as follows:

1. **WHAT** is the action desired?
2. **WHO** will do the action?
3. **WHEN** will the action begin and be completed?
4. **WHERE** will the action start? finish?
5. **WHY** is the action important?
6. **HOW** will you know the action was successful?

The "Plan for Action" Field Organizer is used in conjunction with the "LIST" Field Organizer. Actions are taken from the "LIST" and developed in the "Plan for Action" Field Organizer through the use of the 5 Ws & an H questions. For example, the first long-term action in "LIST" is "Prepare a list of materials needed for teaching nose blowing." For this action ask the six questions listed above. See the responses to these questions recorded in the first cell at the top of the "Plan for Action" Field Organizer. Practice using the "Plan for Action" Field Organizer by working with a partner. Assume the roles of Louise and the teacher.

DIRECTIONS

1. Begin with the Long-Term Actions. Read WHAT action is desired for Long-Term Action #2, and respond to questions 2–6. Do the same for Long-Term Action #3. Use the answers provided for Long-Term Action #1 to model your responses.
2. Turn to the Intermediate Actions and answer questions 2–6 for Intermediate Actions #2 and #3. Refer to the responses provided for Intermediate Action #1.
3. Respond to questions 2–6 the Short-Term Actions #2 and #3. Refer to the responses provided for Short-Term Action #1.

FIELD ORGANIZER

"Plan for Action"

Long-Term Actions

Long-Term Action #1

1. **WHAT** is the **action** desired? *Prepare a list of materials needed for teaching nose blowing.*

2. **WHO** will do the **action**? *Louise and the teacher*

3. **WHEN** will the **action** start? *4th week* finish? *4th week*

4. **WHERE** will the **action** take place? *At school in a brainstorming session*

5. **WHY** is the **action** important? *To identify any supplies that might need to be ordered ahead of time*

6. **HOW** will you know the **action** was successful? *A list is generated.*

(continued)

Long-Term Actions

Long-Term Action #2

1. **WHAT** is the **action** desired? *Gather the materials needed for teaching nose blowing.*

2. **WHO** will do the **action**?_____

3. **WHEN** will the **action** begin and be completed?_____

4. **WHERE** will the **action** take place? _____

5. **WHY** is the **action** important? _____

6. **HOW** will you know the **action** was successful? _____

Long-Term Action #3

1. **WHAT** is the **action** desired? *Teach nose blowing activities.*

2. **WHO** will do the **action**?_____

3. **WHEN** will the **action** start? _____ finish? _____

4. **WHERE** will the **action** take place? _____

5. **WHY** is the **action** important? _____

6. **HOW** will you know the **action** was successful? _____

Intermediate Actions

Intermediate Action #1

1. **WHAT** is the **action** desired? *Develop a computerized matrix form to record children's baseline nose blowing performance.*

2. **WHO** will do the **action**? *Louise*

3. **WHEN** will the **action** start? *2d week* finish? *2d week*

4. **WHERE** will the **action** take place? *Computer terminal*

5. **WHY** is the **action** important? *Spreadsheet (matrix form) will facilitate data collection.*

6. **HOW** will you know the **action** was successful? *Spreadsheet will be ready to use.*

Intermediate Action #2

1. **WHAT** is the **action** desired? *Gather baseline data on the children's nose blowing skills.*

2. **WHO** will do the **action**?_____

Intermediate Actions

3. **WHEN** will the **action** start? _____ finish? _____

4. **WHERE** will the **action** take place? _____

5. **WHY** is the **action** important? _____

6. **HOW** will you know the **action** was successful? _____

Intermediate Action #3

1. **WHAT** is the **action** desired? *Develop a plan how to sequence the nose blowing activities based on the analysis of the baseline data.*

2. **WHO** will do the **action**? _____

3. **WHEN** will the **action** start? _____ finish? _____

4. **WHERE** will the **action** take place? _____

5. **WHY** is the **action** important? _____

6. **HOW** will you know the **action** was successful? _____

Short-Term Actions

Short-Term Action #1

1. **WHAT** is the **action** desired? *Check references for developmental information about nose blowing.*

2. **WHO** will do the **action**? *Louise*

3. **WHEN** will the **action** start? *1st week* finish? *1st week*

4. **WHERE** will the **action** take place? *Pediatric textbooks*

5. **WHY** is the **action** important? *Provides a reference point to use when setting goals for the preschool children with hearing impairments*

6. **How** will you know the **action** was successful? *Will either have developmental levels for nose blowing or know that no such data have been published*

Short-Term Action #2

1. **WHAT** is the **action** desired? *Make appointments to visit local child care centers.*

2. **WHO** will do the **action**? _____

3. **WHEN** will the **action** start? _____ finish? _____

(continued)

"Plan for Action" *(Continued)*

4. **WHERE** will the **action** take place? _____

5. **WHY** is the **action** important? _____

6. **HOW** will you know the **action** was successful? _____

Short-Term Action #3

1. **WHAT** is the **action** desired? *Observe children at child care centers.*

2. **WHO** will do the **action**? _____

3. **WHEN** will the **action** start? _____ finish? _____

4. **WHERE** will the **action** take place? _____

5. **WHY** is the **action** important? _____

6. **HOW** will you know the **action** was successful? _____

To complete the exercise, you used six actions from the LIST. Had this been a real therapy experience, you would need to pose the 5 Ws and an H question for every action you wish to pursue. Therapy guides develop the habit of routinely asking the 5 Ws and an H question about their proposed actions before integrating the actions into the therapy expedition.

After using the 5 Ws and an H question to uncover the general details about your proposed actions, increase your perspective by envisioning them with as much detail as possible. Ideally, your future vision should include all of the things that you anticipate will "go right" with the action plan as well as those things that may "go wrong."

Looking into the Future: Four Thinking Keys Revisited

In Section 3 you were introduced to four Thinking Keys that sharpen your skills at looking into the future. You will use them again in the Focusing Phase of Acceptance Finding and apply them to the Nose Blowing Expedition. You may recall that each of these Thinking Keys offers a unique method of systematically projecting your thinking into the future to broaden the perspective of the actions you are about to take. The four Thinking Keys you will revisit here are:

- "What's Next? Question Series"
- "If–Then"
- "What If . . . ? Question Series"
- "Think Positive"

"What's Next? Question Series." This Thinking Key provides a mental structure for sequencing actions into the future.

Imagine that you are the therapy consultant in a third grade classroom; you consult on several children in the class once a month. On this particular day, you are scheduled to observe Jennifer's handwriting while she is engaged in her written work. The teacher asked for a consultation because Jennifer is slower than the other children in completing her assignments.

You note that Jennifer keeps changing her grasp on the pencil as she writes and several times, during the brief observation, the pencil drops from her hand altogether. You speculate that perhaps if she used a different kind of pen or pencil, she might be more successful at holding onto it and her penmanship might improve. You introduce several different sizes and weights of pens and pencil grasp holders to Jennifer, and she agrees to try two different ones.

"What's next?" you ask yourself. You know that you will need to check back with Jennifer and her teacher within the next few weeks to evaluate the effectiveness of the pen and pencil grip Jennifer chose.

When you ask "What's next?" following each client-directed action, you develop the habit of connecting one action to the next. As the actions become embedded within the therapy expedition's story, they sequentially connect with one another. Asking "What's next?" continually directs your thinking towards follow-up actions you will take with the client. The follow-up actions are what makes your initial actions meaningful. Practice using the "What's Next? Questions Series" Thinking Key in the Field Organizer that follows, with reference to the Nose Blowing Expedition.

DIRECTIONS

1. Read the proposed actions recorded in column A.
2. For each action, ask, "What's next?"
3. In column C, rows 5–6, record an action that might logically follow from the proposed action listed in column A. Use the examples in column C, rows 1–4 to model your responses.

 FIELD ORGANIZER

"What's Next? Question Series"

A Describe *one part* of the therapy plan	B Ask, "What's next?"	C Respond to the question, "What's next?"
1. Teach the children how to blow through a straw placed in one inch of water.	"What's next?"	Measure how high the children can make the water bubbles go in their cup by marking progress with markings inside the cup.
2. Teach the children how to use their noses to blow lightweight objects (e.g., cotton ball, feather) across a piece of paper.	"What's next?"	Measure how far the children can make the cotton ball travel across the paper.
3. Inform parents of the nose blowing program using a fun-to-read outline with a couple of nose blowing related pictures.	"What's next?"	Follow up with an assignment that links the children's school activities (nose blowing) with home activities (i.e., children demonstrate to their parents their nose blowing skills)
4. Inform the principal of the overall program plan for the nose blowing program.	"What's next?"	Invite the principal to a Nose Blowing Graduation Ceremony in which the children receive their nose blowing certificates—a nose with their name on it.
5. Make plans with the teacher to integrate nose blowing into the school routine.	"What's next?"	
6. Promote future therapy referrals by sending directors of preschool and kindergarten programs a flyer describing the success of the nose blowing program.	"What's next?"	

Note in the above sequence of proposed actions that Louise could easily have stopped after the action described in row 3. But by inviting the principal to a nose blowing graduation ceremony, she helps insure support for nose blowing programs in the future. The ceremony gives the principal an opportunity to see first hand the success of the program and paves the way toward future referrals for therapy services within the school program.

"If–Then." This Thinking Key helps to structure the hypothesis that provides future direction to the therapy expedition. Practice using the "If–Then" Thinking Key in the Field Organizer that follows, with reference to the Nose Blowing Expedition.

DIRECTIONS

1. Read the hypotheses in column A.
2. Complete the "Then" portion of the hypotheses in column B, rows 5–6. Use the examples in column B, rows 1–4 to model your responses.

FIELD ORGANIZER

"If–Then"

A IF...	B THEN...
1. **IF** the children learn how to blow air out through their mouths	**THEN** they would be prepared to learn how to blow air out through their noses.
2. **IF** the children learn how to blow air out through their noses during games	**THEN** they would have the necessary motor skills to blow into a tissue.
3. **IF** the parents were informed of the nose blowing program at school	**THEN** they could reinforce the nose blowing skills at home.
4. **IF** the principal knew of the success of the nose blowing program	**THEN** she could share with other administrators the value of asking the occupational therapist to teach nose blowing as a benefit to both students and teachers.
5. **IF** the teacher integrated nose blowing into the school routine	**THEN**
6. **IF** Louise published a fun-filled booklet on how to teach nose blowing	**THEN**

The "If–Then" Thinking Key and the "What's Next? Question Series" Thinking Key may be used together or independently. The main difference between the two is that the "What's next? Question Series" helps sequentially project your thoughts into the future and the "If–Then" Thinking Key helps to develop a hypothesis statement based on the causal relationship between two events.

"What If . . . ? Question Series." This Thinking Key may be used with the "If . . . Then" Thinking Key and the "What's Next? Question Series" or independently. The "What If . . . ? Question Series" also helps you think into the future. The unique function of the "What If . . . ? Question Series" is that it helps you to consider possible outcomes of taking a certain action. Most therapy-related actions have many possible consequences. Asking

"What if . . . ?" stimulates you to think about the worst- and best-case scenarios when planning an action or a series of actions. The more consequences you can anticipate from a proposed action, the better prepared you are when you enter the situation. Practice using the "What If . . . ? Question Series" Thinking Key in the Field Organizer that follows, with reference to the Nose Blowing Expedition.

DIRECTIONS

1. Read the "What if . . . ?" questions in column A.
2. Identify one consequence of the "What if . . . ?" questions in rows 3–4.
3. Record your responses in column B. Use the examples in rows 1–2 to model your responses.

FIELD ORGANIZER
"What If . . . ? Question Series"

A "What If . . ."	B Worst- and Best-Case Scenario
1. **What if** the children practice their blowing skills by using whistles and straws?	◆ Children share toys after they have put them in their mouths. ◆ Children love the activities and ask for the toys often.
2. **What if** some children have a cold during the nose blowing activity program?	◆ Children infected with colds could spread germs during blowing games and relay races. ◆ Children with a cold could greatly benefit from the program.
3. **What if** some of the children in the group are already proficient at nose blowing?	◆ ◆
4. **What if** every child had his or her own personalized tissue box in the classroom?	◆ ◆

"Think Positive." This Thinking Key can be used throughout the planning and implementation of the therapy expedition. Use the "Think Positive" Thinking Key whenever you find yourself saying "I can't" to an idea that you would really like to pursue. "Think Positive" helps replace thoughts of "I can't" with "How might I?" Practice using the "Think Positive" Thinking Key in the Field Organizer below, with reference to the Nose Blowing Expedition.

DIRECTIONS

1. Read rows 1–2, from column A to column B, to see how "I can't" statements are transformed into "In what ways might" questions.
2. Transform the "I can't" statement in column A, row 3, into three questions beginning with "In what ways might" that create a possibility for accomplishing the desired action.
3. Record your responses in column B, row 3. Use the examples in rows 1–2 to model your responses.

A I can't . . .	B In what ways might . . . ?
1. **I can't** *figure out how to make a chart on the computer to document the children's baseline nose blowing performance.*	1. **In what ways might** *a family member, colleague, or friend make a computer chart for me?* 2. **In what ways might** *I make a chart using grid paper and a ruler?* 3. **In what ways might** *an existing graphic table be adapted to a chart to record the children's baseline performance?*
2. **I can't** *get approval from the principal to buy supplies for the nose blowing activity program.*	1. **In what ways might** *the school supply materials such as straws, cotton balls, and tissues?* 2. **In what ways might** *parents purchase a personalized packet of oral motor blow toys?* 3. **In what ways might** *the school's parent teacher association (P.T.A.) provide financial support for supplies for the Nose Blowing Program?*
3. **I can't** *get as much time as I think is necessary to assess the children and conduct the nose blowing activities.*	1. **In what ways might** 2. **In what ways might** 3. **In what ways might**

When you use the "Think Positive" Thinking Key you are actualizing the familiar phrase "Where there is a will there is a way." Once a therapy guide has the determination to find a way to reach a goal, she isn't easily deterred. A goal is the vision that fuels the therapy expedition to continue moving forward.

"Action Plan Adoption Checklist"

As you finalize the action plan, there are five factors to consider. Each factor plays an integral role in determining whether the client will support the plan. The five factors are listed below, each followed by a question for you to ask yourself that relates the factor to the action plan.[5]

1. **Advantages.** What advantages does the proposed plan have over actions taken in the past? Note: Consider the factor "advantages" only for clients who have received therapy services in the past. Skip it for a client who, for example, is receiving therapy services following a traumatic injury or corrective medical intervention from a newly diagnosed problem.
2. **Compatibility.** In what ways is the plan compatible with the client's operating paradigm and value system?

3. **Complexity.** Is the complexity of the plan consistent with the anticipated time frame of the therapy expedition? How easily can it be understood by others? How easily can it be implemented?
4. **Trialability.** Are there parts of the plan that might warrant an evaluative, trial period before including them in the therapy expedition routine?
5. **Visibility.** In what ways are the outcomes of the plan clearly visible to those who share ownership in the client's problem?

The **"Action Plan Adoption Checklist" Thinking Key** helps to finalize your plan of action by addressing its advantages, compatibility, complexity, trialability, and visibility. Turn to the "Action Plan Adoption Checklist" Field Organizer, below. To use this Thinking Key, ask the two questions under each of the factors to help you examine the effectiveness of the therapy plan. Practice using the "Action Plan Adoption Checklist," with reference to the Nose Blowing Expedition. (As you work, you may want to refer to the list of five factors and the questions they raise.)

DIRECTIONS

1. Read the two questions in column A for each of the five factors.
2. Record your responses in column B, row 2, for each factor. Refer to the examples in row 1 for each factor to model your responses.

 FIELD ORGANIZER

"Action Plan Adoption Checklist"

A Question	B Response
Advantage	
1. What are the benefits to the client and the client's support group for accepting the plan?	*The children, their families, school personnel, and all persons the children come in contact with will benefit from not being exposed to cold germs if the children learn to blow their noses.*
2. How is this action plan better than previously tried actions?	
Compatibility	
1. In what ways is the plan consistent with the client's paradigm (values, experiences, needs)?	*Children relate to learning about life through play. Learning how to blow their noses through games motivates children to participate.*
2. Who among the client's support group will agree with the plan?	
Complexity	
1. In what ways can the plan be clearly communicated to others?	*Mount a huge poster board nose with a tissue attached to it in the classroom as a daily reminder to encourage independence in nose blowing.*

(continued)

"Action Plan Adoption Checklist" (Continued)

A Question	B Response
Complexity (continued)	
2. In what ways can the plan be simplified?	
Trialability	
1. In what ways can the plan be first implemented on a trial basis?	*Try several games with the children to assess their responses to blowing games.*
2. In what ways can the plan be modified and still accomplish the goal?	
Visibility	
1. In what ways are the outcomes of the plan visible to all involved with the plan?	*Children demonstrate their new skill every time they need to blow their noses.*
2. In what ways can the outcomes be made easy for others to see and understand?	

"Preparing to Seek Feedback"

Therapy guides continuously monitor the progress of an action plan to confirm that it is effective and on target. As a therapy guide vigilantly monitors the therapy plan, the question that remains uppermost in his mind is, "Is the client making progress toward reaching the goals set forth in the action plan?" To answer this question the therapy guide must collect feedback from everyone involved in the therapy expedition. Feedback sources can include the client, family members, and all other individuals who have contact with the client.

Use the "Preparing to Seek Feedback" Thinking Key to organize your thoughts as you go about gathering data about the effectiveness of the action plan. The Field Organizer for the **"Preparing to Seek Feedback" Thinking Key** uses the 5 Ws and an H question set to trigger your thoughts.

Practice using the "Preparing to Seek Feedback" Thinking Key with reference to the Nose Blowing Expedition. You can either pair up with a partner or do the activity alone. Doing the activity with a partner allows you to see that there are many answers to each question, depending on the respondent's point of view.

DIRECTIONS

1. Read the questions in column A.
2. Record the responses in column B. To get you started, possible answers have been included in column B, row 1. See whether you can generate more responses to those provided in row 1 before moving on to rows 2–5.

FIELD ORGANIZER

"Preparing to Seek Feedback"

A The 5 Ws & an H Question	B Responses
1. **Who** might provide feedback?	*the teacher* *the teacher's aide* *the children* *the parents*
2. **What** feedback will I seek?	
3. **When and where** are the best times to seek feedback?	
4. **How** might I acquire the feedback?	
5. **Why** do I want to acquire the feedback?	

Seeking feedback about a client's progress, from members of the expedition, allows the guide to assess whether change, brought about as a result of the therapy process, is observed by others. Feedback from others helps a therapy guide make adjustments in the itinerary in order to ensure that the plan of action is on the right course. Acknowledgment from members of the expedition that they do observe changes in a client's daily performance ensures that the efforts of the therapy team are focused on producing functional outcomes.

Evaluating the Action Plan by Monitoring Flow

In addition to gathering feedback, a guide monitors the effectiveness of the action plan through direct observation of the client. Direct observation helps you determine whether the activities provide the client with the just right challenge. The just right challenge refers to the right activity, selected for the client at the right time. It is also called the Flow experience or simply Flow.[6]

Flow describes the sense that one's skills are perfectly matched with the demands of the situation. During a Flow experience, all self-consciousness disappears. You are oblivious to time and absolutely absorbed in the activity of the moment. The Flow experience is analogous to a finely balanced scale. The right amount of challenge is matched with the right amount of skill. When the scales tip toward one direction or the other, the quality of the experience is altered and the Flow experience becomes disrupted. Either boredom or anxiety results. See Figure 11.2. When a person's skills are not matched with the challenge he is about to face, he feels anxiety. And when a person's skills are too great for the challenge, she feels boredom. Thus Flow is a state of mind that can be described as a point delicately poised between boredom and anxiety.

An activity that brings one into the Flow state must meet the following seven criteria:

1. The individual has the *appropriate skills* with which to engage in the task.
2. The task has the *potential of completion.*
3. The individual has the *ability to concentrate* on the task because action and awareness are merged. Concentration on the task is possible when the following two conditions are met: the individual has clear goals about the outcome of the activity, and the activity provides immediate feedback about how the individual is doing.
4. The individual is able to engage in the activity with a deep, *effortless involvement* that removes everyday anxieties or frustrations. The task is fun to do.
5. The individual has a *sense of control* over personal actions.
6. The individual is so involved in the activity that he or she experiences a *loss of the sense of self*, yet paradoxically, the sense of self emerges stronger after the Flow experience is over.
7. The individual is so involved in the activity that he or she experiences an *altered sense of time*.

Let's now relate each of the criteria for a Flow experience to the therapy process. To help you internalize the concepts of Flow, as you read each section below, you will be asked to complete a journal entry that reflects on past experiences.

Appropriate Skills. Think back to the time that you learned to ride a bicycle. First you learned how to mount the bike. As you adapted your balance reactions to the narrow, odd-shaped seat, you tried moving the pedals. Perhaps you fell off several times before you learned how to successfully maneuver the vehicle by pedaling and steering. After some practice, you were able to make the necessary adjustments to stay upright while steering. Eventually you were able to ride your bike to where you wanted to go.

At each step along the way you demonstrated proficiency at attaining the skills that were necessary for meeting the next challenge. Mastering the sequence of all of the steps culminated in your learning to ride a bicycle. Had any of your skills in the sequence failed to appropriately match the task (e.g., you consistently fell off of the bike; you ran into objects) you might not have persisted in your efforts to learn to ride. Attaining the necessary skills each step of the way allowed you to successfully meet each challenge of learning to ride a two-wheeled vehicle.

Plotting out a therapy plan is similar to teaching someone to ride a bike. The difficulty level of the therapy experience must match the client's skill level. Therapy guides finely tune a therapy plan to include activities that challenge and motivate the client to participate and, at every level of accomplishment, bolster his self-esteem.

Figure 11.2. *The Flow Experience Continuum*

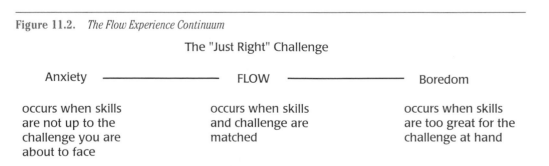

The "Just Right" Challenge

Anxiety ——————— FLOW ——————— Boredom

| occurs when skills are not up to the challenge you are about to face | occurs when skills and challenge are matched | occurs when skills are too great for the challenge at hand |

You can monitor the therapy plan by asking yourself the following sequence of questions:

1. Am I presenting activities matched to the client's skill level?
2. What challenge do the activities offer the client? (i.e., is the challenge too little, too great, or just right?).

Activities that are not challenging may lead to boredom. Conversely, activities that are too challenging may raise the client's state of arousal and lead to undue anxiety. Focused on promoting successful therapy outcomes, therapy guides plan activities that provide the right amount of challenge for the person's skill level. And because therapy guides are risk takers, they enter each therapy situation with the mindset that every activity they select may not be a match for every client the first time. Their confidence in experimenting allows them to patiently grade activities up or down until they find the "just right" challenge level for the client.

Successes help the client develop the confidence that is necessary to take risks. Each success increases the client's feeling of confidence. By building one success on another, a client gradually learns new skills. Little by little, as the client's repertoire of skills increases, the motivation to interact in ever more challenging situations increases, further expanding the client's comfort zone for tackling new and challenging situations. This ever-widening spiral of success leading to comfort and comfort leading to success can occur only when "the challenges are balanced with the person's capacity to act."[7]

Potential of Completion. In order for a therapy plan to be effective, a client's goals must be achievable within a realistic time frame. Establishing clear end points within each therapy session strengthens a client's motivation to move forward.

The worth of an activity is enhanced when it has a well-defined end point. Likewise, engaging in therapeutic activities that have a tangible point of completion develops an internal sense of completion within the client because he can visualize the target to which he is moving. The definitive end point also provides the client with a way to measure how far she is into the task and how much more she needs to do before completing it. The following scenario relates the concept of Flow to a therapy situation.

Imagine that you are working with Devin, a seven-year-old second grader. His therapy goals include developing age appropriate skills in printing, dressing, and using scissors. Because you want Devin to work at his optimal performance level, you structure the therapy experience in such a way that he feels a sense of completion throughout each element of the therapy process. You learned from Devin's mother that Devin has an active imagination. He likes to pretend that he is a building contractor, like his uncle. So you use that information in designing his therapy expedition. Devin's therapy expedition will center on your "hiring" Devin as a contractor to build your new house using blocks, scraps of wood, and construction paper for "roofing material."

The imaginary context of each session relates to the life of a building contractor working in the field. Devin begins each therapy session by changing into his "work clothes." He puts on an oversized pair of pants and a shirt that require snapping, zipping, and buttoning. When Devin is ready for "work," he receives his "construction" schedule for the session.

The activities planned for the first session include constructing the foundation, the walls, and the roof. The activities for the next sessions involve detailing the inside of the house. Whatever the activity, every session has a clearly defined beginning, middle, and end.

Upon completion of each "workday," Devin changes his clothes again (more practice with dressing skills) as he prepares to go home. He then evaluates his progress. He plans for the next session by making some brief notes on the "construction schedule" (printing skills), which he then cuts out (scissor skills) and glues into his logbook. The logbook is a reporting system for his parents. Devin carries it from home to therapy each session and uses it to communicate therapy progress to his parents. His parents use the logbook to reinforce Devin's skill development at home. Because Devin knows what the goal of each session is, he looks forward to coming to each session, and he expects to complete building his house.

The "potential of completion" concept has implications for client home programs. You will increase the probability of a client's active participation in an activity prescribed for completion at home when you present the activity in straightforward, easy-to-understand language. Each activity also must have meaning and relevance to the client's daily routine. For example, design a program to increase the child's proficiency in dressing skills that includes activities to be practiced when the child is normally engaged in dressing and undressing. Present home activities with indicators that clearly specify when the activity is complete and the goal has been met. If "putting on a front button shirt" is a goal, the therapist should specify that the home program has been completed when the child can put on a shirt and button all of the buttons without assistance.

Clients who receive home programs while they are actively engaged in therapy are more likely to participate in home activities than if they are handed a home program on their last day of treatment. If the client is actively participating in a therapy program, the therapy guide can monitor the client's home program and clearly specify the goals of each activity. The "potential of completion" then becomes a relevant part of the home program. When home activities are integrated into the therapy program from the initiation of the therapy program, the home program can be reinforced during every therapy session.

Ability to Concentrate. The ability to concentrate on a task elicits the Flow state when actions and awareness are merged. A client can concentrate on an activity best when he has a clear idea of the goals of the activity and when he is receiving feedback that he is performing the activity properly.

For a client to derive meaning and enjoyment from activities in therapy, she must be able to focus all her attention on the task. Focusing causes one to filter out irrelevant background information. The following scenario relates the "ability to concentrate" concept to a therapy situation.

Imagine that you are working with Adrienne, who is fifteen months old. Her therapy goals address developing skills in self-feeding. Your short-term goal is to teach your young client to reach for finger foods. To accurately reach for finger food Adrienne must first look at the food item for which she is reaching.

You observe that Adrienne does not seem to attend to or sustain eye contact on most objects for longer than three seconds. Hence, you add a goal that addresses Adrienne's need to look at the food as she reaches for it. You decide to begin the feeding program with Adrienne's favorite food, pretzel sticks. While pretzel sticks may not provide optimum nutrition for Adrienne, they will be a greater motivation for achieving a "look and reach for" goal than a food item in which she is not interested.

Your strategy with Adrienne is to provide her with immediate feedback each time she looks at the pretzel stick. Your plan is to lightly brush the pretzel on the palm of her hand followed by placing a small piece of the pretzel on her lips. As Adrienne's awareness and resulting concentration on the pretzel increases, you will vary the opportunities (i.e., placement of the pretzel; length of time the pretzel is placed on her palm) for her to look at and reach for the pretzel. With consistency and repetition, Adrienne learns that looking at food is the precursor to reaching for and eating it.

Adrienne learns to broaden her concentration on the food by first visually attending to it—the goal or objective of the self-feeding activity—and then reaching for it. Her reaching for the food provides immediate feedback from looking at the food.

When a client is engaged in an activity which holds meaning for him he is more likely to focus his attention on it. Tap into a client's internal interest in an activity and you tap into a reservoir of focused attention.

Effortless Involvement. One's effortless involvement in an activity contributes to the Flow state. When you are mindful of a client's interests and skill level, you are more likely to provide activities at which the individual can succeed. When the therapy guide continually engages the client in successful experiences, the client moves toward a state of Flow, enjoying the activity.

Think of an activity that you learned that required a moderate to high level of motor coordination, such as a sport or dance, then complete the following thoughts:

1. I remember the first time I learned to . . .

2. The first time that I learned the activity, I remember feeling . . .

3. I started to really enjoy the activity once I . . .

Activities become fun and enjoyable for a client when she has the necessary skills to cope with the challenges of the activity. Activities that are geared to a client's interests and skill level avoid putting stress on the client by requiring her to make moment-to-moment decisions while executing the activity. When a client is freed from physically or psychologically expending energy in thinking "What do I do?" "How do I do it?" and "Am I doing what I ought to be doing?" she can experience a sense of enjoyment or Flow from engaging in the activity. She is able to participate with effortless involvement. The following scenario illustrates the concept of "effortless involvement" in therapy.

Imagine that you are Andre's therapist. Andre is eight years old and in third grade. He receives weekly therapy at a private out-patient center. Each session is 90 minutes and is scheduled after school. He was referred to therapy because his teacher noticed that he has problems with both fine and gross motor coordination. His coordination problems affect his performance at school, his social interactions, and his performance of his home chores.

Andre lives on a small farm and is expected to help his older brothers and sisters perform daily chores around the farm. Since Andre has trouble coordinating his movements, he has many problems carrying out his share of the work. Andre's family is very supportive of his need to move slowly when executing his chores and motivates him to work hard to overcome his problems. But Andre gets frustrated with his own clumsiness.

As you plot out the therapy expedition, you plan to engage Andre in activities that will allow him to experience effortless involvement. Andre's father previously told you about Andre's vivid imagination and interest in books. You use this information to create therapy activities around the stories that Andre loves to act out. He is particularly intrigued with a fantasy story about a wizard and a group of dwarfs traveling with a hobbit.[8] The story's hobbit character is helping the dwarfs recover gold and silver taken by a horrible dragon.

The therapy expedition that you design for Andre challenges Andre to take on the role of the hobbit. You help Andre imagine ways to help the dwarfs recover their lost treasure. In your plan, Andre will "travel" through the "land" on a pony disguised as a scooter board. He will begin his journey by traveling through the dark and misty haunted forest. The haunted forest is created by large plastic traffic cones, bolsters, and hoola hoops that are covered with cardboard trees taped to them.

During one therapy session, to reach the mountain where he can help the dwarfs, Andre practices his skill maneuvering through the forest and then through a series of tunnels. The tunnels are created by floor mats set up like pup tents. Andre must pass through the tunnels very quietly as he tries to avoid bumping into the tunnel walls. If he hits a tunnel, he risks being captured by the trolls, who will "roast him for their supper." Once he gets through the tunnels and arrives at the mountain, Andre must find a way to help the dwarfs recover their stolen treasure.

To recover the stolen treasure, Andre must engage in a series of visual motor activities that include many challenges. He must decipher a secret code that opens the concealed door to the mountain and place a set of shapes into a form board before a timer goes off. He also must "return to his homeland" with the silver and gold treasure before he is captured by the evil force. The treasure is tucked away in a backpack, filled with weighted objects, that Andre straps to his body.

During another therapy session, Andre returns to visit the forest. The forest has thickened and the trees have grown closer together. Andre must alter the speed of his movement around the trees. The closely spaced trees mandate that he move slowly to avoid being caught by the evil tree roots that lurk close to the surface.

Andre's challenge is increased by the addition of a weighted backpack, the threat of being caught by an evil force, and trees that are closer together. Andre experiences effortless involvement because the activity is supported by his desire to return safely to his homeland.

Andre's mystical adventure also met the first three criteria for a Flow experience. Andre had the appropriate skill to explore the magical land. You the therapist built a sense of completion into each phase of the activity; for example, Andre's goals included maneuvering around the tunnels and trees without touching their sides and returning home safely from the journey without being caught. The clearly stated goals provided immediate feedback to Andre. He knew whether he had achieved his goal according to the designated criteria. Establishing these criteria helped Andre concentrate and focus on the activity.

And Andre had fun. He was completely absorbed in the activity. From your perspective as the therapy guide, Andre's adventure was the just right challenge that allowed him to develop an accurate sense of how his body moves in space and through time. His knowledge of how to move his body contributed to the development in his brain of a "map" of his movements. This "map" is his body percept or body scheme. An accurate body percept contributed to Andre's motor planning abilities and an improved ability to carry out his daily tasks (play, self-care, school activities, and chores).

Sense of Control. One's ability to exercise a sense of control over one's own actions contributes to the Flow state. When a client has the opportunity to make choices during therapy, she can assume some control over her own therapy process. Whenever possible, provide the client with an opportunity to exercise control over the choice of activities and to participate in the goal selection process. The client who is allowed to exercise a sense of control in the therapy process is more likely to enjoy therapy than if she is a passive recipient.

REFLECTIVE JOURNAL ENTRY 11.9

Complete the following thoughts:

1. *My most recent experience of feeling "in control" of a situation was when . . .*

2. *At the time of the experience described above, I felt this way because . . .*

Therapy guides value the client's need to make choices during the therapy session. Allowing the client to make choices during therapy taps into the client's inner drive to participate. Through the act of making a choice, the client is taking responsibility for her own actions. Clients who are empowered to make choices during therapy gain confidence in creatively solving their own problems outside the therapy setting.

REFLECTIVE JOURNAL ENTRY 11.10

Reflect on Andre's adventure and identify three ways he might exercise a sense of control over his actions while acting out his storybook fantasy, then complete the following thoughts:

Andre might increase his feeling of being "in control" of the adventure by . . .

a.

b.

c.

Some ways in which Andre might increase his feeling of being "in control" during his fantasy include the following: Andre could control the direction of the path through the enchanted land by arranging the position of the trees; he could control the speed at which he was to travel by increasing or decreasing the spacing of the trees in the forest and the width of the tunnel; he could control the length of time it would take him to go through the forest; he could control the position he chose to ride his pony (scooter board).

Loss of the Sense of Self. Losing one's sense of self within an activity contributes to the Flow state. When you observe young children playing, laughing, and acting silly, their actions clearly demonstrate a loss of the sense of self. Young children easily lose themselves in play because they do not engage in self-scrutiny. They have not yet developed the inner voice of judgment that causes adults to be self-conscious. They are experts at becoming totally absorbed in whatever activity they are involved in at the moment.

REFLECTIVE JOURNAL ENTRY 11.11

Complete the following thoughts:

1. The last time that I became completely absorbed in an activity was when . . .

2. At the time of the activity described above I felt . . .

3. After completing the activity described above I felt . . .

A client will more likely become absorbed in a therapy plan that is designed around his interests, has clearly delineated goals, and is well organized than one that is imposed on him. Let's consider how Andre's therapy plan (previously described) could allow him to experience a loss of his sense of self.

Andre can get lost in the atmosphere of excitement and suspense embedded in the design of his adventure. As the therapy guide, you can sustain and encourage the fun and excitement of the activity by entering into Andre's fantasy world and limiting the amount of control exerted over him while he is engaged in the activity. If Andre can put forth psychic energy independently during his adventure, he will derive more enjoyment and benefit from the therapy experience when it has ended.

Altered Sense of Time. An altered sense of time results in a Flow state. When one has a Flow experience the rhythms of the activity define the time. Reference points outside of the event such as the duration of time measured by a clock seem to have little meaning. Time becomes distorted and hours pass in what seems like minutes. Research studies on Flow experiences show that when one is in a state of Flow one's perception of time fails to match the actual duration of time in which the event occurs.

REFLECTIVE JOURNAL ENTRY 11.12

Complete the following thoughts:

1. *The last recollection I had when time seemed to "fly" by was when I . . .*

2. *While I was involved in the activity described above I felt . . .*

3. *After completing the event described above I felt . . .*

The adage "Time flies when you're having fun" fits the Flow experience. When a client asks, "We're done already?" or exclaims, "It can't be time to go already!" or "Oh, please, just a little bit longer!" more than likely your client has experienced a state of Flow.

Triggering Elements of Flow

Clients benefit greatly from therapy sessions that involve Flow experiences. Their desire to learn and to take on more new challenges increases. While you may not be able to bring all seven elements of Flow into each therapy experience, you will increase the client's productivity by promoting as many elements of Flow as possible.

To orchestrate a Flow experience for a client, identify the client's interests and abilities and use your observation skills. Imagine that you are working with Ana Maria, a fifteen-year-old adolescent who demonstrates profound deficits in cognition and movement. She is limited in her ability to interact with objects and people. To guide your thinking as you work with Ana Maria, ask yourself the following questions:

1. What little things make her smile?
2. What movement stimulates her to vocalize?
3. What object stimulates her to reach?
4. If she reacts to a stimulus, what is the duration of the reaction?
5. When the stimulus is removed, does she notice that it is no longer present?
6. Does she manifest any observable signs of searching for the stimulus after it is removed from her view?

These are the kinds of questions that a therapy guide might ask herself when trying to determine the capabilities of a client who lacks expressive communication skills. Your goal is to discover the elements within the environment that you perceive bring happiness and enjoyment to the client. The next step is to build on those elements by incorporating them into the therapy session.

A therapy session that taps into the client's inner drive will motivate the client to perform optimally in mind, body, and spirit. The path to optimal experiences must begin with a meaningful activity.

REFLECTIVE JOURNAL ENTRY 11.13

Reflect on a personal experience and complete the following thoughts:

1. A meaningful activity that I recall within the past year was . . .

2. I can recount the following five details surrounding the activity:

   a.

   b.

   c.

   d.

   e.

3. I still remember feeling . . .

The details of the activity seem to be carved into your memory as though it just happened yesterday. Because you were deeply involved with the situation at the time, you were actively committed to each of the conditions and the outcome of the situation.

"Flow Checklist"

Now let's return to Louise's Nose Blowing Expedition and analyze her therapy plan using the **"Flow Checklist" Thinking Key** Field Organizer, which appears below. The Field Organizer has two columns. Column A lists the seven criteria of the Flow experience; column B explains how the criteria is present in the activity being analyzed.

Practice using the "Flow Checklist" Thinking Key by completing the Field Organizer with reference to the Nose Blowing Expedition. This activity may be done in pairs or individually. When you complete the Field Organizer with a partner, you have the advantage of expanding your way of looking at each item on the checklist.

DIRECTIONS

1. Read the Flow Criteria in column A.
2. Think "off the page" to infer what activities might have occurred to cause a Flow state in Louise's expedition.
3. In column B, record one indication that each criteria for the Flow state in rows 2–7 was present in the activities during Louise's therapy expedition.

FIELD ORGANIZER

"Flow Checklist"

A Flow Criteria	B Indication That Flow Criteria Was Present
1. Possesses the *appropriate skills* to perform the activity.	*Children were successful at a series of nose blowing activities that were developmentally sequenced for them.*
2. Indicated a sense of the *potential of completion* (goal directed) of the activity.	

(continued)

A **Flow Criteria**	B **Indication That Flow Criteria Was Present**
3. *Able to concentrate* on activity.	
4. Evidence of *effortless involvement* while participating in activity.	
5. Experience a *sense of control* while participating in activity.	
6. Indication of *loss of self* (became absorbed) while performing activity.	
7. Indication that the *sense of time was altered* while participating in activity.	

The Nose Blowing Expedition qualifies as a Flow experience. The Flow experience evolved out of a series of steps that took Louise through many creative (Generating Phase) and critical thinking (Focusing Phase) processes. Some of the elements of Flow are explicitly stated, while others are conjectured.

Both creative and critical thinking processes are necessary to develop a successful action plan. Creative thinking (used in the Generating Phase) helps build a vision. Critical thinking (used in the Focusing Phase) helps develop a plan to carry out the vision. Both types of thinking are crucial to creating an action plan that is interesting and well thought out.

In Section 13 you will have an opportunity to further develop the knowledge and skill you have gained using CPS in Sections 1–11.

Symbol for Acceptance Finding

The picture of two hands embraced in a handshake represents Acceptance Finding. The handshake symbolizes the process of gathering support from the therapy expedition travelers for the action plan. Acceptance and support for the action plan contributes to the success of the action plan. Whenever you see the handshake icon, you are being reminded to use Acceptance Finding.

Mind Map Guidelines

1. Place the section's main concept in the center of the space using pictures or words or both.
2. Radiate ideas from the central thought.
   - Use images (be sure to use color).
   - Headline text—one or two words per line.
   - Print text (for easy reading).
3. Link the main concepts and generate more ideas from the linkages.
4. Have fun!

Remember, the more linkages that you generate between elements, the greater your ability to see how all the elements relate to one another.

Section 11
SELF-ASSESSMENT

Now that I have completed the eleventh part of my journey, I can:

○ explain the purpose of identifying forms of "support" and "resistance" when planning a therapy expedition

○ use the "Potential Sources of Support and Resistance" Thinking Key to identify the supporters and resisters of the action plan

○ identify the factors that influence how people deal with change

○ identify the two kinds of change that influence therapy outcomes

○ describe mindsets that support change and those that are barriers to change

○ identify three context-related factors that support change

○ develop an action plan with the "Generating Potential Actions" Thinking Key

○ use the "LIST" Thinking Key to organize actions into long-term, intermediate, and short-term plans

○ develop an action plan using the "Planning for Action" Thinking Key

○ develop an action plan with the "What's Next? Question Series," "If–Then," "What If . . . ? Question Series," and "Think Positive" Thinking Keys

○ finalize a plan using the "Action Plan Adoption Checklist" Thinking Key

○ explain how to gather feedback about an action plan using the "Preparing to Seek Feedback" Thinking Key

○ use the "Flow Checklist" Thinking Key to evaluate a treatment plan

NOTES

1. Stephen Covey, *First Things First* (New York: Simon & Schuster, 1994).
2. There are inventories that measure various aspects of a person's personality profile. One such inventory is the Myers-Briggs Type Indicator (MBTI). The MBTI is based on Carl Jung's theory of psychological types. The inventory renders a profile on four scales: introverted or extroverted, sensing or intuitive, thinking or feeling, and judging or perceiving. I. B. Myers and M. H. McCaulley, *Manual: A Guide to the Development and Use of the Myers-Briggs Type Indicator* (Palo Alto, Calif.: Consulting Psychologists Press, 1985).
3. R. M. Kanter, *The Change Masters: Innovation for Productivity in the American Corporation* (New York: Simon & Schuster, 1983).
4. There is some evidence based on research findings that once you engage in a new task or activity, the partially completed efforts become part of your subconscious. The incomplete efforts haunt you more than those tasks that are on your "to do" list of items not yet begun. Alex Osborn refers to this "haunting" feelings as the "incubation period." Once the idea starts to incubate, your conscious mind starts to search for additional facts and tentative ideas. Soon a concentration of thoughts and feelings develop and an automatic flow of associated ideas begins to emerge and give birth to even more ideas. According to Osborn, "through strenuous effort we indirectly induce 'idle' illumination" of ideas (*Applied Imagination*, 3d ed. rev. [New York: Charles Scribner's Sons, 1963], 117).
5. E. M. Rogers, *Diffusion of Innovations* (New York: Free Press, 1983).
6. Mihalyi Csikszentmihalyi, *Flow: The Psychology of Optimal Experience* (New York: HarperCollins, 1991). Csikszentmihalyi, a psychologist at the University of Chicago, studied the phenomena of optimal experience. He was primarily interested in finding out what makes an activity so genuinely satisfying that a person wants to engage only in that activity and nothing else.

He defines Flow as "the [psychological] state in which people are so involved in an activity that nothing else seems to matter; the experience itself is so enjoyable that people will do it even at a great cost, for the sheer sake of doing it" (4).

7. Ibid., 52.
8. Tolkien, J. R. R. *The Hobbit* (New York: Ballantine Books, 1937).

Show and Tell: Test Your Knowledge of CPS

Itinerary #12

At the end of the twelfth part of your journey, you will be able to:

✓ evaluate your knowledge of CPS

Now it's time to evaluate your knowledge of CPS by playing Show and Tell. Show and Tell is a team game that will let you see what you have learned about CPS. The game has 11 parts, referred to as rounds. Each round represents a section in Unit I and consists of 20 items. In each round you and your team will answer a series of questions targeting the main points in each section.

Look over this section before you begin. You will find game directions followed by Show and Tell Rounds 1–11 and the CPS Scoreboard. All answers are in Appendix A. The game can be played in teams of two or more. If you are playing alone, use the game as a study guide.

DIRECTIONS

1. Divide into Team A and Team B. Team A will begin the game.
2. Each team designates a Referee; at the end of each round, the team selects a new Referee. The Referee determines whether responses offered by the group members match the answers in the Show and Tell Reference Guide in Appendix A.
3. Start with Show and Tell Round 1, question 1, in the column labeled Questions for Team A. Begin the game with both teams reading the question. Team A responds first. The two Referees then compare the team's answer to the answer in Appendix A. If they agree that the answer is "correct," the Team A Referee records one point in the column labeled A directly to the right of the question. If Team A is unable to respond correctly to the question, Team B has an opportunity to answer. If the Referees agree that Team B's response is correct, the Referee for Team B records one point in the column labeled B to the right of the question.
4. If neither Team A nor Team B responds correctly, a Referee reads the correct answer and neither team scores.
5. Team B continues the game by answering question 1 in the column labeled Questions for Team B. If Team B answers the question correctly, they receive a point. If Team B is unable to answer the item, Team A has a chance to answer the item and score a point.
6. The game continues with Team A followed by Team B responding to the questions in their respective columns.
7. When all questions have been answered, the Referees add the points in all four columns and record the subtotals. The Referee for Team A adds up the points in both A columns and enters the total in the space marked Total for Team A. The Referee for Team B adds up the points in both B columns and enters the total for Team B.
8. The Referees record the points each team received for the round on the CPS Scoreboard. The team with the highest score at the end of the round receives a star in the Ta-Dah column.
9. Continue playing Rounds 2–11, following steps 3–8.

Show and Tell Round 1 (Section 1)

Questions for Team A	A	B	Questions for Team B	A	B
1. Name the term currently used to describe the simultaneous thought processes of a therapist.			1. Name the two authors of *Clinical Reasoning: Forms of Inquiry in a Therapeutic Practice.*		
2. Explain how balancing plates on vertical rods can be used as a metaphor to describe how a therapist processes information.			2. What do the authors of *Clinical Reasoning: Forms of Inquiry in a Therapeutic Practice* call the kind of clinical reasoning that has three parts: procedural, interactive, and conditional.		
3. Thinking strategies are used for what purpose?			3. Explain how the metaphor of riding a train to get to the light at the end of a tunnel can be used to describe what a skilled therapist does.		
4. What is the name for thinking strategies in this field book?			4. What does the acronym CPS stand for?		
5. Why does the word *clinical* in "clinical reasoning" fail to accurately describe what therapists do in practice?			5. Why does the word *reasoning* in "clinical reasoning" fail to describe accurately what therapists do in practice?		
6. What is the difference between creative solutions and ready-made solutions?			6. When therapists begin to solve a problem why should they first check to see if a ready-made solution will work?		
7. Give one example of the use of creativity in therapy.			7. Give one example of the use of creativity in therapy.		
8. What does it mean to think out of the box?			8. What innate ability helps you to think out of the box?		
9. Name one way children begin questions when they are wondering about the nature of things.			9. Name one way children begin questions when they are wondering about the nature of things.		
10. Why are CPS skills needed when change is a constant?			10. Why is it necessary for a therapist to think on his or her feet?		
Subtotals			*Subtotals*		
Total for Team A			*Total for Team B*		
Score *9–10 Clear as a bell.* *7–8 You did well.* *6 and ↓ It's time to excel.*			*Score* *9–10 Clear as a bell.* *7–8 You did well.* *6 and ↓ It's time to excel.*		

Show and Tell Round 2 (Section 2)

Questions for Team A	A	B	Questions for Team B	A	B
1. The problem solving model presented in this field book is based on the research of what three researchers?			1. Name the two originators of the CPS model.		
2. Name the originator of the term *brainstorming*.			2. Osborn believed that ideas flow best in the absence of either positive or negative _____ . (Complete the sentence.)		
3. Name the phenomenon that invites illumination or sudden flashes of brilliance after a period of purposeful relaxation.			3. Name the three components in the CPS process presented in this field book.		
4. What two-word phrases describe the three components of the CPS process?			4. Name the three stages in Get Ready to understand the problem.		
5. Name the "finding" stages in Get Set to find a solution and Go Forward with an action plan.			5. Is there a prescribed sequence for the components and stages of the CPS process? Explain.		
6. Why does each stage of the CPS process end with the word *finding*?			6. What does the star shape symbolize in the CPS model presented in this field book?		
7. What are the three parts of the OT process that correspond to Get Ready to understand the problem in the CPS process?			7. Identify the four parts of the OT process that correspond to Get Set to find a solution and Go Forward with an action plan in the CPS process.		
8. Describe how a diamond shape can represent the Generating and Focusing Phases.			8. Distinguish between Deferred Judgment and Affirmative Judgment.		
9. Describe the relationship between the two guidelines used in the Generating Phase.			9. Distinguish between "hitchhiking" and "free-wheeling."		
10. Name and explain the three guidelines used in the Focusing Phase.			10. Explain the use of a "doability" scale.		
Subtotals			Subtotals		
Total for Team A			Total for Team B		
Score 9–10 Clear as a bell. 7–8 You did well. 6 and ↓ It's time to excel.			Score 9–10 Clear as a bell. 7–8 You did well. 6 and ↓ It's time to excel.		

Show and Tell Round 3 (Section 3)

Questions for Team A	A	B	Questions for Team B	A	B
1. Describe the two kinds of journeys described in this field book.			1. How do therapy guides use their heads and their hearts to select the right route for a therapy expedition?		
2. Provide an example showing how the "What's Next? Question Series" Thinking Key helps a therapy guide envision the future path of the therapy route.			2. Create a hypothesis using the "If–Then" Thinking Key and explain how generating hypothesis statements helps create an unfolding narrative in the client's therapy expedition.		
3. Name the five qualities associated with the mindset of a therapy guide.			3. Describe two characteristics of a guide who tolerates ambiguity.		
4. Provide an example of examining worst/best-case scenarios using the "What If?" Thinking Key.			4. Why does taking risks involve moving beyond one's comfort zone?		
5. Provide an example of a therapy guide flexibly responding to a change. The example should demonstrate the ability of the therapy guide to see a change as an opportunity.			5. Why is it important for a therapy guide to think positively about a problem?		
6. Describe the role of empathy in a therapy guide's mindset.			6. Why is a therapy guide on a continuous quest for information while on a therapy expedition?		
7. Why is occupational therapy described as a "reflective practice"?			7. What do you "drop" when you use the "Stop, Drop, and Listen" Thinking Key?		
8. What is the importance of watching for cues and looking for patterns on a therapy expedition?			8. How do paradigms provide a filter by which we examine all information?		
9. How does reframing a problem require a paradigm shift?			9. How do the Thinking Keys "Consider Other Viewpoints" and "Think Positive" help you reframe a problem?		
10. Provide an example of how a change in context can influence the paradigm in which a decision is made.			10. How is intuition like having a compass on an expedition?		
Subtotals			*Subtotals*		
Total for Team A			*Total for Team B*		
Score *9–10 Clear as a bell.* *7–8 You did well.* *6 and ↓ It's time to excel.*			*Score* *9–10 Clear as a bell.* *7–8 You did well.* *6 and ↓ It's time to excel.*		

Show and Tell Round 4 (Section 4)

Questions for Team A	A	B	Questions for Team B	A	B
1. Name the paradigm that unifies all areas of occupational therapy practice.			1. Name the three categories of Performance Areas.		
2. Why does a therapy guide look at each client from the broad scope of all three performance areas?			2. What influence does context have on a person's occupational performance?		
3. Provide an illustration where a problem that is solved under one set of circumstances (context) can become a new problem when the context changes.			3. How does a therapy guide determine whether a client's referral to therapy falls within the realm of occupational therapy services?		
4. Explain the difference between Performance Areas and Performance Components.			4. Identify the uniform system used to communicate the three domains of occupational therapy practice adopted by AOTA.		
5. What are the three domains used in Uniform Terminology?			5. Depending upon the perspective, a therapy guide may choose to place a client's occupational performance in one main area or another. Explain.		
6. What are the three categories within the domain of Performance Components?			6. What are the two categories within the domain of Performance Contexts?		
7. Name eight of the subcategories under the Performance Area ADL?			7. What are the four subcategories under Performance Areas: work and productive activities?		
8. What are the two subcategories under Performance Area: play and leisure?			8. What are the three subcategories under Performance Components: sensorimotor component?		
9. What are the three subcategories under Performance Component: psychosocial skills?			9. What are the five subcategories under Performance Components: cognitive integration and cognitive components?		
10. What are the four subcategories under Performance Contexts: temporal aspects?			10. What are the three subcategories under Performance Contexts: environment?		
Subtotals			*Subtotals*		
Total for Team A			*Total for Team B*		
Score *9–10 Clear as a bell.* *7–8 You did well.* *6 and ↓ It's time to excel.*			*Score* *9–10 Clear as a bell.* *7–8 You did well.* *6 and ↓ It's time to excel.*		

Show and Tell Round 5 (Section 5)

Questions for Team A	A	B	Questions for Team B	A	B
1. What are the seven Thinking Keys designed to help a therapy guide prepare to use the CPS process?			1. Explain how individual differences play a role in the process of solving problems.		
2. What does it mean to share ownership of a problem while on a therapy expedition?			2. Identify four criteria that help to determine whether an individual is a candidate to share in the ownership of a problem.		
3. Why does a client need to recognize that there is a gap between "what is" and "what should be"?			3. Why must a client be able to measure the gap in order to know when progress is made in solving his or her problem?		
4. Why must a person have a need to solve a problem in order to solve it?			4. What kinds of resources must a person have access to in order to solve a problem?		
5. Provide an illustration of a therapy guide seeing a problem from a client's perspective (developing a shared vision).			5. State three questions that will help you understand a client's problem.		
6. How might a therapy guide collaborate with a client in an effort to build "bridges" of understanding?			6. Provide an example of a well-structured problem.		
7. What is the difference between a well-structured problem and an ill-structured problem?			7. What are the three characteristics of a ill-structured problem?		
8. Provide an example of a ill-structured problem.			8. Why was Louise's problem on the Nose Blowing Expedition an ill-structured problem?		
9. How was Louise like an explorer on the Nose Blowing Expedition?			9. What steps are taken in "Highlighting" Part 2?		
10. Identify what the acronym PACC stands for.			10. What can the "PACC" Thinking Key be used for on a therapy expedition?		
Subtotals			*Subtotals*		
Total for Team A			*Total for Team B*		
Score *9–10 Clear as a bell.* *7–8 You did well.* *6 and ↓ It's time to excel.*			*Score* *9–10 Clear as a bell.* *7–8 You did well.* *6 and ↓ It's time to excel.*		

Show and Tell Round 6 (Section 6)

Questions for Team A	A	B	Questions for Team B	A	B
1. CPS is a flexible problem solving model. Explain.			1. How can Opportunity Finding help you to better understand a client's needs?		
2. How does the name Opportunity Finding place a positive frame around the client's problem?			2. State four questions that identify the broad challenges, concerns, and opportunities within the problem during Opportunity Finding.		
3. When can you skip Opportunity Finding and move directly to Data Finding?			3. What does the invitational stem "WIBGI . . ." mean and how does it expand your thinking about the situation?		
4. What does the word *visionizing* mean?			4. Your goal in Opportunity Finding is to capture the scope of the client's problem, not to define the problem. Explain.		
5. Why should WIBGI questions be kept broad and brief?			5. How does using the invitational stem "WIBGI . . ." create a positive mindset to seek opportunities?		
6. How do you know when you have generated enough WIBGI questions?			6. Explain how to use the "Head and Shoulders Test" Thinking Key.		
7. In what situation would you use the "Highlighting" Thinking Key rather than the "Head and Shoulders Test"?			7. What does it mean to cluster information?		
8. What are the "Hits" used in the "Highlighting" process?			8. What occurs in Part 1 of the "Highlighting" process?		
9. What occurs in Part 2 of the "Highlighting" process?			9. What occurs in Part 3 of the "Highlighting" process?		
10. Get Ready to understand the problem represents 1/4, 1/2, or 3/4 of the CPS process?			10. What is the symbol used in Opportunity Finding?		
Subtotals			*Subtotals*		
Total for Team A			*Total for Team B*		
Score *9–10 Clear as a bell.* *7–8 You did well.* *6 and ↓ It's time to excel.*			*Score* *9–10 Clear as a bell.* *7–8 You did well.* *6 and ↓ It's time to excel.*		

Show and Tell Round 7 (Section 7)

Questions for Team A	A	B	Questions for Team B	A	B
1. Data Finding always precedes Opportunity Finding. True or False? Explain.			1. What are the three stages of the component Understanding the Problem?		
2. What is the focus of Data Finding?			2. How does a person qualify as a resource person on a therapy expedition?		
3. Provide two examples of therapy expeditions that illustrate how resource people vary from one expedition to the next.			3. How is a resource person like a flashlight's light beam?		
4. Why is it important to record everyone's thoughts during Data Finding?			4. How is the wish statement generated in Opportunity Finding like the tip of the iceberg?		
5. Provide an example of the kind of data derived from asking "What" questions.			5. Provide an example of data derived from asking "How" questions.		
6. How does being familiar with the context in which the problem occurs help you be more adept at identifying creative solutions?			6. What is the reason for performing the "5 Ws & an H?" and the "5 Ws & an H else?" Thinking Keys within a group?		
7. How are the "5 Ws & an H" and the "5 Ws & an H else" Thinking Keys related?			7. Compare the Focusing Phases of Opportunity Finding and Data Finding.		
8. Why is only Part 1 of "Highlighting" used in the Focusing Phase of Data Finding?			8. What is the main use of the "Storytelling" Thinking Key?		
9. For what do you use the "Storytelling" Thinking Key?			9. What is the value of extracting a theme from each story element?		
10. How does the data generated during Data Finding serve as a reference point throughout CPS?			10. How does the symbol of the computer and the heart on the computer screen represent the Data Finding stage?		
Subtotals			*Subtotals*		
Total for Team A			*Total for Team B*		
Score *9–10 Clear as a bell.* *7–8 You did well.* *6 and ↓ It's time to excel.*			*Score* *9–10 Clear as a bell.* *7–8 You did well.* *6 and ↓ It's time to excel.*		

Show and Tell Round 8 (Section 8)

Questions for Team A	A	B	Questions for Team B	A	B
1. Distinguish between Opportunity Finding and Problem Finding.			1. How does having a vision on a therapy expedition relate to goal setting?		
2. What does the phrase "begin with an end in mind" mean to a therapy guide on a therapy expedition?			2. How does having a vision help a client get back on "course" after taking a detour during an expedition?		
3. What does it mean to restructure or reframe a problem?			3. What effect does using the invitational stem "IWWM" have on your thinking?		
4. How do you combine the invitational stem "IWWM . . ." with the phrase "Who does what" to generate problem statements?			4. How does formulating a problem statement using the "IWWM . . . Who–Does–What?" Thinking Key create thoughts toward formulating a future vision?		
5. What is the purpose of the "Substitution" Thinking Key?			5. What is the function of the word "Who" in the "IWWM . . . Who–Does–What?" Thinking Key?		
6. What does the word "Does" in the "IWWM . . . Who–Does–What?" Thinking Key cause you to think about?			6. What does the "What" in the "IWWM . . . Who–Does–What?" Thinking Key cause you to think about?		
7. How does the "Substitution" Thinking Key help to create alternative wording for a problem statement?			7. What does asking "Why" questions do to a problem statement?		
8. How does asking "How" questions narrow a problem statement?			8. What are the two Thinking Keys used in the Focusing Phase of Problem Finding?		
9. What is the function of the "Hits" in the Focusing Phase of Problem Finding?			9. What part of the "Highlighting" process is dedicated to looking for relationships among the Hits?		
10. When you restate a Hot Spot, why do you want to avoid making the restatement too broad or too narrow?			10. Why does the magnifying glass symbolize the Problem Finding stage?		
Subtotals			*Subtotals*		
Total for Team A			*Total for Team B*		
Score *9–10 Clear as a bell.* *7–8 You did well.* *6 and ↓ It's time to excel.*			*Score* *9–10 Clear as a bell.* *7–8 You did well.* *6 and ↓ It's time to excel.*		

Show and Tell Round 9 (Section 9)

Questions for Team A	A	B	Questions for Team B	A	B
1. How many stages make up the component Get Ready to find a solution?			1. Is the emphasis in Idea Finding on the Generating or the Focusing Phase?		
2. Identify three sources you rely on when you generate ideas.			2. How does quantity breed quality?		
3. Why is it important to look for value in some part of every idea?			3. What are four qualities associated with creative performance?		
4. Which quality of creative performance does the "Brainstorming" Thinking Key help to develop?			4. Why is it important not to judge and evaluate during brainstorming?		
5. What effect does internal evaluation have on the flow of ideas?			5. What is the name given to the leader of a brainstorming session?		
6. What benefit is derived from using self-sticking notes during a brainstorming session?			6. What effect does eliciting help from others have on your point of view?		
7. Which quality of creative performance does the "CAMPERS" Thinking Key help to develop?			7. What does the acronym "CAMPERS" stand for?		
8. Which quality of creative performance does the "Force Fit" Thinking Key help to develop?			8. How does adding a new stimulus to a problem solving session help the mind get unstuck?		
9. What are three sources you can use to identify a random stimulus when using the "Force Fit" Thinking Key?			9. Which quality of creative performance does the "Attribute Listing" Thinking Key help to develop?		
10. How do you use the Thinking Key "Attribute Listing"?			10. What is the purpose of the "Reach for the Sky/Stick to the Basics" Criteria Guide?		
Subtotals			*Subtotals*		
Total for Team A			*Total for Team B*		
Score *9–10 Clear as a bell.* *7–8 You did well.* *6 and ↓ It's time to excel.*			*Score* *9–10 Clear as a bell.* *7–8 You did well.* *6 and ↓ It's time to excel.*		

Show and Tell Round 10 (Section 10)

Questions for Team A	A	B	Questions for Team B	A	B
1. Go Forward with an action plan is made up of what two stages?			1. Is the emphasis in Solution Finding on the Generating or the Focusing Phase?		
2. Why does a therapy guide need to evaluate the criteria used to make decisions on a therapy expedition?			2. How does the "Will It . . . ?" Thinking Key work?		
3. What does the acronym TRACS stand for?			3. How do you use the "TRACS" Thinking Key to expand your thinking about the time, resources, acceptability, cost, or space requirements of an option?		
4. How do you use the "Make an Idea More Acceptable" Thinking Key?			4. When you use the "In-tuit" Thinking Key what source of criteria do you use?		
5. What value is derived by blending the emotional with the rational mind?			5. How do therapy guides build their confidence using intuition to make decisions?		
6. What does the acronym AL-O stand for?			6. How can a therapy guide use the "AL-O" Thinking Key to help overcome a limitation of a proposed action?		
7. What is the purpose of the "Evaluation Matrix" Thinking Key?			7. What are two different kinds of rating scales that can be used in the "Evaluation Matrix"?		
8. How does the evaluation matrix help prevent you from becoming biased toward your favorite options?			8. Compare the "Evaluation Matrix" and the "PCA" (Paired Comparison Analysis) Thinking Keys.		
9. When can a rule of thumb become a mindtrap?			9. What are the three subcategories of the "Availability" Rule of Thumb?		
10. What does the "Anchoring and Adjustment Phenomenon" Rule of Thumb relate to?			10. Provide an example that shows how the "Representativeness Bias" Rule of Thumb can become a mindtrap.		
Subtotals			Subtotals		
Total for Team A			Total for Team B		
Score 9–10 Clear as a bell. 7–8 You did well. 6 and ↓ It's time to excel.			Score 9–10 Clear as a bell. 7–8 You did well. 6 and ↓ It's time to excel.		

Show and Tell Round 11 (Section 11)

Questions for Team A	A	B	Questions for Team B	A	B
1. Distinguish between Solution Finding and Acceptance Finding.			1. Distinguish between sources of support and sources of resistance.		
2. Provide an example of how one person can be both a source of support and a source of resistance on a therapy expedition.			2. What three factors influence the extent to which a person is able to accept change?		
3. Identify the two broad kinds of change a therapy guide might be faced with on an expedition?			3. What are the five pairs of mindsets used in the "Check the Mindset" Thinking Key?		
4. What three context-related factors support change?			4. What questions do you answer when you use the "Generating Potential Actions" Thinking Key?		
5. Why does a therapy guide want to begin an expedition with an end in mind?			5. What does the "LIST" Thinking Key help you do?		
6. What six questions does the "Plan for Action" Thinking Key use to help you develop the specific actions for the therapy plan?			6. What Field Organizer is used in conjunction with the "Plan for Action" Thinking Key?		
7. What four Thinking Keys can you use in Acceptance Finding to project your thinking into the future by broadening your perspective of the actions you are about to take?			7. What are five factors to consider as you finalize the action plan?		
8. Why is it essential that a therapy guide gather feedback from members of the therapy expedition?			8. What is another name for the "just right challenge"?		
9. Why is it necessary to design therapy activities that are matched to the client's skill level and have the possibility of completion?			9. How is a client's ability to concentrate on an activity related to the ability to experience effortless involvement in the activity?		
10. Why is it important for a client to have a sense of control over the activities he or she performs in therapy?			10. What value is derived from triggering elements of Flow on a therapy expedition?		
Subtotals			*Subtotals*		
Total for Team A			*Total for Team B*		
Score *9–10 Clear as a bell.* *7–8 You did well.* *6 and ↓ It's time to excel.*			*Score* *9–10 Clear as a bell.* *7–8 You did well.* *6 and ↓ It's time to excel.*		

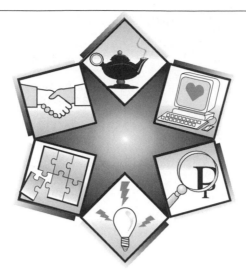

CPS Scoreboard

Team A			Team B		
Round	Ta-Dah	Points Received	Round	Ta-Dah	Points Received
1			1		
2			2		
3			3		
4			4		
5			5		
6			6		
7			7		
8			8		
9			9		
10			10		
11			11		
Total			Total		

Practice Applying CPS to the Occupational Therapy Process

*I*n Unit II, you will have an opportunity to practice using CPS by applying the Thinking Keys to two of the three stories provided about people who received occupational therapy. Two of the stories are about young children. The first child, Sam, is a preschooler with neurodevelopmental and sensory processing problems. The second child, Kaitlyn, is a toddler with a congenital amputation. The third story is about Mary, an adolescent with developmental disabilities; her therapy expedition leads her to planning for her future—prevocational training. You are invited to join Sam's therapy expedition in Section 13. In Section 14, you will choose either Mary's or Kaitlyn's story and design your own therapy expedition.

As you travel through Sections 13 and 14, you will have four kinds of learning experiences associated with each story.

Learning Experiences in Sections 13 and 14

Story: Distill information from the story that relates to the occupational therapy process and CPS.

Reflective Journal Entries: Recognize your personal thoughts, feelings, and insights about the story through the process of journaling.

Mind Mapping: Link information from the story to the therapy expedition "itinerary" by relying on the creative potential of a Mind Map; develop skill at connecting information from your mind to the "outside world" of the story.

Thinking Keys and Field Organizers: Develop skill using the Thinking Keys and Field Organizers to expand your thinking and creatively solve problems.

Story

The stories that you will read in Sections 13 and 14 were selected because they are outstanding examples of problems that were solved creatively within the context of occupational therapy practice.

"Sam Finds Help and Hope" is told by Sam's mother, Anne Miller. Sam's therapy expedition sensitizes you to some of the issues that face occupational therapists who work with children. What is most important is that the child's family (or primary caregiver) is an integral part of the therapy process. Sam's story provides a detailed account of his mother's perceptions of life with a child with severe sensory processing problems. She describes her

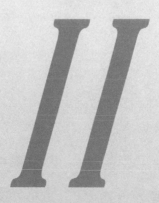

U N I T

II

feelings about and frustrations with her son, the creative way she worked with occupational therapists, and the steps she took to ameliorating his sensory processing difficulties.

This story presents a historical perspective of Sam from birth through his entry into the school system. The therapy frames of reference or paradigms for this story are neurodevelopmental and sensory integration therapy. Sam's story will be referred to in Section 13 as "Sam's SI (Sensory Integration) Expedition."

"Putting Cosmetic Prostheses to Work" describes how Victor Espinoza, an occupational therapist working in a skilled nursing facility, taught a toddler how to use a cosmetic hand prosthesis. This story, told from the therapist's perspective, exemplifies the mindset of a therapy guide. You will see how the operating paradigm plays a role in the therapist's ability to solve problems creatively. Espinoza draws on an occupational science frame of reference to develop a functional plan for this young client.

You will meet Mary in "When Mary Finishes High School." Mary is a 16-year-old who has a developmental disability. Diana Bal, Mary's therapy guide, describes Mary's quest to learn a vocational skill. You will read about how Mary acquired new skills through graded activities that Diana created along Mary's path to developing the skill of sorting mail. Diana relies on a transfer of training approach when she structures the therapy goals and activities for Mary.

Reflective Journal Entries

In Unit I, the goal of each Reflective Journal Entry is to help you understand new concepts about CPS by embedding the ideas in your personal experiences and paradigms. In Unit II, the Reflective Journal Entries serve a slightly different purpose. Each entry targets your perception of the primary challenges of the therapy expedition.

In each section there are three Reflective Journal Entries. You will make the first journal entry immediately after reading the story. You will make the second and third journal entries at the end of the section after you have had an opportunity to apply the Thinking Keys to the story. Recall that the purpose of each Thinking Key is to "unlock" your mind and expand your thinking about the situation. Therefore, in the last journal entry in each section you will be asked to evaluate your responses in the first two journal entries and determine whether your perceptions of the individuals in the story changed as a result of your experience using the Thinking Keys.

Mind Mapping

You were introduced to mind mapping in Unit I as an alternative to outlining the content of a section. In Unit II, you will also be making Mind Maps. In contrast to the Mind Maps you created in Unit I, however, the Mind Maps you will create in Unit II, Sections 13 and 14, will be a visual representation of the client's therapy expedition. They will help you identify the problematic situations within the story that you perceive can best be solved by using CPS.

Mind Maps in Unit II will be created in the following manner: First you will be asked to read the story through once completely to become familiar with its content and to gain first impressions of the people in the story. Next, you will be asked to reread the story to extract information to include in the Mind Map. Determine which information in the story has relevance to an occupational therapy expedition.

Thinking Keys and Field Organizers

As you practice using CPS in Unit II, you will rely on your imagination to expand on the content of each story. First you will use seven Thinking Keys to prepare to use CPS within the occupational therapy process. Next, you will use the Thinking Keys associated with CPS to generate a future vision for the client described in the story. Finally, you will design an action plan that will effectively transform that vision into a reality.

For instructional purposes, you will practice using the Thinking Keys in the same order that you learned them in Unit I. Once you become comfortable with CPS, adapt the order that you use the Thinking Keys to the context of the situation. Keep in mind when using

CPS that the three components and six stages are descriptions of their contribution to ways to solve problems creatively; they are not prescriptive steps and are not meant to be used in a predetermined sequence.

To help you get started in Section 13, several ideas have been recorded in each Field Organizer. Your task will be to complete the Field Organizers as you did with Louise's Nose Blowing Expedition.

Because the application of CPS to the occupational therapy process depends entirely on the context in which the problem occurs, solutions are beyond the answers found in published literature, such as textbooks and periodicals. Suggested responses to some of the Field Organizers in Section 13 are provided in Appendix A as a demonstration of *possible* ways to think about the elements of the story. They are not absolute answers. We recommend that you look at the options in Appendix A only after you have completed your Field Organizers. The thoughts and options that you choose to include in each field organizer will undoubtedly be different than ours. Bear in mind that your responses reflect your paradigm; and, your paradigm is defined by your life experiences, comfort zone, and ability to visionize into the future, and by your resources, assumptions, intuition, and value system.

Practice Using CPS in the Context of Occupational Therapy Services

Itinerary #13

At the end of the thirteenth part of your journey, you will be able to:

✓ describe the therapy expedition route of Sam, a child with sensory processing problems

✓ extract relevant information from Sam's story that relates to the occupational therapy process and CPS

✓ use journaling to identify personal thoughts, feelings, and insights about Sam's story

✓ use mind mapping to link information in Sam's story to the therapy expedition itinerary

✓ use Thinking Keys and Field Organizers to creatively solve Sam's therapy-related problems

Sam's Sensory Integration (SI) Expedition

In this section you will meet Sam and travel with him on his therapy expedition, using all of the Field Organizers you learned in Unit I. Begin Sam's SI Expedition by reading through Sam's story, written by his mother, Anne Miller. Next, reread paragraphs 1–17 of the story and complete Reflective Journal Entry 13.1 from the perspective of Sam's therapy guide. You will then begin a Mind Map of Sam's SI Expedition.

Sam Finds Help and Hope: An SI Success Story

Anne Miller

1 The doctor said he'd been a real fighter. Four weeks premature and sick with infection, our infant son had fought death and won! Fifteen days after birth, we took Sam home. My husband Barry and I were so excited! Little did we know the battle had just begun.

2 Sam cried constantly. The pediatrician said Sam had colic. Sam's "colic" lasted several years. Instinctively I cuddled him, but he was inconsolable. Even while breastfeeding, Sam nursed as fast as he could, his little body rigid and resistant to being snuggled.

3 Any skin exposure at all sent him into hysterics, making bathing, dressing, and even diaper changes a nightmare. Haircuts and nail-clippings were even worse. Sam obviously felt terrorized.

4 Sam never played with baby toys and rattles. He never initiated even the simplest of activities. Yet he wasn't satisfied to be a passive observer.

5 By trial and error, I eventually discovered two remedies to stop the crying. One was to bounce him vigorously on my knees. The other was to flex and stretch his arms and legs. The only other activity Sam enjoyed were our walks outside with him scrunched up in a knapsack. He became so quiet that I'd frequently peek in on him to be sure he was still breathing. Though he couldn't see out, his eyes were wide open. These were his only moments of contentment.

6 Because of his emotional fragility, we avoided taking Sam out in public and seldom had visitors. Having people in or taking Sam out upset him terribly. He cried hysterically for hours following the briefest change in his environment.

7 At 12 months, Sam was diagnosed as having mild cerebral palsy. Consequently, although we shared information about his bizarre behavior with medical professionals (which was much more difficult for us to deal with than his CP), they were unable to see beyond his orthopedic problems. A frequent response to our concerns was, "He's just a strong-willed child."

8 At age 2 and ½, Sam stopped crawling and started to run. He never stopped running. His hyperactivity did not stem from having an overabundance of energy. On the contrary, Sam never slept well at night, awakening between 2 and 5 times a night. He tired easily during the day, and often spaced out, staring into nothing for several moments. Typically, his body was very floppy. He leaned against any nearby object or person for support. I had to take care, whenever I stepped away from him, that he didn't topple over. These "spacing out" periods were usually followed by rapid head-shaking or frenzied running. His wild behavior appeared to be more of an attempt to "rev" himself up than an outlet for excess energy.

9 Even though Sam became more mobile, he continued to be just as difficult. He could not tolerate a bikeseat, stroller, or carseat. Car rides longer than 5 minutes were endured with Sam screaming non-stop. His play was destructive, repetitive, and always puzzling. Frequently and deliberately, he crashed into walls and furniture. At times, he heaved heavy objects and furniture.

10 He had no interest in table-top activities. He avoided puzzles, blocks, and any play which involved putting parts together. I recall one occasion when Barry and I were overseeing a Sunday school class where Sam and several other children his same age were playing with playdough. His classmates created animals, monsters, or pretend food with their dough. After pushing at his dough a short while, Sam picked it up and threw it at them. Later, when the other children started to color pictures, Sam made a brief attempt to draw too, then wadded his paper up and tore it to pieces. He was at a total loss as to how to be constructive or creative, and our attempts to demonstrate didn't help him.

11 Sam never played with toys. He demanded my constant attention. I begged him to watch TV—if I could have just 10 minutes to prepare dinner while he watched "Sesame Street." But Sam would have nothing to do with TV, radio, or noise of any sort. Even the noise of Barry and me engaged in normal conversation always upset him. It seemed that the only noises he could tolerate were those he made himself. Paradoxically, in response to these other noises, Sam got louder and louder himself.

12 Especially nerve-wracking to me was his aversion to engaging in any new activity. He would get in a rut and was completely satisfied to remain there. I was continually and unsuccessfully trying to draw him into new activities. Sometimes I sat with him while he turned all the switches in our car on and off, over and over again, for hours. It was preferable to his screaming. One hot summer, when Sam was 4, I spent hours each day walking alongside him as he pushed a cartload of concrete blocks around the neighborhood. Day after day, always the same activity and always the same path. When I tried to alter things just slightly, he became outraged.

13 My greatest heartache was Sam's hostility toward me. He wanted my total attention, but none of my affection. Barry would come home each evening and rough-house with Sam. He would spin Sam around, throw him up in the air, bounce him on the bed, and wrestle him on the floor. At times I thought he was being too rough. But Sam adored him. I was grateful for their close relationship. But Sam's deep affection for Barry, in contrast to his intense dislike for me, hurt me all the more. I did not love Sam with my heart. My heart could feel no warmth for this cold, hostile person. But I did love Sam deeply with all of my will and my strength.

14 We couldn't figure Sam out. He insisted on having his arms and legs covered up, refusing to wear anything but long-sleeved shirts and pants, even in the middle of summer. Anything touching him was an extreme irritant. Yet he touched everything! In his impulsivity, nothing and no one was off limits. Before we could stop it, his hands were in our food at the dinner table, or all over another person's hair.

15 Sam seemed almost impervious to pain. I recall one occasion when I'd decided to break him of his habit of pinching. After repeatedly explaining to him that pinching hurts, I finally decided he needed to be shown how much it hurts. I pinched him lightly. He laughed. I pinched a little harder, being careful not to really hurt him. I needn't have worried. After several unsuccessful attempts, I finally pinched him as hard as I could. He still didn't feel it.

16 With other children, Sam was extremely aggressive. Since rough physical treatment felt good to him, he couldn't understand how his physical aggression could be a threat to others. Also, being around other children compounded the problems he already had. Because he was unable to direct his own activities constructively, he had no idea how to enter into the play activities of others. If he didn't get his way, he became hysterical.

17 To counter Sam's aggression, obstinacy, and other inappropriate behaviors, we tried all the traditional disciplinary techniques—timeouts, spankings, rewards, and removal of privileges. Nothing worked. Most of the time Sam was like a wild animal out of control. We had no idea how to tame him.

18 When Sam was age 4 and ½, we experienced a breakthrough. Sam had just received orthopedic surgery for his CP. Following this, he entered the Rehabilitation Institute of Chicago as an inpatient for 2 months of intensive physical and occupational therapy. While at the Institute, I shared with Sam's OT some of his bizarre behaviors. She arranged to have her supervisor, Jeanne, test Sam for possible sensory integration dysfunction. She also loaned me the book *Sensory Integration and the Child*, by Jean Ayres.

19 As I read the book, I wept. I couldn't believe that someone else could know my son so well. Yet there Sam was, with all his peculiarities, on every page! Ayres obviously understood Sam. Incredible! And most wonderful of all, she opened that door of understanding to me. For the first time we were hopeful that our family could be helped. Sam needed help so desperately, and so did we.

20 The sensory integrative approach to therapy was begun immediately and continued for the remaining 1 and ½ months we were at the Institute. At first I was concerned that much less time was being given to skills development. It was difficult for me to imagine how swinging on a bolster or being squeezed between mattresses could help Sam in any way. To my amazement, the sensory integrative approach had a profound effect.

21 By the end of Sam's short stay, I had witnessed him doing things he'd never been able to do before. After 20–30-minute periods of intense treatment, I watched Sam initiate a table-top activity. He then proceeded to duplicate the pattern of several blocks arranged by the therapist. In prior screenings, he had not even been able to put 3 blocks together in the correct pattern! Then I watched as he correctly copied the designs she had drawn. As incredible as it seemed, there had to be a connection between the therapy he had just received and his newly acquired abilities. Sam had begun to grasp the concept of putting parts together to make a meaningful whole. I was impressed. By the time we returned home, I knew without a doubt that SI treatment was essential for Sam's continued progress and success in life.

(continued)

22 We began meeting regularly with our local school district's special education director, and with the staff and administrators of the school our son attends. Through teleconference, Jeanne also participated in one of these meetings. We discussed how foundational sensory integration is to education, and we shared our desire that Sam's therapy and classroom programs incorporate a strong sensory integrative approach. Five months later, our local district hired Liz [an OT] to consult with the staff at our son's school for one year. Additionally, I developed a home program based upon Liz's and Jeanne's recommendations.

23 Since Sam's testing at the Institute 3 years ago, the results of his home and school programs have been dramatic in every way. Physically, it soon became apparent that many of Sam's difficulties, which had been attributed to his CP, were actually a result of his sensory integrative dysfunction. Sam was constantly bumping into people and objects and tripping over curbs and cracks in the sidewalk. He couldn't walk just a few yards without falling. Now Sam almost never falls or bumps into things. He has a much clearer perception of his position in relation to other people and objects.

24 Sam's sense of balance has vastly improved, too. At one time, he couldn't sit on our porch swing without support. Now, not only does he sit on it without holding on, but he target shoots while I send the swing flying.

25 Sam's sense of directionality is clearer too. He no longer loses his orientation during games involving bases and goal lines. His posture is more erect. And his ability to use both sides of his body is much improved.

26 Just this past winter, Sam underwent a thorough gait study at Children's Memorial Hospital in Chicago. Based upon the results of this study as well as observations, it became apparent that Sam's gait pattern was substantially better without his leg braces. Consequently he no longer wears braces. From observation it appears that his gait is continuing to improve. Previously, when wearing his braces, Sam often used his left leg like a straight peg and dragged it along. It's been interesting to notice that he now uses it much more naturally, flexing and extending it as appropriate.

27 It is a joy watching the excitement in Sam's eyes as he experiments with his body to discover all the ways he can perform various actions. No longer is he merely satisfied to jump. Now he jumps up feet together and lands feet spread wide apart. No longer is it enough to climb across the monkey bars, one bar to the next. Now he must skip every other bar. As he achieves one goal, he sets up another, each more challenging than the one before. At last unencumbered, Sam feels unlimited and free to explore. He is surprised and delighted by all his new accomplishments.

28 Academically, it became apparent that many of Sam's problems were due to sensory integration dysfunction rather than CP. A striking example was in handwriting. By the end of kindergarten, Sam still could not form even the simplest of letters. Because it was thought that his CP was preventing him from acquiring handwriting skills, the traditional follow-the-dots approach was used to teach him. He learned to do this expertly. Unfortunately though, when presented with a blank piece of paper, he had not even the slightest idea how to begin.

29 During the following summer, I continued our home program. It consisted of much physical movement and no writing practice. Then one day in early August, on his own initiative, Sam sat down and started to write "S A M." In amazement he looked up at me and said, "Mom, I can't believe it! I'm writing!" That fall, when Sam returned to school, not only was he writing, he was reading too.

30 Now as Sam is about to complete the 2nd grade (he is fully mainstreamed into a regular division classroom), he has a clear understanding of all his subjects. He seems to grasp new concepts quickly and easily. At home, one of his favorite toys are his Legos. This past week, he put together a new set consisting of 80 pieces. He was able to figure out the correct location and position of each piece. Only a few times did he ask me for help due to problems with finger dexterity.

31 A continuing concern is the area of organization—his desk at school is usually in a state of disarray, and he has difficulty remembering to bring home the proper materials. However, he is making progress. A couple of years ago, Sam didn't even notice when I'd totally rearrange a room. And he was completely oblivious to disorder. He had little conscious awareness of the objects in his environment. Now I often discover that he has picked up his room without being asked. Although he sometimes has trouble establishing it, orderliness has become very important to him.

32 Emotionally, Sam is not nearly as fragile as he used to be. His extreme mood swings have lessened considerably, as have his extremes in activity level. He no longer runs everywhere. He rarely gets "hyper" and his stamina has increased greatly. Usually he is constructive, content, and self-directed in his play, alternating between quiet and more lively activities. Last fall, for the first time in 7½ years, Sam started sleeping though the night.

33 Skin exposure no longer bothers him either. This spring, Sam could hardly wait until it became warm enough for him to fling off his pants and put on shorts. He tolerates noise much better, but at times is still overwhelmed by too many sounds. He enjoys TV and limited conversation, but simultaneous conversation can distress him.

34 In the past year, Sam has become increasingly in touch with his nervous system needs. Sometimes, when bordering on overstimulation, he will initiate his own "timeouts" saying "Mom, I need some time alone for a while." Once he did this when he had an especially noisy friend over. He went to his bedroom for about 10 minutes of quiet time. When Sam does lose control, he can now normally be reasoned with.

35 Sam still copes best when in routine, but no longer goes "off the deep end" when it is altered. We used to be annoyed when he asked us endless questions about future plans and events. Now, since learning that this is his way of preparing his nervous system, we try to answer his questions as best we can. It really makes a difference in his ability to successfully handle a new situation.

36 Especially precious has been the healing of Sam's relationship with me. He finally knows that I never meant to torment him in his early years, and that I loved him as best I knew how. Deep down I think he realizes and greatly appreciates his mother's unique acceptance and understanding of him. He knows that I have always loved him. And he loves me back with lots of hugs and "I love you's."

37 The next school year will be an exciting one for Sam. This fall of '93, he will start attending school in our home district. Recently our district sponsored an in-service, conducted by Liz on sensory integrative dysfunction. About 50 people attended. Not only will Sam benefit, but many other students as well.

38 We have many people to thank for Sam's progress. We are especially grateful to Jeanne and Liz. They treat Sam as the unique person he is, with unique therapeutic needs, sensory as well as orthopedic. I dare not think where we'd be today without their tremendous help and encouragement. Their vast knowledge and open-mindedness has made all the difference.

39 Perhaps all things are possible for Sam. He believes so.

Reprinted with permission from Sensory Integration International, 1602 Cabrillo Ave, Torrance, CA 90501; *Sensory Integration Quarterly*, fall 1993. 12–15.

Now you know about Sam's early life and experiences on his therapy expedition. But you may be thinking, "What's the rest of his story?" Life goes on for Sam. Following several years of special services directed at ameliorating his sensory processing problems, he continues to develop and be a joy to his parents (see Figure 13.1). The following epilogue was written by Sam's mother in spring 1997, when Sam turned 12 years old.

Figure 13.1. *Left, Sam at the age of 12; right, Anne, Barry, and Sam*

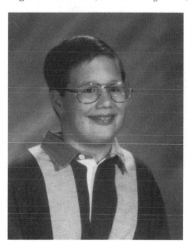
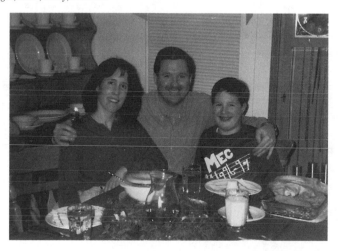

Sam at Age Twelve Years: An Epilogue

Anne Miller

It is three and a half years later. Sam just turned 12 and is completing the sixth grade. In preparation for writing this sequel, I reread the story I had written about his early years. I had not read it in a long time. I am relieved that Sam has come so far. Yet given his difficult start in life, I can hardly believe it!

Beginning in third grade, Sam was fully mainstreamed into the local school. He had formerly been bused to a school about 12 miles away in another community. At this time, I had to make a difficult decision. We had to continue his strengthening and stretching exercises to treat his cerebral palsy. Should I also continue our home program to intensively address his sensory integration (SI) needs as I had done for the past three years? The SI home program had produced such magnificent results. Or should I redirect my efforts and focus primarily on his social needs and skills development? I chose the latter. There wasn't time or energy to work on everything. And I overloaded him and frustrated myself by trying to do too much. Although I knew Sam could further benefit from a continuing emphasis on SI, I also realized that the returns for our time spent on this approach would diminish. Also, we had already laid a good if not complete SI foundation for Sam's ongoing development and knew he would continue to progress in the area of SI through his participation in other activities.

To address Sam's social needs in his new school, we immediately began a campaign to invite almost every boy from his class over to our house at least once during the school year. It soon became apparent to us that this was one of the wisest things we could ever have done for our son. We didn't sit back and wait for friendships to develop. From the very start we worked at providing an environment in which friendships would develop. Within a month, Sam became a very popular child, with all the boys actually competing to see who would be invited over to his house next.

To better ensure that these outreaches would be successful, I telephoned the mothers of the boys ahead of time to explain about Sam's cerebral palsy and asked that they pass on the explanation to their sons. I then helped Sam set up a rough schedule of specific activities that the boys might do together. Given Sam's prior problems with structuring time, and also his need for predictability and some measure of control in a situation, this preplanned schedule was especially important. Then too, we kept the time together short. I am delighted to say that as Sam has matured; we no longer need these safeguards. He is now able to go with the flow and to give and take and share with others.

Acquiring specific skills was another important part of Sam's development. When we had tried previously to teach Sam various skills, we had been successful. A sufficient SI foundation had not been laid. By this time, however, Sam had had three years of therapy incorporating a strong SI approach. Sam was ready to move on.

There were two main areas of skills we chose to address. We needed to address daily living skills to increase Sam's ability to function independently. We also needed to enhance skills related to his social development and those skills that would promote natural strengths he already had in order to build his self-esteem.

Over the years, Sam has pursued a variety of interests, including drawing, self-defense, and basketball. Learning to play basketball has been especially valuable because this is an activity he can enjoy with his friends. We had enrolled Sam in programs to give him training in these and have not discouraged him. At the same time, however, his father and I had encouraged him to pursue interests and develop skills in areas in which we believe he has the greatest potential for success. Sam took archery lessons from a former Special Olympics champion. Sam is a gifted writer of short stories. Some of these we have submitted for possible publication. He has also been taking piano lessons for the past two years. Even with his hemiplegia affecting his left arm and fingers, he has made tremendous progress. He enjoys piano and has a keen ear for music. If Sam continues to demonstrate an interest or would like to compose music, we will buy him a synthesizer to help him progress. Then he can first record the left hand part by playing it with his right hand. We want him to know that his cerebral palsy need not limit him.

More recently we have been encouraging Sam in the area of public speaking. He has a natural ability to speak to a group of people. We have exposed him to live drama and to several well-known motivational speakers and are encouraging him to enroll in classes that will help him develop his public speaking abilities. Recently Sam was selected to be the master of ceremonies for a performance at school. He is beginning to realize that he need not be a super athlete to make an impact on this world. Through the spoken word, he can make a powerful contribution.

Sensory integration dysfunction is no longer a concern for Sam. This is quite incredible considering that his sensory integrative deficits had been so devastating to our family. Only rarely are we not reminded that SI deficits were a major problem, such as when we visited Grandma and Sam refused to take off his socks because he could not stand the feeling of her plush carpet on his bare feet. Or when he needed a little more home tutoring to help him understand his geometry. Overall, Sam is doing very well. He has lots of friends, he is emotionally stable, and he is an honor-roll student.

Sam's therapy needs continue to change. Important parts of his therapy program now include working out with Nautilus and on the treadmill for strengthening and weight control. As Sam has grown, these activities have become increasing concerns in countering the effects of his cerebral palsy. And although Sam is less than enthusiastic about his workout program, it helps his perspective to realize that working out is an activity for a lifetime and one we should all be doing.

To be honest, I often feel guilty about all that I don't do with Sam. Too often I neglect his floor exercises and exercises to improve the function of his left arm. I choose instead to play basketball or cards with Sam, or we go for a walk together after a freshly fallen snow. These times together are important, but I sometimes wonder how much he has lost because of my neglect of his home therapy. But then I marvel at what he has gained. Time goes by, and so much is left undone. The weight of the responsibility to make the right choices for my son's well-being is great.

As Sam is about to enter his teenage years, I look forward to watching him grow into a young man. I have no doubt that we'll encounter some challenging times in the years ahead, but I have no dread. We have a close relationship. I believe Sam trusts me to understand him as no one else can. And he shares his thoughts with me, often and deeply. I truly like the person he is becoming. And he likes himself. Raising Sam has given me great joy. I am privileged to be his mother.

Reflective Journaling: First Stop

REFLECTIVE JOURNAL ENTRY 13.1

Imagine that you are the therapy guide who will consult with Sam and his mother on Sam's SI Expedition and complete the following thought:

I feel the primary challenges of Sam's SI Expedition are . . .

Create Layer 1 of your Mind Map for Sam's SI Expedition. Include information from paragraphs 1 through 17 that you consider to be important to an occupational therapy expedition. Begin with Layer 1. Use your black pen or marker.

Create a Mind Map of Sam's SI Expedition

Mind Map Guidelines

1. Place the story's main concept in the center of the space using pictures or words or both.
2. Radiate ideas from the central thought.
   - Headline text—one or two words per line.
   - Print text (for easy reading).
3. Use the following color code for each layer:
   Layer 1 — black
   Layer 2 — green
   Layer 3 — blue
4. Link the main concepts and generate more ideas from the linkages.
5. Have fun!

Remember, the more linkages that you generate between elements, the greater your ability to see how all the elements relate to one another.

Preparing for CPS Within an Occupational Therapy Paradigm

The domain of occupational therapy covers many services. To ensure that the referral for services is appropriate, you will use the "Watch for Cues and Look for Patterns" and "PACC" Field Organizers. Use these two Field Organizers now to begin "Sam's SI Expedition." They provide the necessary structure to guide the first level of therapy-related decision making— "to treat" or "not to treat." The first part of the "Watch for Cues and Look for Patterns" Field Organizer helps you extract relevant data from the client's story. The second part directs you to conceptualize the data into patterns related to the client's global needs.

The "PACC" Field Organizer explicitly frames the elements of the story within an occupational therapy paradigm. Before you go on an expedition you need to pack your bags. Think of the "PACC" as a tool for packing the information from the story into an occupational therapy frame of reference. The structure of the "PACC" provides you with a format to analyze the story data, point by point, with Uniform Terminology.

"Watch for Cues and Look for Patterns." Use the "Watch for Cues and Look for Patterns" Field Organizer to uncover cues in paragraphs 1–17 of Sam's story. Select cues that give insight about Sam and his relationship with his family and others. Record the cues and describe your perception of them; next look for patterns. Recall that patterns are made up of repeating elements that form a distinct concept. The patterns that emerge from the cues will give you a picture of Sam and the challenges he faces in performing his daily occupational performance. To help you get started, the Field Organizer has example cues and perceptions from paragraphs 1–5.

DIRECTIONS

1. Read through the examples in Part I for story paragraphs 1–5.
2. Identify the cues in paragraphs 6–17. Briefly state the cues in a headline format in column A. You may find more than one cue in each paragraph. (Hint: there are at least two cues in paragraphs 8, 12, 13, 14, and 16, and three cues in paragraph 11.)
3. Describe your perception of the cue in terms of its relevance to you as a therapy guide in column B. Use the examples for paragraphs 1–5 to model your responses.
4. Move to Part II and look for patterns among the cues you found in paragraphs 2–17 by asking yourself the question, "What elements of the story seem to reoccur?" Record the patterns you found and identify the paragraphs in which you found the cues for each pattern. Note: Cues can be used more than once. Use the example for paragraphs 2–5 to model your responses.

FIELD ORGANIZER

"Watch for Cues and Look for Patterns"

Part I: Cues		
Story Paragraph #	**A Cue**	**B What might this cue mean?**
1	Birth history	Sam's birth history is important information. Prematurity at birth brings to mind the consequences related to being, and the developmental patterns of, a full-term vs. a premature infant. Fifteen days in the hospital—is that extraordinary for a preemie or is that the average hospital stay? I wonder whether Sam had other complications in addition to the prematurity. He certainly seems to have been a fighter.

(continued)

"Watch for Cues and Look for Patterns" (Continued)

Part I: Cues		

Story Paragraph #	A Cue	B What might this cue mean?
2	Inconsolable crying	Sam cried constantly; the pediatrician may have told the mom that Sam was colicky. From an occupational therapy perspective, I question whether something else was going on within his ability to process sensory information. His mom related that she had difficulty consoling Sam, even when she cuddled him. Cuddling, or firm touch pressure, should have a calming influence on an infant. Something else must be occurring with this infant since the ordinary methods of calming him did not work. The mom related that Sam nursed as fast as he could. When nursing, his body became rigid. I wonder about his ability to synchronize his breathing with his sucking. I wonder whether his dyschrony between sucking and breathing caused him so much stress that he went into an extension pattern as a consequence of this apparent stress.
3	Low tolerance for passive touch	Sam's constant crying brings to question his ability to take in sensory information from the environment and make sense out of it. His low tolerance for haircuts and nail-clippings is indicated by his mom's impression that Sam felt "terrorized." The information related to how he responds to any stimulus that touches his skin further supports a sensory processing problem. His problem seems to be related to the tactile system.
4	Avoided toys	Sam never played with baby toys or initiated activities. Yet he appeared to be dissatisfied being a passive observer. I wonder how the mom recognized that he didn't enjoy being a "passive observer"—what other behaviors did he exhibit? Was he unable to initiate activities because of motor problems, muscle tone, coordination problems—or, did he have difficulty processing sensory information and it appeared to his mom that he was frustrated with being a passive observer? Based on this information, Sam seemed to be bright and was making comparisons between what he thought he could do and what he actually was able to do.
5	Mom was a creative problem solver	Sam's mom seems to be creative and open to trying new ways to manage the crying. Without having a theoretical model on which to base her reasons for bouncing Sam to stop the crying, she intuitively imposed vestibular and proprioceptive input on his apparently disorganized central nervous system (CNS). His mom recognized that his only moments of contentment were when he was "scrunched up in a knapsack" during walks. Sam's mom's understanding of why Sam stopped crying when he was "scrunched up in a knapsack" during walks will be a good starting point for family education about the mechanisms that integrate the sensory-motor system.
6		
7		

"Watch for Cues and Look for Patterns" (Continued)

Part I: Cues		
Story Paragraph #	**A Cue**	**B What might this cue mean?**
8		
9		
10		
11		
12		
13		
14		
15		
16		
17		

(continued)

"Watch for Cues and Look for Patterns" (*Continued*)

Part II: Patterns

Story Paragraph #	Patterns that emerged from cues found in the story
2–5	*Early signs of a sensory processing problem*

"PACC" (Performance Areas, Components, and Contexts). With this Thinking Key, you will decide whether you can pack the elements of Sam's story into an occupational therapy frame of reference. The "PACC" Thinking Key helps to guide your thinking toward whether the elements of Sam's story are a match with the occupational therapy domains of concern (Performance Areas, Performance Components, and Performance Contexts). The "PACC" Field Organizer has three parts, one for each domain of concern.

DIRECTIONS

Materials: yellow, green, and blue highlighters

1. Reread Sam's story and highlight the story elements that relate to each area of the "PACC." Color code the story elements using the same color system you used in Section 4, Story Writing. (Anchor the color code in past experiences.)

   Yellow: Performance Areas

   Green: Performance Components

   Blue: Performance Contexts

2. Begin with the yellow highlighted elements. Record the paragraph number of each Performance Area element in the Story Paragraph # column opposite the appropriate activity of daily living in Part 1.

3. In the Story Element column, describe each element or copy it verbatim from the story. In some cases, you may need to read between the lines and think off of the page to respond. Use the examples in Part 1 to model your responses to all three parts of the "PACC" Field Organizer.

   Note: Create a future vision for Sam. Tap into your intuition to complete the "PACC." Not every Performance Area, Component, or Context will have a matched story element. Some categories and subcategories will have more story data than others. For example, in Sam's story, the Performance Area activities of daily living has many more elements related to Sam than does the Performance Area work and productive activities.

4. Repeat steps 2 and 3 for Part 2 (Performance Components elements with green highlighting) and Part 3 (Performance Contexts elements with blue highlighting).

Part 1: Performance Areas

Performance Area	Story Paragraph #	Story Element
A. Activities of daily living		
1. Grooming	3	
2. Oral hygiene	3	*Any skin exposure sent Sam into hysterics during self-care activities*
3. Bathing/showering	3	
4. Toilet hygiene	3	
5. Personal device care		
6. Dressing		
7. Feeding and eating	3	
8. Medication routine		
9. Health maintenance		
10. Socialization		
11. Functional communication	6	*Parents avoided visitors or taking Sam out in public*
12. Functional mobility		
13. Community mobility	9	*Sam ran all over; difficulty modulating motor control; couldn't tolerate car rides, bike seat, or stroller*
14. Emergency response		
15. Sexual expression		
B. Work and productive activities		
1. Home management		
a. Clothing care		
b. Cleaning		
c. Meal preparation and cleanup		
d. Shopping		
e. Money management		
f. Household maintenance		
g. Safety procedures		
2. Care of others		
3. Educational activities	10	*No interest in table-top activities—pre-readiness school activities*
4. Vocational activities		
a. Vocational exploration		
b. Job acquisition		

(continued)

Part 1: Performance Areas

Performance Area	Story Paragraph #	Story Element
c. Work or job performance		
d. Retirement planning		
e. Volunteer participation		
C. Play and leisure		
1. Play and leisure exploration	9	*Could not tolerate bike seat or stroller; heaved heavy objects*
2. Play and leisure performance	9	*Sam's play was destructive, repetitive*

Part 2: Performance Components

Performance Component	Story Paragraph #	Story Element
A. Sensorimotor component		
1. Sensory		
a. Sensory awareness		
b. Sensory processing		
(1) Tactile		
(2) Proprioceptive		
(3) Vestibular		
(4) Visual		
(5) Auditory		
(6) Gustatory		
(7) Olfactory		
c. Perceptual processing		
(1) Stereognosis		
(2) Kinesthesia		
(3) Pain response		
(4) Body scheme		
(5) Right-left discrimination		
(6) Form constancy		
(7) Position in space		
(8) Visual-closure		

Part 2: Performance Components

Performance Component	Story Paragraph #	Story Element
(9) Figure ground		
(10) Depth perception		
(11) Spatial relations		
(12) Topographical orientation		
2. Neuromusculoskeletal		
a. Reflex		
b. Range of motion		
c. Muscle tone		
d. Strength		
e. Endurance		
f. Postural control		
g. Postural alignment		
h. Soft tissue integrity		
3. Motor		
a. Gross coordination		
b. Crossing midline		
c. Laterality		
d. Bilateral integration		
e. Motor control		
f. Praxis		
g. Fine coordination/ dexterity		
h. Visual-motor integration		
i. Oral-motor control		
B. Cognitive integration and cognitive components		
1. Level of arousal		
2. Orientation		
3. Recognition		
4. Attention span		
5. Initiation of activity		
6. Termination of activity		
7. Memory		
8. Sequencing		

(continued)

Part 2: Performance Components

Performance Component	Story Paragraph #	Story Element
9. Categorization		
10. Concept formation		
11. Spatial operations		
12. Problem solving		
13. Learning		
14. Generalization		
C. Psychosocial Skills		
1. Psychological		
a. Values		
b. Interests		
c. Self-concept		
2. Social		
a. Role performance		
b. Social conduct		
c. Interpersonal skills		
d. Self-expression		
3. Self-management		
a. Coping skills		
b. Time management		
c. Self-control		

Part 3: Performance Contexts

Performance Context	Story Paragraph #	Story Element
A. Temporal aspects		
1. Chronological		
2. Developmental		
3. Life cycle		
4. Disability status		
B. Environment		
1. Physical		
2. Social		
3. Cultural		

"Problem Ownership Checklist." To benefit from the therapy process the potential client must first be aware that a problem exists. The "Problem Ownership Checklist" Thinking Key helps the therapy guide determine whether the client is aware that he has a problem. The four questions posed in the Field Organizer target the potential client's awareness of the existence of a problem and the desire and access to resources needed to solve the problem.

To apply the "Problem Ownership Checklist" to Sam's story, replace the word "person" in the checklist with the words "Sam's parents." Because Sam is a child, his primary caregivers—his parents—are as much a "client" to the therapy process as Sam is.

DIRECTIONS

1. Answer questions 2–4 with a check in the appropriate box.
2. Briefly describe your rationale in the space under the question. Use the example provided to model your response.

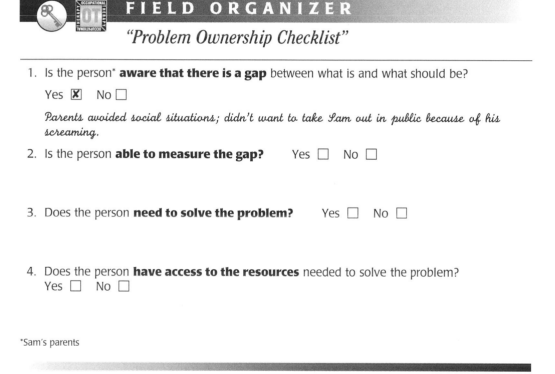

FIELD ORGANIZER
"Problem Ownership Checklist"

1. Is the person* **aware that there is a gap** between what is and what should be?

   Yes ☒   No ☐

   Parents avoided social situations; didn't want to take Sam out in public because of his screaming.

2. Is the person **able to measure the gap?**   Yes ☐   No ☐

3. Does the person **need to solve the problem?**   Yes ☐   No ☐

4. Does the person **have access to the resources** needed to solve the problem?
   Yes ☐   No ☐

*Sam's parents

"Stop, Drop, and Listen." The "Stop, Drop, and Listen" Thinking Key reminds you to keep an open mind and to listen to what the client is saying. To be receptive to all information, you need to drop assumptions that may filter the information as you are listening to it. The "Stop, Drop, and Listen" Thinking Key also provides you with an opportunity to evaluate what is behind the words of the person who is speaking to you. In Sam's story, you will apply the "Stop, Drop, and Listen" Thinking Key to comments made by Sam's mother. Use your intuition and empathy to think beyond the scope of the explicit words in the story.

The story paragraphs have been preselected for this practice session. Refer to paragraphs 3, 4, and 8 of Sam's story to complete the "Stop, Drop, and Listen" Field Organizer. Note that columns B and C have been completed for paragraph 1.

1. Read the comments in column A for paragraphs 3, 4, and 8.
2. In column B record any preconceived assumptions that you may have about the comments in column A.
3. In column C describe your *perception* of what Sam's mother was really saying.

FIELD ORGANIZER

"Stop, Drop, and Listen"

Story Paragraph #	A WHO said WHAT?	B Assumption to Be Dropped	C Behind these words or actions the person is saying . . .
1	Mother said, "Our infant son had fought death and won."	Mother exaggerated.	Do you understand how critically ill Sam was and how happy we were that he lived?
3	Mother said, "Any skin exposure at all sent him into hysterics."		
4	Mother said that Sam never played with baby toys, yet he wasn't satisfied being a passive observer.		
8	Mother said, "Sam never slept well at night, awakening between 2 and 5 times a night."		

"What Paradigm Is Operating?" A client's paradigms have a pervasive influence on the way the client values the therapy process (i.e., how well she keeps appointments and follows through with home program suggestions, and how openly and honestly she shares information about therapy-related issues). Use the "What Paradigm Is Operating" Thinking Key to help you focus in on what paradigms a client might be operating under during the therapy process.

In Sam's story, Sam's mother, Anne, explicitly details Sam's reactions to many kinds of sensory stimulation from the environment. Her emotionally laden descriptors ("My *greatest heartache* was Sam's hostility toward me." "I *begged* him to watch TV." "Especially *nerve-wracking* to me was his aversion to engaging in any new activity.") are an indication of the paradigms Anne was using at the time that she wrote about her son. Anne was operating under a definitive set of assumptions that influenced her expectations of Sam's behavior. It was her operating paradigm or set of assumptions about how a young child should behave that caused Anne grief and sadness over Sam's behavior. The following assumptions were most likely among Anne's thoughts: Sam should bond with me; Sam should not be hostile toward me; young children enjoy watching children's television programs.

Practice identifying the paradigm that might be operating within four situations described in Sam's story using the "What Paradigm Is Operating" Thinking Key. As for previous Field Organizers, story paragraphs were preselected for this practice session. You may wish to analyze additional paragraphs.

1. Read the behaviors in column A and identify the operating paradigm that could explain the behavior.
2. In column B, describe the paradigm from Sam's mother's point of view. To get you started, the first row has been completed.

FIELD ORGANIZER

"What Paradigm Is Operating?"

Story Paragraph #	A Record a behavior to be analyzed.	B Identify the operating paradigm that could explain the behavior described in column A.
2	"Sam cried constantly. . . . Instinctively I cuddled him, but he was inconsolable. Even while breastfeeding, Sam nursed as fast as he could, his little body rigid and resistant to being snuggled."	Sam is my son. I must love and care for him even if he cannot demonstrate that the loves me back.
3	"Sam obviously felt terrorized" by routine skin exposure, including having his nails clipped and hair washed.	
5	"By trial and error, I eventually discovered two remedies to stop the crying. One was to bounce him vigorously on my knees. The other was to flex and stretch his arms and legs."	
6	"Because of his emotional fragility, we avoided taking him out in public and seldom had visitors."	
12	"I was continually and unsuccessfully trying to draw him into new activities."	

"Consider Other Viewpoints." Therapy guides actively seek to understand a situation from more than one perspective. Use the "Consider Other Viewpoints" Thinking Key to expand your understanding of a situation or a person's behavior.

In Sam's story, you will apply the "Consider Other Viewpoints" Thinking Key to Anne's (Sam's mother) comments about Sam's behavior. For instructional purposes the perspective of the therapy guide is being considered as the alternative viewpoint. Note: the use of this Thinking Key is not limited to exploring the perspective of the therapy guide. It may also be used in any situation in which you wish to expand your understanding of a situation or a person's behavior.

1. Read Anne's statements (preselected and recorded in column A) and respond with an explanation (point of view) for Sam's behavior derived from an occupational therapy paradigm.
2. Record your responses in column B. To get you started responses have been provided to the first four entries in column A.

"Consider Other Viewpoints"

Source	**A** It is (was) _____'s (record name of person) perspective that _____ (record target view).	**B** On the other hand _____ (record name of other person) perceives that perhaps_____ (record other person's perspective).
Story Paragraph #	**It was *Anne's* perspective that . . .**	**On the other hand, *you* perceive that perhaps . . .**
2	*Sam nursed as fast as he could, his little body rigid and resistant to being snuggled.*	*Sam had a problem with having his skin lightly touched, a normal occurrence during breastfeeding.*
12	*when Sam played, he got into a rut and stayed there, never venturing into any new activities.*	*Sam's repetition of familiar activities felt good to him; new activities upset him because they were too much of a challenge.*
13	*Sam was hostile toward his mother when he didn't have her full attention.*	*Sam had developed such a strong dependence on his mother that when her attention was diverted away from him he felt vulnerable.*
13	*Sam's father played too rough with Sam.*	*some of Sam's sensory needs were satisfied through the roughhousing with his father (e.g., being tossed in the air, bounced on the bed, and play-wrestled on the floor).*
14	*Sam insisted on having his arms and legs covered at all times.*	
15	*Sam was almost impervious to pain.*	
16	*Sam was extremely aggressive with other children.*	

"Well-Structured vs. Ill-Structured Problem Checklist." Use the "Well-Structured vs. Ill-structured Problem Checklist" Thinking Key to determine whether a problem is well-structured or ill-structured. Recall that when a therapist is faced with a well-structured problem it is to her advantage—in saving both time and money—to use a ready-made solution that has routine procedures and a predictable outcome. When a therapist has an ill-structured problem he can use CPS to find a solution.

Apply the "Well-Structured vs. Ill-Structured Problem Checklist" Field Organizer to Sam's story.

DIRECTIONS

1. Analyze the content of the first 17 paragraphs in terms of each of the three categories listed on the checklist: information, outcome, and solutions.
2. Check the appropriate box in rows 2–3 and describe the rationale for your decision next to the box you checked. Use row 1 as a model.

FIELD ORGANIZER

"Well-Structured vs. Ill-Structured Problem Checklist"

Well-Structured Problem	Ill-Structured Problem
1. ☐ Sufficient information	☒ Insufficient information *Many questions remain regarding why Sam behaves the way he does.*
2. ☐ Predictable outcome(s)	☐ Unpredictable outcome(s)
3. ☐ Ready-made solutions(s)	☐ Custom-made solution(s)

Applying CPS to the Occupational Therapy Program of a Child with Sensory Processing Problems

CPS is an appropriate thinking structure to use for organizing Sam's therapy expedition because his therapy-related needs meet the criteria for an ill-structured problem. CPS will help map out Sam's therapy expedition route, which consists of his long-term, intermediate, and short-term therapy goals. Establishing goals and seeing that they are carried out involves engaging traveling companions to join you on the therapy expedition. The traveling companions are all the people, in addition to Sam and his parents, who share ownership in Sam's problem, whose lives, in any way, are impacted by the quality of Sam's occupational performance.

In the first component of CPS, Get Ready to understand the problem, your task is to determine Sam's *real problem*. His occupational performance profile is complex and reveals a multitude of therapy-related needs. No doubt you identified numerous areas of concern as you read Sam's story and used the "Watch for Cues, Look for Patterns" Thinking Key. Begin Sam's therapy expedition with the Generating Phase of Opportunity Finding as you seek to understand the scope of Sam's problem. (To review Opportunity Finding, see Section 6.)

Get Ready to Understand the Problem: Opportunity Finding

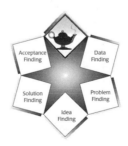

Opportunity Finding: The Generating Phase

"WIBGI . . . ?" To organize your thinking in the Generating Phase of Opportunity Finding use the "WIBGI . . . ?" Thinking Key. This key will help you identify the broad challenges, concerns, and opportunities within Sam's problem.

Note: The "WIBGI . . . ?" and the "Highlighting" Thinking Keys are paired in the following Field Organizer. Wish statements developed during the Generating Phase of Opportunity Finding are recorded in the first column, under the invitational stem "Wouldn't it be great if . . ." The columns on the right side of the Field Organizer, Parts 1 and 2 are for the "Highlighting" Thinking Key, which is used in the Focusing phase of Opportunity Finding.

To generate wish statements using the "WIBGI . . . ?" Thinking Key think about all three areas of Sam's occupational performance (ADL, work and productive activities, and play and leisure). To generate the list of wish statements work in small groups, with each member of the group assuming the role of someone who shares ownership of the problem (e.g., the therapy guide, Sam's parents, Sam's teacher). One person should assume the role of therapy guide and direct the activities. Note that the Field Organizer has spaces for 20 wish statements. Don't limit yourself to the spaces in the Field Organizer. If you generate more than 20 statements, record them on another sheet of paper. The more ideas you generate, the more you increase the potential for arriving at great ideas. Quantity breeds quality.

DIRECTIONS

1. Generate as many wish statements as you can. As you generate wish statements, envision who will be on Sam's SI Expedition and include those individuals in your wish statements. Be mindful of generating wish statements that are broad and brief.
2. Record your wish statements in the first column. In the true spirit of brainstorming, be sure to record *every* wish that the group suggests. To get you started, 10 wish statements have been recorded.

FIELD ORGANIZER

"WIBGI . . . ?"/"Highlighting"

Generate			**Focus**			
			Part 2: Clustering Hits into Hot Spots			
	Wouldn't it be great if . . .	**Part 1: Hits**	**A Performance Area**	**B Performance Area Subcategory**	**C Location**	
1.	Sam played with puzzles and blocks.	●	Play and leisure	Play and leisure performance	Home and school	
2.	Sam engaged in imaginative play.	●	Play and leisure	Play and leisure performance	Home and school	
3.	Sam enjoyed bath time.					
4.	Sam looked forward to stroller and car rides.	●	ADL	Community mobility	Home and school	
5.	Sam demonstrated age appropriate eating skills.	●	ADL	Feeding and eating	Home and school	
6.	Sam participated in Sunday School activities.					

			Part 2: Clustering Hits into Hot Spots		
	Generate		*Focus*		
	Wouldn't it be great if . . .	**Part 1: Hits**	**A Performance Area**	**B Performance Area Subcategory**	**C Location**
7.	Sam played with children in a friendly manner.	⬤	ADL	Socialization	Home and school
8.	Sam loved to play on playground equipment.	⬤	Play and leisure	Play and leisure performance	Home and school
9.	Sam enjoyed listening to stories read to him.	⬤	Work and productive activities	Educational activities	Home and school
10.	Sam and his parents took family vacations.				
11.					
12.					
13.					
14.					
15.					
16.					
17.					
18.					
19.					
20.					

Opportunity Finding: The Focusing Phase

"Head and Shoulders Test." Use the "Head and Shoulders Shoulders Test" to determine if one wish among the group of wishes stands head and shoulders above the rest. Since the school system is funding Sam's therapy services on this expedition, a school-related option is the target of the "Head and Shoulders Test." To complete the next Field Organizer you will need to refer to the wish statements recorded in the "WIBGI . . . ?"/"Highlighting" Field Organizer and work in the same group.

DIRECTIONS

1. Review the list of wishes to determine whether the client (in this context the client is represented by those persons who share ownership of the problem, including Sam's parents and teacher) prefers one wish over all the rest.
2. Record the client's wish statement in the space provided.

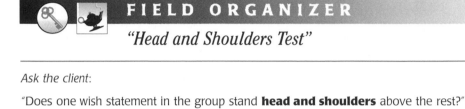

FIELD ORGANIZER

"Head and Shoulders Test"

Ask the client:

"Does one wish statement in the group stand **head and shoulders** above the rest?"

If the client is very interested in pursuing one of the statements or a combination of statements at this point, confirm the wish statement with the client and write it on the line below.

WIBGI _____?

Proceed to Data Finding using this wish statement.

Practice using the "Highlighting" Thinking Key as if you had not found one wish statement that you like better than all the rest.

"Highlighting." In situations where one wish statement does not stand head and shoulders above the rest, use the "Highlighting" Thinking Key in the "WIBGI . . . ?"/"Highlighting" Field Organizer to evaluate each wish statement. The "Highlighting" Thinking Key will help you decide which wish statements you would like to pursue in the Data Finding stage.

"Highlighting" has three parts:

Part 1: Hits are identified.

Part 2: Hits are clustered into Hot Spots and labeled.

Part 3: The label for each Hot Spot is restated to reflect the essence of the Hits clustered in that Hot Spot.

Recall that a Hit is a promising option that the client is interested in pursuing because it feels right, it "sparkles"; it is realistic, understandable, workable, intriguing, or appropriate. Recall, too, that the "Highlighting" Thinking Key is paired with the "WIBGI . . . ?" Thinking Key so that you can identify the Hits and then cluster them without having to rewrite them.

Turn back to the "WIBGI . . . ?"/"Highlighting" Field Organizer and note that Part 1 is for identifying the Hits, and Part 2 is for clustering the Hits.

For your convenience, for Sam's SI Expedition, as for Louise's story in Unit I, you will practice clustering the wish statements using preselected categories. The categories include Performance Area, Performance Area subcategory, and Location. "Performance Area" refers to the Performance Areas identified in the Uniform Terminology dictionary: (1) activities of daily living (ADL), (2) work and productive activities, and (3) play and leisure. "Performance Subcategory" refers to all the specific activities listed in the Uniform Terminology dictionary under each category of Performance Areas, such as grooming and oral hygiene under the category ADL. (When you use Performance Subcategories to cluster Hits you get a more detailed breakdown of wish statements than when you use Performance Areas.)

"Location" refers to the context in which the wish statement will be implemented. The category Location was selected for Sam's SI Expedition because of the desire to identify options that Sam's parents and the school could work on together. In Sam's story, home and school are likely locations for the wish statements to occur. Use the labels home and school together in column C if a Hit can be worked on both at home and at school; use the labels individually if a Hit is best worked on only at one location or the other.

In this Field Organizer you will cluster each Hit in all three of the categories offered (columns A, B, and C). But in actual practice, when clustering Hits, you may select only one main category for each Hit. Note that in the process of clustering the Hits and labeling the Hot Spots, the client may find a Hot Spot that is head and shoulders above the rest.

To complete the "WIBGI . . . ?"/ "Highlighting" Field Organizer, continue working with the group that represents the people who share ownership of the problem (including Sam's parents and the teacher). The person role playing the therapy guide should direct the activity. To get you started we identified seven of the 10 wish statements as Hits, that is, promising options that might support Sam's educational goals.

DIRECTIONS

Part 1

Materials: orange adhesive dots

1. Review the list of wishes in the left column with the client (in this context the client is represented by those persons who share ownership of the problem including Sam's parents and teacher).
2. Direct the client (in this case a group) to identify the Hits (promising options) by placing the orange dots in the Hits column. Your role is to support the client during the selection of the Hits.

Part 2

1. Look for relationships among the Hits (only those options that have been identified with an orange dot) and cluster them into "Hot Spots."
2. Create three labels that capture the theme of each hot spot. Record the labels for each hit in columns A, B, and C. To get you started, labels have been assigned in columns A–C for each of the seven Hits identified from among the first 10 "WIBGI . . . ?" options provided.

Turn to the "Highlighting" Part 3 Field Organizer below and note that it has three parts (areas). Each area features Hot Spots from one of the columns (A, B, C) in "Highlighting" Part 2. You will record Hots Spots in Area I of each part. You will restate the wish statements in Area II of each part.

DIRECTIONS

Part 3

1. Transfer all the Hits from column A, Performance Areas ("Highlighting" Part 2) into their respective Hot Spot in "Highlighting" Part 3. The Hot Spots are:

   Hot Spot One: Play or leisure

   Hot Spot Two: ADL

   Hot Spot Three: Work and productive activities

   To get you started the seven Hits identified out of the first 10 options provided have been transferred in one of the three Hot Spots listed above.
2. Analyze the Hits in each Hot Spot (cluster) and restate the label of the Hot Spot as an opportunity statement. When you restate the Hot Spot, avoid making the restatement too restrictive. The restatement should reflect the main ideas stated in the cluster. For example, a restatement of the label ADL for Hot Spot One that reflects the Hits clustered

under that label could be: "WIBGI Sam could enjoy a wide range of play activities typical of a child Sam's age?" Record the Hot Spot restatements in Area II of the Field Organizer. A short version of the restatement listed above has been recorded.

3. Decide which restatement (new opportunity statement) reflects your top priority. You will explore this new opportunity statement in Data Finding. Time permitting, other opportunity statements can be worked through CPS.

4. Repeat the procedure described above in steps 1–3, for columns B and C in "Highlighting" Part 2. Transfer all Hits into their respective Hot Spots according to their label. Note: Spaces have been provided for additional performance subcategory Hot Spots (column B) that might emerge from the Hits you generate. A sample restatement has been provided for Hot Spot Cluster One for columns B and C.

FIELD ORGANIZER

"Highlighting" Part 3

Hot Spots from Column A: *Using* Performance Areas *to Cluster Hits*

Area I: Clusters

Cluster One Labeled: *Play and leisure*

WIBGI . . .

1. Sam played with puzzles and blocks?

2. Sam engaged in imaginative play?

8. Sam loved to play on playground equipment?

Cluster Two Labeled: *ADL*

WIBGI . . .

4. Sam looked forward to stroller and car rides?

5. Sam demonstrated age appropriate eating skills?

7. Sam played with children in a friendly manner?

"Highlighting" Part 3 (Continued)

Cluster Three Labeled: *Work and productive activities (educational)*

WIBGI . . .

9. *Sam enjoyed listening to stories read to him?*

Area II: Restatements

Hot Spot One: WIBGI *Sam could enjoy a wide range of typical play activities?*

Hot Spot Two: WIBGI

Hot Spot Three: WIBGI

FIELD ORGANIZER

"Highlighting" Part 3

Hot Spots from Column B: Using Performance Subcategories to Cluster Hits

Area I: Clusters

Cluster One Labeled: *Play and leisure performance*

WIBGI . . .

1. *Sam played with puzzles and blocks?*

2. *Sam engaged in imaginative play?*

8. *Sam loved to play on playground equipment?*

Cluster Two Labeled: *Community mobility*

WIBGI . . .

4. *Sam looked forward to stroller and car rides?*

(continued)

Hot Spots from Column B: *Using* **Performance Subcategories** *to Cluster Hits*

Area I: Clusters

Cluster Three Labeled: *Feeding and eating*

WIBGI . . .

5. *Sam demonstrated age appropriate eating skills?*

Cluster Four Labeled: *Socialization*

WIBGI . . .

7. *Sam played with children in a friendly manner?*

Cluster Five Labeled: *Educational activities*

WIBGI . . .

9. *Sam enjoyed listening to stories read to him?*

Area II: Restatements

Hot Spot One: WIBGI *Sam could enjoy a wide range of typical play activities?*

Hot Spot Two: WIBGI

Hot Spot Three: WIBGI

Hot Spot Four: WIBGI

Hot Spot Five: WIBGI

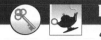

Hot Spots from Column C: Using Location to Cluster Hits

Area I: Clusters

Cluster One Labeled: *Wishes that can be worked on at home and school*

WIBGI...

1. *Sam played with puzzles and blocks?*

2. *Sam engaged in imaginative play?*

5. *Sam demonstrated age appropriate eating skills?*

7. *Sam played with children in a friendly manner?*

8. *Sam loved to play on playground equipment?*

9. *Sam enjoyed listening to stories read to him?*

Cluster Two Labeled: *Wishes best worked on at school*

WIBGI...

Cluster Three Labeled: *Wishes best worked on at home*

WIBGI...

4. *Sam looked forward to stroller and car rides?*

(continued)

Hot Spots from Column C: Using **Location** to Cluster Hits

Area II: Restatements

Hot Spot One: WIBGI *a unified approach to helping Sam develop skills and abilities could be used with Sam at home and at school?*

Hot Spot Two: WIBGI

Hot Spot Three: WIBGI

If, after using the "Highlighting" Thinking Key, the client continues to require guidance in prioritizing the Hot Spots, use either the "Evaluation Matrix" or the "PCA" Thinking Key (see Section 10).

Get Ready to Understand the Problem: Data Finding

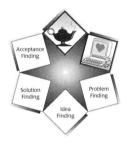

Data Finding: The Generating Phase

"5 W's & an H" and "5 W's & an H else" You have just completed Opportunity Finding and have recorded one wish statement that you will expand on in the Generating Phase of Data Finding. You will use the "5 Ws & an H" and the "5 Ws & an H else" Thinking Keys to systematically gather data about the wish statement and place the data into natural clusters.

The "5 Ws & an H" and the "5 Ws & an H else" and "Highlighting" (Part 1) Thinking Keys are joined together in one Field Organizer. The "5 Ws & an H" Thinking Key is in column A. The wide column (C) on the right side of the Field Organizer represents the "5 Ws & an H else" Thinking Key. Columns B and D are reserved for Part 1 of "Highlighting." You will be directed to use the "Highlighting" Thinking Key in the Focusing Phase of Data Finding.

To practice using the "The 5 W's & an H" and "The 5 W's & an H else" Thinking Keys you will expand upon the following wish statement: "WIBGI Sam enjoyed kindergarten?" To expand on this wish statement use:

- information from Sam's entire story as you did when you generated WIBGI . . . statements, as well as
- your imagination to push beyond the information provided in the story.

For the next Field Organizer, work in a small group, like the one formed for Opportunity Finding, with different members of the group assuming the roles of the people who share the responsibility for bringing about change on the therapy expedition. Before beginning review the list below and refer to it when responding to the questions posed in the "5 Ws & an H"

Thinking Key as they relate to Sam's Expedition. Recall that when you add *else* to the 5 Ws & an H, as in "Who else?" "Where else?" "What else?" and so on, you are pushing beyond the information you uncovered when using the "5 Ws & an H" Thinking Key.

The "5 Ws & an H" Reference List

Who   Identify people who are or could be involved (directly or indirectly) in creating opportunities to solve Sam's therapy-related problems.

Where   Name places and events to consider where opportunities could be found to help Sam's "wish" come true.

What   Identify what is involved in creating opportunities to help Sam's wish come true.

When   Explore time frames and duration related to when opportunities could be found to help Sam's wish come true.

Why   Explore the reason Sam's problem has to be solved.

How   Identify opportunities (such as methods or activities) that are possible and probable as well as those that may seem improbable in helping Sam's dream come true.

DIRECTIONS

"5 Ws & an H"

1. Add a minimum of four pieces of data to the information already listed in each of the six sections in column A (Generate). Each section is for one of the questions posed in the "5 Ws & an H" Thinking Key. Use the question at the top of each section to trigger your thoughts. There are more than five spaces left in each section, so don't limit yourself.

    Collect data with the intention of *thoroughly* exploring the wish statement you selected in the Focusing Phase of Opportunity Finding. This statement is like the tip of the iceberg for Sam's SI Expedition. To help make this wish a reality you will need to delve below the surface to uncover more information about this opportunity statement as well as the problem it is trying to solve.

2. Complete the "5 Ws & an H" Thinking Key before starting the "5 Ws & an H else" Thinking Key.

"5 Ws & an H else"

3. Add at least four pieces of data to the information already listed in each of the six sections in column C (Generate). Each section is for one of the questions posed in the "5 Ws & an H else" Thinking Key. Use the question at the top of each section to trigger your thoughts. There are more than five spaces left in each section, so don't limit yourself.

 FIELD ORGANIZER

"5 Ws & an H"/"5 Ws & an H else"/"Highlighting" Part 1

Wish Statement: WIBGI *Sam enjoyed kindergarten?*

A Generate	B Hits	C Generate	D Hits
Who might be involved in the opportunity?		**Who *else* might be involved in the opportunity?**	
1. *Sam's mother (Anne)*	●	1. *Sam's grandparents*	

(continued)

"5 Ws & an H"/"5 Ws & an H else"/"Highlighting" Part 1 (Continued)

A Generate	B Hits	C Generate	D Hits
Who might be involved in the opportunity?		**Who *else* might be involved in the opportunity?**	
2. Sam's father (Barry)	●	2. extended family (aunts, uncles, cousins)	
3. kindergarten teacher	●	3. neighbors (adults and children)	
4. school physical education teacher	●	4. family friends	
5. occupational therapy consultant	●	5. Sunday School teachers	
6. school classmates	●	6. Sunday School classmates	
7. social worker, school district		7. children's librarian in community	
8. psychologist, school district		8. community play group coordinator	
9.		9.	
10.		10.	
11.		11.	
12.		12.	
13.		13.	
14.		14.	
What is involved in the opportunity?		**What *else* is involved in the opportunity?**	
1. Review therapy reports from the rehabilitation center (initial evaluation and discharge summary).	●	1. Help Sam develop the emotional stability needed to attend to the learning activities he is exposed to at school and at home.	●
2. Help Sam sort out and make sense of sensations from his environment.	●	2. Help Sam learn about his body through classroom, gym, and playground activities.	●
3. Understand what kinds of touch, sound, movement, and visual experience calm Sam and what kinds appear to upset him.	●	3. Identify Sam's current baseline performance in the following areas: hygiene, dressing, eating, play, and fine and gross motor skills.	

What is involved in the opportunity?		What *else* is involved in the opportunity?	
4. Observe Sam at home.	●	4. Seek out a contact for the local parent support group.	
5. Observe Sam at school.	●	5. Inquire about Sam's interests.	
6. Identify Sam's coping strategies.	●	6. Identify the parents' methods for dealing with Sam when he becomes upset.	
7. Help Sam expand on his current coping strategies for dealing with changes in the environment.		7. Videotape Sam's performance on selected tasks throughout the therapy expedition to monitor change.	
8. Analyze Sam's performance with regard to how he processes sensory information.		8. Obtain resource materials on sensory processing problems.	
9.		9.	
10.		10.	
11.		11.	
12.		12.	
13.		13.	
14.		14.	

Where might opportunities occur to work on the wish?		Where *else* might opportunities occur to work on the wish?	
1. kindergarten classroom	●	1. restaurant	●
2. location of hanging equipment (school and at home)	●	2. grandparents' homes	
3. gym class	●	3. grocery shopping with mother	●
4. backyard of home	●	4. homes of neighbors and friends	
5. kitchen	●	5. school playground	●
6. local play indoor playlot	●	6. library	

(continued)

Where might opportunities occur to work on the wish?		Where *else* might opportunities occur to work on the wish?	
7. bathroom at school	●	7. community play center	
8. traveling to/from school in the car	●	8. homes of classmates	
9.		9.	
10.		10.	
11.		11.	
12.		12.	
13.		13.	
14.		14.	
When might there be an opportunity to work on the wish?		**When *else* might there be an opportunity to work on the wish?**	
1. gym class	●	1. bathroom periods at school	●
2. recess time on the playground	●	2. snack time at school	●
3. using hanging equipment at home and school	●	3. during nail care	●
4. listening to stories	●	4. when riding in the stroller or car	●
5. water and sand play time	●	5. holiday family get-togethers	
6. art activities at school (using crayons, paste, clay)	●	6. when Sam is watching television	
7. removing/putting on coat at school	●	7. bath time at home	●
8. playing with blocks, puzzles, and other manipulative toys	●	8. meal preparation at home	●
9.		9.	
10.		10.	

"5 Ws & an H"/"5 Ws & an H else"/"Highlighting" Part 1 (Continued)

When might there be an opportunity to work on the wish?		When *else* might there be an opportunity to work on the wish?	
11.		11.	
12.		12.	
13.		13.	
14.		14.	
Why is it important to look for opportunities in this area?		**Why *else* is it important to look for opportunities in this area?**	
1. to help Sam develop the readiness skills he needs to go into first grade	●	1. because Sam needs to learn how to cope with changes in life in order to grow and develop his full potential	●
2. Sam's parents need information in order to better understand Sam's behaviors.	●	2. If Sam could enjoy kindergarten he could participate in activities that will help him learn about his body and in turn help him cope.	●
3. Knowledge of Sam's special needs will better help his teacher understand Sam's unique behaviors.	●	3. If Sam had more accurate knowledge of his body he could experiment with different play activities that involve motor planning and coordination of both sides of his body.	●
4. Participating in kindergarten (and home) routines can help Sam develop the eye-hand coordination and visual perception needed to be successful in first grade.	●	4. If Sam could develop his concentration for performing tasks and his ability to organize himself he would enjoy learning and growing.	●
5. In the light of Sam's apparently high threshold for pain, he may bring injury to himself if his needs are not addressed.		5. so that Sam could develop social relationships and the necessary academic skills needed to function confidently in school	
6. Sam needs to develop friendships with peers.	●	6. so Sam will want to go to school every day	●
7. so that Sam can be better prepared for learning how to read and write	●	7. so that Sam demonstrates competence in bathroom skills by managing his clothing	●
8. to enhance Sam's self-esteem and self-concept, so that he feels good about himself	●	8. so that he can develop his imagination and creativity	
9.		9.	
10.		10.	

(continued)

"5 Ws & an H"/"5 Ws & an H else"/"Highlighting" Part 1 (Continued)

Why is it important to look for opportunities in this area?		Why *else* is it important to look for opportunities in this area?	
11.		11.	
12.		12.	
13.		13.	
14.		14.	
How will you make this wish a reality?		**How *else* will you make this wish a reality?**	
1. Parents fill out a checklist of Sam's sensory preferences in regard to touch, movement, visual, auditory, olfactory, and gustatory sensations.	●	1. Explore with Sam's parents sensory experience that could be part of Sam's play time at home.	●
2. Arrange to meet with Sam's parents to review the data from the sensorimotor history.	●	2. Explore Sam's response to deep pressure used on his legs and arms to make him less defensive to touch.	●
3. Correlate the data from the sensorimotor history with results from an assessment of Sam's occupational behavior.	●	3. Explore with the teacher the use of a quiet space that Sam (and the other kindergartners) could use when they get upset.	●
4. Correlate the data from the sensori-motor history with how Sam copes with stress (e.g., when he gets upset does he curl up with a blanket [tactile] or jump up and down [proprioceptive]).	●	4. Explore with the teacher the use of an energy space in a corner of the room where kids can do exercises to either rev up their energy levels or tap off a little excess energy.	
5. Use Sam's most adaptive coping strategy and brainstorm with parents ways to help Sam use that strategy in stressful situations.	●	5. Explore whether a movable air cushion (designed originally for adult office workers) could meet some of his need for movement stimulation.	
6. Explore with parents those things that Sam is most interested in and brainstorm on ways to incorporate those interests in a therapy plan.	●	6. Explore with parents strategies for incorporating movement experiences into their daily routine.	
7. Arrange a time to observe Sam at home and in the community.	●	7. Explore with Sam's teacher and parents strategies that can be used both at home and at school to help Sam cope with change.	●
8. Arrange a meeting time with Sam's teacher and parents to review the findings from the occupational therapy assessment process.	●	8. Model to adults working with Sam different ways to engage him in play.	

"5 Ws & an H"/"5 Ws & an H else"/"Highlighting" Part 1 (Continued)

How will you make this wish a reality?		How *else* will you make this wish a reality?	
9.		9.	
10.		10.	
11.		11.	
12.		12.	
13.		13.	
14.		14.	
15.		15.	

Data Finding: The Focusing Phase

"Highlighting." In Data Finding, only Part 1 of the "Highlighting" Thinking Key is used because the emphasis of the Highlighting process in this stage is on identifying all the Hits from the list of options that could help make Sam's SI Expedition a success. In contrast, the function of Highlighting in Opportunity Finding is to identify one wish statement that can be explored in Data Finding.

Before returning to the "5Ws . . ." Field Organizer to complete "Highlighting" Part 1, reorganize the group so that one person is the therapist and the others are playing the role of the client. The therapist facilitates the client's critique of the data generated.

DIRECTIONS

"Highlighting" Part 1

1. Direct the client to indicate the Hits by placing an orange dot in the Hits column to the right of each piece of information (columns B and D).
2. Complete Part 1 of the "Highlighting" Thinking Key before moving on to the "Storytelling" Thinking Key.

"Storytelling." The "Storytelling" Thinking Key will help you find relationships among Hits identified in the six sections for who, what, when, where, why, and how and the six sections for the 5 Ws & an H else. The Hits will be joined into a story that will help you think about how to make Sam's wish come true.

Practice using the "Storytelling" Thinking Key working with the same group, with one person in the role of the therapist and the others as the client. Each group member should have a completed copy of the "5 Ws & an H"/"5 Ws & an H else"/"Highlighting" Part 1 Field Organizer. Note that there is a sample "Storytelling" Field Organizer to help you get started. You will complete the second, blank version that follows the sample.

1. Ask the client to look for relationships among the Hits.
2. Begin the story by recording a portion of the wish statement selected from Opportunity Finding on the line at the top of the blank "Storytelling" Field Organizer. Drop the "WIBGI" from the wish statement and begin the statement with "If," as in "If Sam enjoyed kindergarten. . . ."
3. Complete this phrase by adding a Hit from the "5 Ws . . ." Field Organizer. Record the complete statement in row 1. Use the response in row 1 of the sample Field Organizer to model your response. "If Sam enjoyed kindergarten *he would develop the readiness skills he needs to go into first grade.*"
4. Develop the story by continuing to create and record sentences that incorporate Hits from the "5 Ws . . ." Field Organizer. Refer to the sample Field Organizer, which illustrates Hits that have been organized in such a way as to tell a story.
5. Place each story element on a line and create a linking phrase between one statement and the next such as "For this to occur . . ." or "If this could occur . . ." The arrows between the lines indicate the links between the story elements. As Hits are incorporated into the story, place the name of the section and the number associated with the Hit in parentheses. (See row 1 of the sample.) Recording where each Hit was drawn from will help you track the items as they are sequenced into the story and avoid duplication of Hits. You can create one long story or multiple short stories.
6. Next, direct the client to identify the theme that emerged from each story element (each area between arrows) and record the theme in the corresponding space at the bottom of the Field Organizer in Part B.

FIELD ORGANIZER

"Storytelling" (Sample)

Part A

Wish Statement: *If Sam enjoyed kindergarten . . .*

1. *he would develop the readiness skills he needs to go into first grade (Why #1).*

   In order for this to occur . . .

2. *Sam needs to learn to sort out and make sense of sensations from his environment (What #2). In order to help Sam make sense of his environment we need to understand what kinds of touch, sound, movement, and visual experiences calm Sam and what kinds appear to upset him (What #3). We need to observe Sam in his daily activities, in school and at home (What #4 and #5). If Sam's parents could fill out a checklist of Sam's likes and dislikes (sensorimotor history) such information would be very useful (How #1).*

   If these activities could occur . . .

3. *we could begin to analyze Sam's performance with regard to how he processes sensory information (What #8). With this knowledge we could help Sam expand on his current coping strategies for dealing with changes in the environment (What #7). Greater comfort with environmental changes (imposed by people or objects) could help Sam develop the emotional stability needed to attend to the learning activities he is exposed to at school and*

Part A

Wish Statement: *If Sam enjoyed kindergarten . . .*

at home (What else #1). Sam's ability to cope with change (coping strategies) is related to his knowledge of his body and how to move in space (Why else #2).

For this to occur . . .

4. Sam needs to learn about his body through the gross motor activities (e.g., swinging, rolling, spinning, and jumping) that are incorporated into gym class, and classroom, home, and playground activities (What else #2; When #1–3; Where #1, 3; Where else #5). In order to gear activities to Sam's ability level it will be necessary to work closely with Sam's parents, gym teacher, and kindergarten teacher (Who #1–4). If Sam had more accurate knowledge of his body he could experiment with different play activities that involve motor planning and coordination of both sides of his body (Why else #3).

If this could occur . . .

5. Sam would enjoy participating in school and home routines, i.e., mealtime, dressing, hygiene, grooming, and playing with blocks, puzzles, and other manipulatives during art activities (When #1–8; When else #1, 2, 10; Where #1–7; Where else #3). Participating in kindergarten and home routines can help Sam develop his eye-hand coordination and visual perceptual skills (Why #1, 3, 5, 7–8; Why else #7).

If this could occur . . .

6. Sam would be better prepared for learning how to read and write (Why #7). Successes from learning to read and write will help him further develop his self-concept and self-esteem (Why #8).

If this could occur . . .

7. it would help Sam develop social relationships and the necessary academic skills needed to function confidently in school (Why else #5). Then Sam would want to go to school every day (Why else #6).

Part B: Themes from Sam's Story

1. Develop readiness skills needed for first grade.
2. Sort out and make sense of sensory information.
3. Accept change.
4. Feel confident to try new activities.
5. Be successful in daily routines (using eye-hand coordination and visual perception).
6. Build self-control, self-esteem, and self-concept through successes at school.
7. Develop social relationships and academic skills.

FIELD ORGANIZER
"Storytelling"

Part A

Wish Statement: _____
_____

1. _____
_____
_____

↓

2. _____
_____
_____

↓

3. _____
_____
_____

↓

4. _____
_____
_____

↓

5. _____
_____
_____

↓

6. _____
_____
_____

7. _____

_____

_____

Part B: Themes from Sam's Story

1. _____

_____

2. _____

_____

3. _____

_____

4. _____

_____

5. _____

_____

6. _____

_____

7. _____

_____

Hits identified in the "5 Ws . . . " Field Organizer that are not incorporated into a story element may spark an idea you can use in another stage of CPS.

Get Ready to Understand the Problem: Problem Finding

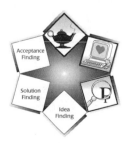

Problem Finding: The Generating Phase

In the Problem Finding stage you will identify the route you and the client will take for the remainder of CPS. To locate the most appropriate route, you will identify the *specific* gap between "what is" and "what should be," in the client's occupational performance. (Recall that in Opportunity Finding you identify a client's challenges broadly.)

The following three Thinking Keys will help you focus in on the gap by viewing the client's problem from many different perspectives: "IWWM . . . Who–Does–What?" "Substitution," and the "Ladder of Abstraction." As you generate problem statements in this stage remain mindful of the Hits identified in Data Finding so that the data can be incorporated as needed.

Each of the three Thinking Keys listed above is paired with Part 1 of the "Highlighting" Thinking Key in its respective Field Organizer. In the "IWWM . . . Who–Does–What?" Field Organizer, Part 1 of the "Highlighting" Thinking Key is located on the right side in the column labeled Focus. In the "Substitution" Field Organizer, Part 1 of "Highlighting" is in Part B, on the right side, in the column labeled Hits. In the "Ladder of Abstraction" Field Organizer, the right corner of each box is reserved for identifying Hits during the "Highlighting" process. You will be directed to use the "Highlighting" portion of each of the Field Organizers in the Focusing Phase of Problem Finding.

Practice using the "IWWM . . . Who–Does–What?" "Substitution," and "Ladder of Abstraction" Thinking Keys with the same group you worked with when practicing Opportunity Finding and Data Finding.

"IWWM . . . Who–Does–What?" To complete the Field Organizer for this Thinking Key you will focus on the following wish statement: "WIBGI Sam enjoyed kindergarten?"

DIRECTIONS

Complete the invitational stem "IWWM . . . ?" by filling in the columns for Who, Does, and What. Note: As you generate ideas, try to hitchhike one idea to another. To get you started 10 problem statements have been provided.

FIELD ORGANIZER

"IWWM . . . Who–Does–What?"/"Highlighting" Part 1

Wish Statement: *WIBGI Sam enjoyed kindergarten?*

Generate				Focus
IWWM . . .				
	Who?	**Does?**	**What?**	**Hits**
1.	*Sam*	*handle*	*a full day of kindergarten?*	●
2.	*teacher*	*help*	*Sam to follow directions?*	
3.	*Sam's parents*	*support*	*school routines at home?*	●
4.	*Sam*	*play*	*school with neighborhood children?*	●
5.	*Sam*	*meet with*	*his teacher before school?*	

	Generate			Focus
IWWM . . .				
	Who?	**Does?**	**What?**	**Hits**
6.	Sam	play	school at home?	●
7.	Sam	invite	cousins to his house to play school?	
8.	Sam	play	the teacher with his mother as the student?	●
9.	Sam	set up	his playroom to resemble a kindergarten?	●
10.	Sam	read	about other children who go to kindergarten?	
11.				
12.				
13.				
14.				
15.				
16.				
17.				
18.				
19.				
20.				

"Substitution." Use the "Substitution" Thinking Key to create alternative wording for the problem statement. The "Substitution" Thinking Key has two parts. Note that the following problem statement has been recorded at the top of the Field Organizer: "IWWM Sam learn to follow the daily classroom routines?"

Part A

1. Read the problem statement for which you will find alternative wording.
2. Circle the verb in the problem statement.
3. Take the verb that has been circled and think up as many substitutions for it as you can. Place the alternative verbs in the column labeled Does? rows 5–8. To get you started four substitutions have been recorded.

Part B

4. Write any new problem statements that resulted in rows 5–8 from changing the wording in the original problem statement. Indicate the statements that you reworded by recording the row number of the original statement to the left of the reworded statement. To get you started new problem statements for rows 1–4 have been recorded.

The "Substitution" Thinking Key can also be used to find alternative wording for the Who and the What parts of the problem statement.

FIELD ORGANIZER

"Substitution"/"Highlighting" Part 1

Part A

Problem Statement: *IWWM Sam learn to follow the daily classroom routines?*

IWWM...

	Who?	Does?	What?
1.	Sam's teacher	show	Sam learn to follow the daily classroom routines?
2.	Sam's teacher	support	Sam learn to follow the daily classroom routines?
3.	Sam's teacher	motivate	Sam learn to follow the daily classroom routines?
4.	Sam's teacher	cue	Sam learn to follow the daily classroom routines?
5.	Sam's teacher		Sam learn to follow the daily classroom routines?
6.	Sam's teacher		Sam learn to follow the daily classroom routines?
7.	Sam's teacher		Sam learn to follow the daily classroom routines?
8.	Sam's teacher		Sam learn to follow the daily classroom routines?

Part B

	Hits
1. IWWM Sam's teacher show Sam how to follow the daily classroom routines?	
2. IWWM Sam's teacher support Sam's ability to follow the daily classroom routines?	●
3. IWWM Sam's teacher motivate Sam to take pride in participating in classroom routines?	●
4. IWWM Sam's teacher cue Sam throughout the day to help him participate in classroom routines?	●

Part B

	Hits

"Ladder of Abstraction." This Thinking Key helps you identify a wide range of problem statements by asking questions that begin "How?" and "Why?" When you ask "How?" questions you get answers about the client's problem that are concrete and specific. When you ask "Why?" questions you get answers that are more general and abstract. Thinking about the client's problem in specific terms as well as in broad terms expands the vision you have of the client's problem. You will begin the "Ladder of Abstraction" Field Organizer with the following problem statement: "IWWM Sam learn to follow the daily kindergarten routine?"

DIRECTIONS

1. Locate the initial problem statement in the middle of the Field Organizer.
2. Decide whether you wish to start by moving up in the ladder and make the initial statement more abstract or down in the ladder and make the problem statement more concrete and specific.

Before you fill in your responses be sure to read the "How?" and the "Why?" questions and the answers to these questions, which have been provided in the middle column as well as the "Why else?" and the "How else?" responses in the first row of the respective portions of the field organizer.

The arrows on the field organizer are used to demonstrate the direction of the question and answer process. The arrows that project out from the Field Organizer represent the future possibility of more questions and answers from that point.

 FIELD ORGANIZER

"Ladder of Abstraction"/"Highlighting" Part 1

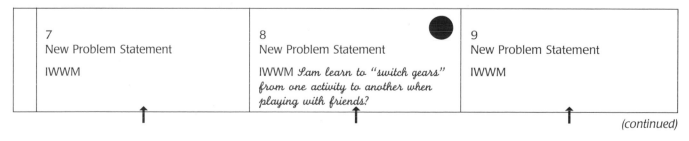

7 New Problem Statement IWWM	8 New Problem Statement IWWM *Sam learn to "switch gears" from one activity to another when playing with friends?*	9 New Problem Statement IWWM

(continued)

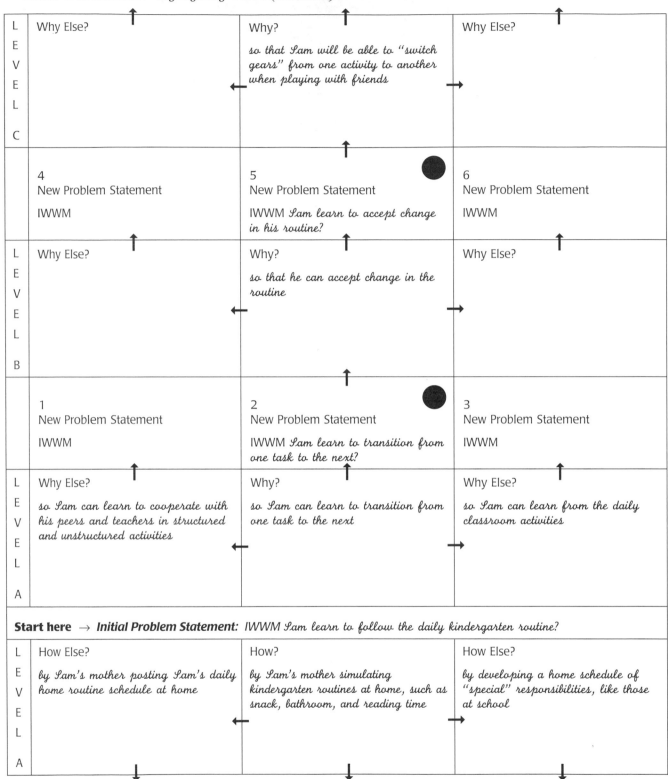

L E V E L C	Why Else?	Why? *so that Sam will be able to "switch gears" from one activity to another when playing with friends*	Why Else?
	4 New Problem Statement IWWM	**5** New Problem Statement IWWM *Sam learn to accept change in his routine?*	**6** New Problem Statement IWWM
L E V E L B	Why Else?	Why? *so that he can accept change in the routine*	Why Else?
	1 New Problem Statement IWWM	**2** New Problem Statement IWWM *Sam learn to transition from one task to the next?*	**3** New Problem Statement IWWM
L E V E L A	Why Else? *so Sam can learn to cooperate with his peers and teachers in structured and unstructured activities*	Why? *so Sam can learn to transition from one task to the next*	Why Else? *so Sam can learn from the daily classroom activities*

Start here → **Initial Problem Statement:** *IWWM Sam learn to follow the daily kindergarten routine?*

L E V E L A	How Else? *by Sam's mother posting Sam's daily home routine schedule at home*	How? *by Sam's mother simulating kindergarten routines at home, such as snack, bathroom, and reading time*	How Else? *by developing a home schedule of "special" responsibilities, like those at school*

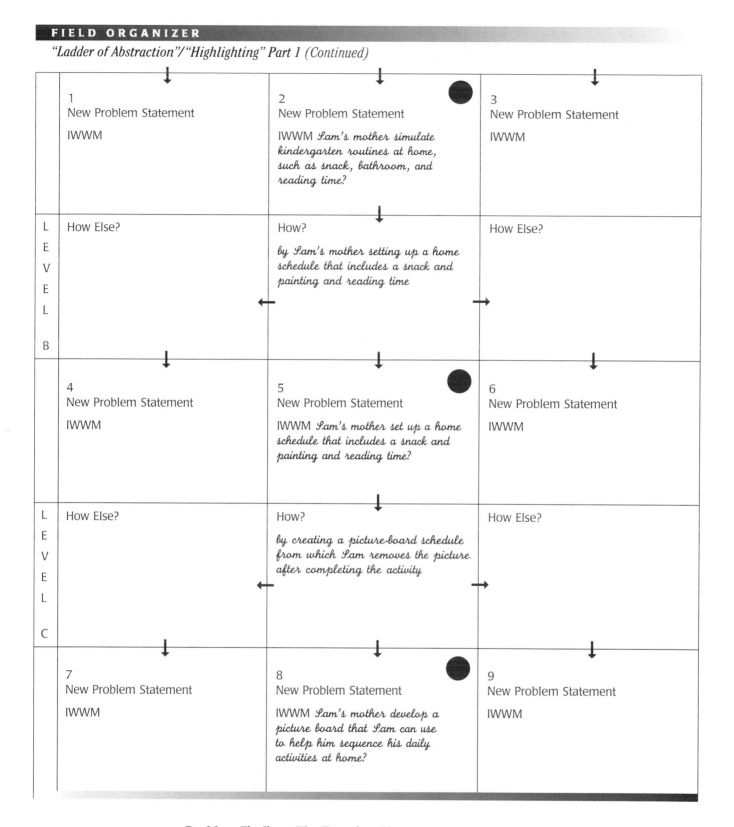

1 New Problem Statement IWWM	**2** New Problem Statement ● IWWM *Sam's mother simulate kindergarten routines at home, such as snack, bathroom, and reading time?*	**3** New Problem Statement IWWM
L E V E L B How Else?	How? *by Sam's mother setting up a home schedule that includes a snack and painting and reading time*	How Else?
4 New Problem Statement IWWM	**5** New Problem Statement ● IWWM *Sam's mother set up a home schedule that includes a snack and painting and reading time?*	**6** New Problem Statement IWWM
L E V E L C How Else?	How? *by creating a picture-board schedule from which Sam removes the picture after completing the activity*	How Else?
7 New Problem Statement IWWM	**8** New Problem Statement ● IWWM *Sam's mother develop a picture board that Sam can use to help him sequence his daily activities at home?*	**9** New Problem Statement IWWM

Problem Finding: The Focusing Phase

"Head and Shoulders Test." Use the "Head and Shoulders Test" to determine whether one problem statement from the "IWWM . . . Who–Does–What?" the "Substitution," or the "Ladder of Abstraction" Field Organizer stands "head and shoulders" above the rest.

Review the list of problem statements to determine whether the client likes one problem statement over all the rest. (In this context the client is represented by those persons who share ownership of the problem, including Sam's parents and teacher.)

FIELD ORGANIZER
"Head and Shoulders Test"

Ask the client:

"Does one problem statement in the group stand **head and shoulders** above the rest?"

If the client is very interested in pursuing one of the statements or a combination of statements at this point, confirm the problem statement with the client and write it on the line below.

IWWM _____

Proceed to Idea Finding using this problem statement.

For instructional purposes, you were asked to select one option for the "Head and Shoulders Test." Now practice using the "Highlighting" Thinking Key as if you had not found one problem statement you liked better than all the rest.

"Highlighting." In situations where one wish statement does not stand head and shoulders above the rest, use the "Highlighting" Thinking Key to evaluate each of the wish statements developed in the Generating Phase. "Highlighting" involves first, identifying Hits; second, clustering the Hits into Hot Spots; and third, restating the Hot Spot labels into new problem statements that reflect the essence of the Hits clustered in each Hot Spot.

Recall that we paired Part 1 of the "Highlighting" Thinking Key into one Field Organizer with each of the three Thinking Keys used in the Generating Phase of Problem Finding so that the Hits can be identified without being rewritten in a separate "Highlighting" Field Organizer. In Problem Finding, a Hit is a problem statement the client wishes to pursue.

You will complete the "Highlighting" process in the next Field Organizer, "Highlighting" Parts 2 and 3. Work with the same group as before with one member as the therapist who facilitates the group process and the others as the client.

DIRECTIONS

Part 1

Materials: orange adhesive dots
1. Review with the client the list of problem statements in the Field Organizers for "IWWM . . . Who–Does–What?" "Substitution," and "Ladder of Abstraction."
2. Direct the client to select the Hits from the list of problem statements by placing an orange dot in the space provided for Hits in each of the three Field Organizers. To get you started some Hits have been identified.

Part 2

1. Transfer the Hits from the "IWWM . . . Who–Does–What?" "Substitution," and "Ladder of Abstraction" Field Organizers to the column labeled Hits in "Highlighting" Part 2. Transfer the Hits from the Field Organizers in any order. The Field Organizer each Hit came from is not important. To get you started all the Hits identified in "Highlighting" Part 1 have been transferred.

2. Look for relationships among the Hits by first identifying the central theme of each Hit. Then record the central theme of each Hit in the right column of the Field Organizer. The themes identified will serve as the label for the Hits when they get clustered into Hot Spots. Three themes emerged from the first 10 problem statements: play school at home, handling change, and school routine.

   How you categorize Hits will depend on where you place the emphasis of the Problem Finding statement as influenced by your paradigm. For example, from one perspective you might categorize the Hit, "Sam's parents support Sam's school routines at home" as "play school at home." From another perspective you might categorize the same statement as "handling change."

3. Record in Area II all of the central themes that were identified. These themes will be used to cluster the Hits into Hot Spots. The three themes identified above have been recorded in the space provided. Add to the three themes listed any other themes that emerge when you analyze the Hits you transfer.

Part 3

1. Transfer all the Hits from Part 2 into their respective Hot Spot in Part 3. Three Hot Spots have been identified:

   Hot Spot One: Handling change

   Hot Spot Two: Play school at home

   Hot Spot Three: School routine

   Space has been provided for you to add Hot Spots that emerge from the Hits you generate.

2. Analyze the Hits in each Hot Spot (cluster) and restate the label of the Hot Spot as a problem statement. The key to restating a Hot Spot is to avoid making the restatement too broad or too narrow. The restatement should reflect the main ideas stated in the cluster. For example, a restatement of the label "Handling change" that reflects the Hits clustered under that label in Hot Spot I could be: "IWWM Sam learn to handle changes in his school and home routines?" Record the Hot Spot restatements in Area II of the Field Organizer in the space provided.

3. Decide which restatement (new problem statement) reflects your top priority. Use that new problem statement for the remainder of CPS. Look for a problem statement that is inclusive of the broadest number of challenges discussed. The more inclusive the problem statement the more comprehensive the solution will be. Keep in mind that the final selection of a problem statement is influenced by the resources available.

 FIELD ORGANIZER

"Highlighting" Parts 2 and 3

Wish Statement: *WIBGI Sam enjoyed kindergarten?*	
Part 2	
Area I: Hits	**Central Theme**
IWWM . . .	
1. *Sam handle a full day of kindergarten?*	*school routine*
2. *Sam's parents support school routines at home?*	*school routine*
3. *Sam play school with neighborhood children?*	*play school at home*
4. *Sam play school at home?*	*play school at home*

(continued)

"Highlighting" (Continued)

Area I: Hits	Central Theme
IWWM . . .	
5. Sam role play the teacher with his mother as the student?	play school at home
6. Sam set up his playroom to resemble a kindergarten?	play school at home
7. Sam's teacher support Sam's ability to follow the daily classroom routines?	school routine
8. Sam's teacher motivate Sam to take pride in participating in classroom routines?	school routine
9. Sam's teacher cue Sam throughout the day to help him participate in classroom routines?	school routine
10. Sam learn to transition from one task to the next?	handling change
11. Sam learn to accept change in his routine?	handling change
12. Sam learn to "switch gears" from one activity to another when playing with friends?	handling change
13. Sam's mother simulate kindergarten routines at home, such as snack, bathroom, and reading time?	play school at home
14. Sam's mother set up a home schedule that includes a snack and painting and reading time?	school routine
15. Sam's mother develop a picture board that Sam can use to help him sequence his daily activities at home?	school routine
16.	
17.	
18.	
19.	
20.	
21.	
22.	
23.	
24.	
25.	
26.	
27.	

Area II: Hot Spots Labels

1. Handling change   4. _____

2. Play school at home   5. _____

3. School routine   6. _____

Part 3

Area I: Hot Spots

Hot Spot I Labeled: Handling change

IWWM . . .

10. Sam learn to transition from one task to the next?

11. Sam learn to accept change in his routine?

12. Sam learn to "switch gears" from one activity to another when playing with friends?

Hot Spot II Labeled: Play school at home

IWWM . . .

3. Sam played school with neighborhood children?

4. Sam play school at home?

5. Sam role play the teacher with his mother as the student?

6. Sam set up his playroom to resemble a kindergarten?

13. Sam's mother simulate kindergarten routines at home, such as snack, bathroom, and reading time?

(continued)

"Highlighting" (Continued)

Hot Spot III Labeled: *School routine*
IWWM . . .
1. *Sam handle a full day of kindergarten?*
2. *Sam's parents support school routines at home?*
7. *Sam's teacher support Sam's ability to follow the daily classroom routines?*
8. *Sam's teacher motivate Sam to take pride in participating in classroom routines?*
9. *Sam's teacher cue Sam throughout the day to help him participate in classroom routines?*
14. *Sam's mother set up a home schedule that includes a snack and painting and reading time?*
15. *Sam's mother develop a picture board that Sam can use to help him sequence his daily activities at home?*
Area II: Restatements
Hot Spot I: IWWM *Sam learn to handle changes in his school and home routines?*
Hot Spot II: IWWM
Hot Spot III: IWWM

Get Set to Find a Solution: Idea Finding

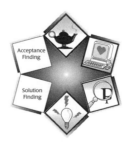

Idea Finding: The Generating Phase

In the Idea Finding stage you focus your efforts on generating many different options for solving the client's problems. In this stage you use the following four Thinking Keys: "Brainstorming," "CAMPERS," "Force Fit," and "Attribute Listing." Each of these Thinking Keys exemplifies a certain quality associated with creative performance. As you develop skill using the Thinking Keys you will learn to select the Thinking Key best suited for the situation.

Thinking Keys That Exemplify Qualities Associated with Creative Performance

"Brainstorming"	**Fluency:** the ability to produce a large quantity of ideas
"CAMPERS"	**Flexibility:** the ability to shift from one method to another or combine methods
"Forced Fit"	**Originality:** the ability to generate novel approaches
"Attribute Listing"	**Elaboration:** the ability to develop ideas by adding details that enrich the original thought

Each of the four Thinking Keys in Idea Finding is paired with Part 1 of the "Highlighting" Thinking Key in its respective Field Organizer. You will be directed to use the "Highlighting" portion of each of the Field Organizers in the Focusing Phase of Idea Finding.

Practice using the Thinking Keys in this section with the same group you worked with when practicing Opportunity Finding, Data Finding, and Problem Finding. The therapy guide should serve as the group facilitator and record all ideas that are generated by the group.

For each of the Thinking Keys in Idea Finding you will be directed to focus on different aspects of the following problem statement: "IWWM a home/school program be developed to help Sam learn how to follow the kindergarten routines?" This problem statement is recorded at the top of each Field Organizer.

In the list below you will find an explanation of what to focus on when using each Thinking Key during Sam's SI Expedition.

Thinking Keys for Sam's SI Therapy Expedition

"Brainstorming":	Generate activities that help remediate Sam's sensory processing problems. Activities should incorporate tactile, proprioceptive, and vestibular input that lead to an adaptive response.
"CAMPERS":	Generate activities that help Sam make the transition from one activity to another.
"Forced Fit":	Force a correlation ("fit") between selected random associations and Sam's home/school program.
"Attribute Listing":	Generate activities that are specifically related to following kindergarten routines, at school, at home, or both.

"Brainstorming." Use the "Brainstorming" Thinking Key when you want to generate a large quantity of ideas. The "Brainstorming" Field Organizer is divided into three main columns (A, C, E) with a narrow column (B, D, F) to the right of each larger column for Part One of "Highlighting." When creating fun activities for Sam's expedition use themes drawn from children's stories, from nature, and from daily happenings in Sam's life. Activities should be designed to be carried out at home (to be incorporated by Sam's parents into their play time with Sam) or to be carried out at school (to be incorporated by Sam's teacher into the classroom routine or with the help of a teacher's aide). The teacher might be given a set of cards, for example, with a single activity printed on each card. She could then include the recommended activities in her weekly lesson plan.

---

1. Generate ideas for the problem statement at the top of the Field Organizer.
2. Refer to the list of Thinking Keys for Sam's SI Expedition for the kinds of activities to generate during "Brainstorming." Indicate in parentheses after each activity which sensory system(s) is most likely stimulated when performing that activity.
3. Record ideas in the spaces provided. Remember to hitchhike one idea on another and record all ideas, even wild and crazy ones. To get you started, 12 brainstorming ideas have been recorded.

 FIELD ORGANIZER

"Brainstorming"

Problem Statement: *IWWM a home/school program be developed to help Sam learn how to follow the kindergarten routines?*

A Idea	B Hits	C Idea	D Hits	E Idea	F Hits
1. Sam imitates a butterfly emerging from a cocoon by trying to wiggle out of a sleeping bag while an adult applies pressure to the top of the bag as resistance to Sam's movements (tactile and proprioceptive).	●	2. Sam imagines himself as a wrestler and play wrestles with an adult on a mat or a carpeted surface. Sam can control the time period of each match (about 10 seconds) (tactile, vestibular, and proprioceptive).	●	3. Sam imagines himself as a burrito (or any other object that rolls such as a wheel, fruit roll-up, dough, yo-yo) by rolling up into a blanket (tactile, vestibular, and proprioceptive).	●
4. Sam and a small group of children lie face down, side by side on a mat with arms extended over their heads. The child at one end of the line rolls up on top of the child next to him and rolls to the end of the line. This continues until all children have rolled over the entire group. When a child rolls over the top of the other children he imagines himself as a baker rolling out dough with the children on the bottom acting as the dough (tactile, proprioceptive, and vestibular).	●	5. Same set up as in #4 with the following adaptation: Instead of the children rolling over one another a mat is placed on top of the children and a big ball is rolled over the group imitating the action of a steam roller (tactile, proprioceptive, and vestibular).	●	6. Sam imagines himself to be a sorcerer with magic powers to fly with the aid of magic dust. Sam rolls a squishy ball over his arms and legs that he pretends is filled with magic dust that is released when the ball is squeezed (tactile and proprioceptive). Using the fundamental idea of rolling the squishy ball to provide tactile and input, the game can be expanded endlessly.	●
7. Sam imagines himself to be a weight lifter sitting in a chair lifting his own weight by using his hands to do a pushup from the seat of the chair. He attempts to increase the amount of time he can maintain his weight off the chair's surface (proprioceptive).	●	8. Sam imagines himself to be a bridge opening up and letting boats pass under by lying on his back and bridging himself up onto his hands and feet (proprioceptive). Once Sam can hold himself he can start moving around.		9. Sam imagines that he is a top spinning to the beat of different rhythms while seated on a scooter board (proprioceptive and vestibular).	●

	A Idea	B Hits	C Idea	D Hits	E Idea	F Hits
	10. *Sam imagines himself to be an Olympic athlete who does squats while holding onto some stable surface (proprioceptive and vestibular).*	●	11. *Sam imagines himself to be Peter Rabbit, who finds a hole to burrow into by sitting in a small tight space filled with cushions or a bean bag chair (proprioceptive and tactile).* *Tight spaces can be created by moving file cabinets away from a wall, using appliance boxes or closet space or pushing desks against a wall so Sam can go under them.*	●	12. *Sam imagines himself to be a muscle-bound weight lifter in training for a match. Sam squeezes and releases different body parts (e.g., face, fists, arms, toes, torso) in response to verbal and tactile cues to do so (e.g., saying "show me the muscles in your arms," "tighten that arm" while touching Sam's arm) (proprioceptive).*	●
	13.		14.		15.	
	16.		17.		18.	
	19.		20.		21.	

"CAMPERS." Use the "CAMPERS" Thinking Key when you want to build flexibility into your thinking. The "CAMPERS" Field Organizer is divided into three columns and seven sections. You will use column C for Part 1 of "Highlighting" in the Focusing Phase of Idea Finding.

DIRECTIONS

1. Generate ideas related to the problem statement listed at the top.
2. Read the questions listed in column A, reflecting on the data gathered about the problem in Data Finding. Note that two questions have been generated for each of the

seven parts of the acronym CAMPERS. To get you started responses have been recorded for the first question in each section.

3. Record responses to the second question in each section.

FIELD ORGANIZER

"CAMPERS"

Problem Statement: *IWWM a home/school program be developed to help Sam learn how to follow the kindergarten routines?*

A Sample questions to develop flexibility in your thinking	B Responses to questions in column A	C Hits
What can I Combine? Can I combine units, purposes, ideas, steps, or different kinds of people, disciplines, or groups? How about a blend or an assortment?	*Routines that are common to kindergarten and home can be put on a simple laminated picture chart (e.g., showing snack, storytime, handwashing, and block play). As routines change Sam could indicate the routine on his board. Washable transparency pens can be used on the laminated surface.*	●
What can I Adapt? Can I use existing materials, processes, or personnel to solve the problem? What or whom can I emulate? What can I use from a past experience? What other activities or things are similar? What other idea does this suggest?	*Kindergarten students could take turns announcing when the group was to move from one activity to another.* *Sam's parents could ask Sam to announce when the family was moving from one activity to another (e.g., moving from setting the table to sitting down and eating).*	●
What can I Modify? What could be added or taken away? What could be made larger or smaller? How can a new twist be added to an obvious situation? How can I increase or decrease the frequency? How can I duplicate, exaggerate, condense, streamline?	*Each time Sam's teacher shifts from one main activity to another she could play music to ready the group for the next activity.*	●

"CAMPERS" (Continued)

A Sample questions to develop flexibility in your thinking	B Responses to questions in column A	C Hits
What can I Put to other uses? In what other contexts might it work? What are some "out-of-the-box" ways to use it? Could its form, weight, or structure suggest another use?	*When Sam is doing errands with his parents, Sam is responsible for announcing the plan for each stop (e.g., "Now we will shop for groceries." "Here we will drop off our dry cleaning.").*	●
What can I Eliminate? Could fewer steps, materials, or people be involved? How can I make less be more?	*Sam's teacher would identify how Sam transitions from one activity to another rather than expect him to readily change every time there is a change in the classroom.*	●
What can I Rearrange? What part of the process can be reversed? Can I interchange things or people?	*Have Sam play the game "Name That Change." To play the game, tell Sam that you are about to change activities but don't tell him what the change will be. Instruct Sam to observe the class as the change takes place. His task is to tell you what change occurred after it takes place.*	●
What can I Substitute? Who else might be recruited? What other ingredients, materials, processes, places, or approaches could be substituted?	*Sam's parents and teacher use puppets to talk to Sam about changing from one activity to another.*	●

"Force Fit." Use the "Force Fit" Thinking Key when you wish to use a trigger from an external stimulus that helps to generate novel or "out-of-the-box" ideas. The "Force Fit" Field Organizer is divided into three columns. You will use column C for Part 1 of "Highlighting" in the Focusing Phase of Idea Finding.

1. Read the six ideas that were generated by forcing a fit between the random input *book* and the problem statement listed at the top.
2. Add a minimum of four ideas using the random input *book* (rows 7–10).
3. Select two additional random input words and record them in column A, rows 2–3. To select a random input, you can:

   ◆ Look around the room for an object

   ◆ Open a dictionary and put your finger on a word

   ◆ Look in a catalogue, telephone book yellow pages, or newspaper advertisements

   ◆ Think of something from nature (e.g., mountain, sunset, river, tree)

   ◆ Think of an animal

4. Consider in what ways the random input may relate to setting up a program to help Sam learn how to follow kindergarten routines. Withhold any concern for the relevance of the input to the problem. "Force" a minimum of five "fits" between each random stimulus and the process of helping Sam learn how to follow kindergarten routines.

FIELD ORGANIZER

"Force Fit"

Problem Statement: *IWWM a home/school program be developed to help Sam learn how to follow the kindergarten routines?*

A Random Input	B Force a Fit Between the Random Input and the Problem at Hand	C Hits
1. *Book*	1. *Read Sam a children's book about a child going to kindergarten (e.g., from the Berenstein Bears collection).*	●
	2. *While reading Sam a book about kindergarten ask Sam how he feels about school.*	
	3. *Use a school-to-home notebook to tell Sam's family about Sam's day at school.*	●
	4. *Arrange for a child from the upper grades to come to Sam's classroom before the end of the day to help him write in his notebook a sentence or two about his day. Sam will bring his notebook home for his parents to read and sign. In the beginning of the year Sam's sentences will be written by the older student with Sam adding a letter or two and a picture. As the year progresses Sam will be expected (and able) to help write some simple words.*	●
	5. *Each time Sam brings home a piece of artwork his mother punches the sheet and puts it into a three-ring notebook. Sam can make a picture for the cover of his notebook.*	
	6. *Sam's parents keep a notebook in which they make an entry on a single page in big letters every time Sam accomplishes a new skill (e.g., "On September 7th Sam put on his coat all by himself—Hooray." "On September 8th Sam cleared his plate from the kitchen table—Hurray," "On September 9th Sam pours his own cereal into his bowl—Hurray! Sam receives a big bear hug with every entry.)*	
	7.	
	8.	

A Random Input	B Force a Fit Between the Random Input and the Problem at Hand	C Hits
1. *Book* (continued)	9. 10.	
2.	1. 2. 3. 4. 5.	
3.	1. 2. 3. 4. 5.	

"Attribute Listing." Use the "Attribute Listing" Thinking Key when you want to elaborate on main elements within the problem statement. The "Attribute Listing" Field Organizer is divided into three columns. Column A identifies three of the main attributes of the problem statement on which you will elaborate. They are *follow, kindergarten,* and *routines.* Column B is for recording the ideas generated, and column C is for Part 1 of "Highlighting."

DIRECTIONS

1. Generate ideas that relate to the problem statement listed at the top.
2. Record your ideas in column B in the space directly to the right of the attributes on which you are elaborating. To get you started five activities have been recorded for each of the three attributes.

FIELD ORGANIZER

"Attribute Listing"

Problem Statement: *IWWM a home/school program be developed to help Sam learn how to follow the kindergarten routines?*

A Attribute	B Elaborate on the Attribute under consideration	C Hits
1. Routine	1. Identify the routines used in Sam's kindergarten.	●
	2. Set up a home routine that incorporates elements of the kindergarten routine (e.g., snack, art, block play, and reading time; hanging up coat on designated hook).	●
	3. Have Sam help make a picture board with home routines that are similar to Sam's kindergarten routines (e.g., snack, art, block play, and reading time; hanging up coat on designated hook).	●
	4. On weekend mornings, instruct Sam to arrange the pictures on his home routine board, according to the order he wants to do his activities.	
	5. Have Sam help make a small board with a pocket to hold a picture of whatever routine activity he is going to begin. As he changes activities, Sam changes his pocket picture.	●
	6.	
	7.	
	8.	
	9.	
	10.	

"Attribute Listing" (Continued)

A Attribute	B Elaborate on the Attribute under consideration	C Hits
2. *Follow*	1. *Ask Sam to follow one-step directions (e.g., "Sam, please hang up your coat." "Sam, please close the door." "Sam, please button your shirt.")*	●
	2. *Have Sam give his mother one-step directions to follow at a designated time in the day (time is marked on a clock in the house so Sam can tell when his time is coming to give directions).*	●
	3. *Make a simple chart of five tasks for Sam to perform (follow) every morning (e.g., eat breakfast, get dressed, brush teeth, get school backpack ready, make bed).*	
	4. *Instruct Sam to put a star on the chart described in #3 for every direction he follows without being told.*	
	5. *Audio- or videotape Sam giving his parents directions that they are to follow. Play back the tape and have Sam listen to himself give directions.*	●
	6.	
	7.	
	8.	
	9.	
	10.	
3. *Kindergarten experience: storytime, snack time, block time, art time*	1. *Set a regular story time in the day to which Sam can look forward.*	●
	2. *During storytime have Sam snuggle up in a sleeping bag (tactile and proprioceptive input) or a blanket next to an adult in a tight space (womblike space).*	●
	3. *Allow Sam to select the storybooks that the teacher will read for the week. Instruct Sam to arrange the books in the order he wants them read.*	
	4. *Encourage Sam to select a story that can be acted out (e.g., "Tom Thumb," "The Three Little Pigs," "Peter Rabbit").*	
	5. *Create a space in Sam's house where his art projects can be displayed.*	
	6.	

(continued)

A Attribute	B Elaborate on the Attribute under consideration	C Hits
	7.	
	8.	
	9.	
	10.	

Idea Finding: The Focusing Phase

"Highlighting." Since the objective in the Focusing Phase of Idea Finding is to identify all those ideas that might help resolve the problem, only Part 1 of "Highlighting" is used. The Hits identified in the Focusing Phase are then further analyzed during Solution Finding.

Recall that each of the Thinking Keys "Brainstorming" "CAMPERS," "Force Fit," and "Attribute Listing" is paired with Part 1 of the "Highlighting" Thinking Key. You will identify the Hits in these Field Organizers before transferring them to the "Highlighting" Part 1 Field Organizer. Continue to work with the "client" group with the "therapist" acting as the facilitator. Recall that in this context the client is represented by those persons who share ownership of the problem, including Sam's parents and teacher.

DIRECTIONS

Materials: orange adhesive dots

1. Review with the client the ideas generated in the following Field Organizers: "Brainstorming," "CAMPERS," "Force Fit," and "Attribute Listing."
2. Direct the client to select the Hits from the list of problem statements by placing an orange dot in the space provided for Hits in each of the four Field Organizers. In Idea Finding, Hits refer to ideas that hold promise for leading the client to a solution.
3. Transfer the Hits from the "Brainstorming," "CAMPERS," "Force Fit," and "Attribute Listing" Field Organizers to the "Highlighting" Part 1 Field Organizer. Transfer the Hits in any order. It is the Hits that are important, not the Field Organizer where they originated.

Problem Statement: *IWWM a home/school program be developed to help Sam learn how to follow the kindergarten routines?*

Hits Transfer

1. *Sam imagines himself in different roles (butterfly, wrestler, burrito, baker, steamroller, sorcerer, weightlifter, Olympic athlete, Peter Rabbit, strong man, spinning top) in which he performs activities designed to enhance his sensory processing.*

Note: Refer to the "Brainstorming" Field Organizer for details on each of these activities.

2. *Routines that are common to kindergarten and home can be put on a simple laminated picture chart (e.g., showing snack time, storytime, handwashing, and block play). As routines change Sam could indicate the routine on his board.*

3. *Kindergarten students could take turns announcing when the group was to move from one activity to another.*

4. *Each time Sam's teacher shifts from one main activity to another she would play music to ready the group for the next activity.*

5. *When Sam is out doing errands with his parents, Sam is responsible for announcing the plan for each stop (e.g., "Now we will shop for groceries." "Here we will drop off our dry cleaning.").*

6. *Sam's teacher would identify how Sam transitions from one activity to another rather than expect him to readily change every time there is a change in the classroom.*

7. *Have Sam play the game "Name That Change." To play the game, tell Sam that you are about to change activities and he has to tell you what the change is after it has happened.*

8. *Sam's parents and teacher use puppets to talk to Sam about changing from one activity to another.*

9. *Read Sam a children's book about a child going to kindergarten (e.g., from the Berenstein Bears collection).*

10. *While reading Sam a book about kindergarten ask Sam about how he feels about school.*

11. *Use a notebook system to communicate between school and home.*

12. *Arrange for a child from the upper grades to come to Sam's classroom before the end of the day to help him write a sentence or two about his day (in his notebook) which Sam will bring home for his parents to read and sign. In the beginning of the year Sam's sentences will be scribed by the older student with Sam adding a letter or two and a picture. As the year progresses Sam will be able to help write some simple words.*

13. *Sam's parents keep a notebook which they make an entry on a single page in big letters every time Sam accomplishes a new skill (i.e., On September 7th Sam put on his coat all by himself—Hurray. On September 8th Sam cleared his plate from the kitchen table— Hurray. On September 9th Sam pours his own cereal into his bowl—Hurray). Sam receives a big bear hug with every entry.*

14. *Identify the routines used in Sam's kindergarten*

15. *Set up a home routine that incorporates elements of the kindergarten routine (e.g., snack, art, block play, and reading time; hanging up coat on designated hook).*

16. *Have Sam help make a picture board with home routines that are similar to Sam's kindergarten routines (e.g., snack, art, block play, and reading time; hanging up coat on designated hook).*

(continued)

Hits Transfer

17. Have Sam help make a small board with a pocket to hold a picture of whatever routine activity he is going to begin. As he changes activities, Sam changes the picture that is in the pocket.

18. Ask Sam to follow one-step directions (e.g., "Sam, please hang up your coat." "Sam, please close the door." "Sam, please button your shirt.")

19. Have Sam give his mother one-step directions to follow at a designated time in the day (time is marked on a clock in the house so Sam can tell when his time is coming to give directions).

20. Audio- or videotape Sam giving directions to his parents which they are to follow. Play back the tape and have Sam listen to himself give directions.

21. Set a regular storytime in the day to which Sam can look forward.

22. During storytime have Sam snuggle up in a sleeping bag (tactile and proprioceptive input) or a blanket next to an adult in a tight space (womblike space).

23.

24.

25.

26.

27.

28.

29.

30.

31.

32.

33.

Hits Transfer

34.

35.

36.

37.

38.

39.

40.

Go Forward with an Action Plan: Solution Finding

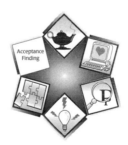

Solution Finding: The Generating Phase

In Solution Finding, the Hits identified during the Focusing Phase of Idea Finding are sorted out and prepared for use in the action plan. You will use criteria to evaluate the ideas that are further developed in Solution Finding, using the following Thinking Keys designed to generate criteria.

"Will It . . . ?" Use the "Will It . . . ?" Thinking Key when you wish to develop criteria by first generating many questions about the proposed ideas, such as, "Will it be understandable?" "It" represents the idea or option under consideration. Completing the question "Will it . . . ?" helps to define concepts that identify specific areas of concern about an idea that can later be translated into criteria. The context in which the proposed action will occur focuses the therapy guide's perception of which criterion generated are the most important to consider.

Complete the "Will It . . . ?" Field Organizer by asking "Will it" questions about the Hit transferred to "Highlighting" Part 1, row 15; "Set up a home routine that incorporates elements of the kindergarten routine (e.g., snack, art, block play, and reading time; hanging up coat on designated hook)." Criteria you generate from the "Will It . . . ?" Thinking Key can be used to evaluate ideas during the Focusing Phase of Solution Finding.

DIRECTIONS

1. Stretch your mind and complete the question "Will it . . . ?" by focusing on possible considerations related to the Hit at the top of the Field Organizer that was identified in Sam's SI Expedition.
2. In column A, rows 7–10, record four questions that have the potential of leading you to a decision about the Hit under consideration. To get you started, questions have been recorded in rows 1–6.
3. In column B, rows 7–10, record the criterion that is embedded in each question in column A.

FIELD ORGANIZER
"Will It . . . ?"

Idea: *Set up a home routine that incorporates elements of the kindergarten routine (e.g., snack, art, block play, and reading time; hanging up coat on designated hook).*

A "Will it . . . ?"	B Criterion
1. be meaningful to the family	Family friendly
2. be practical for the family to implement	Practical
3. tap into Sam's inner drive	Flow experience
4. be easily communicated	Understandable
5. do what it is intended to do	Effective
6. be easy to make adjustments	Adaptable
7.	
8.	
9.	
10.	

"TRACS." The "TRACS" Thinking Key keeps you on track during the therapy expedition. "TRACS" is useful for measuring your proposed action against the five most common categories of criteria within the decision making process. Time, Resources, Acceptance, Costs, and Space. To expand your perceptions about each of the criteria represented in "TRACS," you will use a different criterion for each of the options listed in rows 1–5. (See Section 10 for a review of the definitions of each of these criteria.)

Use the "TRACS" Thinking Key to expand your thinking about five ideas for Sam's SI Expedition (taken from the "Highlighting" Part 1 Field Organizer). Work in pairs or groups of three or four to complete the "TRACS" Field Organizer.

DIRECTIONS

1. Create questions by joining the Hits listed in column A with the "TRACS" criterion listed in the same row in column B.
2. Record your responses in column C. To get you started, three responses have been recorded in row 1 and one response each in rows 2–5. Identify a minimum of two considerations for each of the options listed in rows 2–5.

FIELD ORGANIZER

"TRACS"

A Option	B Criterion	C Considerations
1. If Sam imagines himself in different roles (e.g., butterfly, wrestler, burrito) in which he performs activities designed to enhance his sensory processing . . .	what *time* would be involved?	1. The time it takes for an adult to set up the activity (this would vary from one imaginary situation to another) 2. The time it takes to engage Sam (and classmates where applicable) to enter the imaginary situation. 3. The actual time the activity would take
2. If each time Sam's teacher shifts from one main activity to another she would play music to ready the group for the next activity . . .	what *resources* would be involved?	1. Permanent electronic equipment to play music (record player, tape recorder, CD player) 2. 3.
3. If Sam's teacher would identify how Sam transitions from one activity to another rather than expect him to readily change every time there is a change in the classroom . . .	what *acceptance* issues would be involved?	1. A willingness on the part of Sam's teacher to accept Sam's resistance to change 2. 3.

(continued)

A Option	B Criterion	C Considerations
4. *If routines that are common to kindergarten and home can be put on a simple laminated picture chart (e.g., showing snack, storytime, handwashing, and block play) . . .*	what *cost* would be involved?	1. *Obtain cardboard to use for picture chart* 2. 3.
5. *If Sam's teacher and parents used a notebook system to communicate between school and home . . .*	what *space* would be involved?	1. *Special space identified in kindergarten classroom where notebook would be stored when not being used* 2. 3.

Use the "TRACS" Field Organizer with any Hit you wish to examine systematically according to time, resources, acceptability, cost, or supplies needed to implement the idea.

"Making an Idea More Acceptable." Use the "Making an Idea More Acceptable" Thinking Key when you wish to improve on an idea you do not want to abandon. When you prepare an idea for acceptance with the "Making an Idea More Acceptable" Thinking Key you increase the number of options to contemplate. Use the "Making an Idea More Acceptable" Field Organizer to practice reworking an idea to improve it using the inherent criterion of the idea.

DIRECTIONS

1. Read the two ideas to be improved on in column A, rows 1–2.
2. Read in column B the essential criterion embedded in each of the ideas recorded in column A.
3. Record in column C at least one idea that improves on the original idea, while retaining the essential criterion identified in the idea. To get you started, two ideas are listed in row 1 and one idea in row 2.

"Making an Idea More Acceptable"

A Idea to Be Improved	B Essential Criterion to Consider	C Possible Improvements
1. Kindergarten students could each take a turn announcing when the group was to move from one activity to another.	Announcing when one activity is ending and another will begin.	a. Vary having the children make the announcement with the teacher making the announcement. b. Teacher could turn the lights down as a signal to the students that they should get ready for the next activity by cleaning up. c.
2. When Sam is out doing errands with his parents Sam is responsible for announcing the plan for each stop (e.g., "Now we will shop for groceries." "Here we will drop off our dry cleaning.").	Sam assumes a role where he is in control of making change happen.	a. Sam practices being in charge while in his own home while his parents help him clean up his room. b. c.

Solution Finding: The Focusing Phase

In the Focusing Phase of Solution Finding you will select those criteria you and the client feel are best suited to assess the Hits identified in Idea Finding. The number of ideas being evaluated and the purpose of your evaluation together will determine which of the four Thinking Keys to use when applying your criteria: "In-tuit," "AL-O," "Evaluation Matrix," or "PCA" (the Paired Comparison Analysis). Each Thinking Key uses a different strategy to evaluate Hits. Select a Thinking Key according to the strategy you want to use. Use:

"In-tuit" when you wish to use your intuition to evaluate an idea

"AL-O" when you wish to explore the advantages and limitations (as well as strategies to overcome the limitations) of a limited number of ideas

The "Evaluation Matrix" when you have a set of ideas that you wish to evaluate systematically against criteria you developed in the Generating Phase of Solution Finding

"PCA" (Paired Comparison Analysis) when you wish to rank order a small group of ideas which you feel are of equal value

The ideas you ultimately decide on will be used to develop the plan of action—the itinerary—for the therapy expedition.

"In-tuit." When you use the "In-tuit" Thinking Key to evaluate the merit of an idea, you ask questions such as, "What do I sense about this idea?" or "Does this idea feel right?" Use the "In-tuit" Field Organizer to evaluate five ideas (Hits) from Sam's SI Expedition.

DIRECTIONS

1. Read each idea listed in column A and evaluate it by asking the question on the top, "Do I sense that this idea will help solve the problem?"
2. Consider the potential of each idea for solving the problem and put a check in column B, C, or D according to the following criteria:

   a. If you *feel positive that the idea* has potential for solving the problem, check Yes in column B.

   b. If you sense that *the idea will not help* to solve the problem, check No in column C.

   c. If you feel the idea *has merit but needs to be reworked* using the "Make an Idea More Acceptable" Thinking Key, check "Rework" in column D.

FIELD ORGANIZER

"In-tuit"

A Do I sense that this idea will help solve the problem?	B Yes	C No	D Rework
1. Have Sam play the game "Name That Change." To play the game, tell Sam that you are about to change activities and he has to tell you what the change is after it has happened.			
2. Sam's parents and teacher use puppets to talk to Sam about changing from one activity to another.			
3. Arrange for a child from the upper grades to come to Sam's classroom before the end of the day to help him write a sentence or two about his day (in his notebook), which Sam will bring home for his parents to read and sign. In the beginning of the year Sam's sentences will be scribed by the older student with Sam adding a letter or two and a picture. As the year progresses Sam will be able to help write some simple words.			
4. Have Sam help make a small board with a pocket to hold a picture of whatever routine activity he is going to begin. As he changes activities, Sam changes the picture that is in the pocket.			
5. Set a regular storytime in the day to which Sam can look forward.			

Intuition allows therapy guides to arrive at decisions using their immediate understanding of the situation. Therapy guides who practice using intuition and self-reflection to make decisions learn to trust their intuition in making decisions.

"AL-O." "AL-O" teams your intuition with your logic. Use the "AL-O" Thinking Key when you wish to view the advantage and limitations of an idea as well as consider how to overcome the limitations. You will consider three ideas in the "AL-O" Field Organizer.

1. Read the advantages listed in column A for each idea under consideration.
2. Read the limitations recorded in column B for each idea.
3. Record two strategies in column C for overcoming the limitations described in column B for rows 2–3. To get you started three strategies have been provided in row 1 and one each in rows 2–3.

FIELD ORGANIZER

"AL-O"

Idea: *Sam imagines himself in different roles (butterfly, wrestler, burrito, baker, steamroller, sorcerer, weightlifter, Olympic athlete, Peter Rabbit, strong man, spinning top) in which he performs activities designed to enhance his sensory processing.*

A Advantages	B Limitations	C How to Overcome a Limitation
1. *Sam pretends to do activities that he finds challenging.*	**Limitation:** *Engaging Sam in imaginative play* *The issue becomes: How to engage Sam in imaginative play*	a. *Use stories, ideas, or situations that are of interest to Sam.* b. *Keep activities short and simple.* c. *Reward all attempts to participate in a new activity.*

Idea: *Ask Sam to follow one-step directions (e.g., "Sam please hang up your coat." "Sam, please close the door." "Sam, please button your shirt.")*

2. *Sam practices processing small bits of information to reduce the confusion from being asked to perform multiple steps.*	**Limitation:** *Sam may get frustrated if multiple requests are made of him at one time.* *The issue becomes: How to help Sam learn to follow directions with more than one step*	a. *Once Sam follows through on a few easy steps they can be joined together (e.g., "Sam, please put on your coat and boots.").* b. c.

Idea: *During storytime have Sam snuggle up in a sleeping bag (tactile and proprioceptive input) or a blanket next to an adult in a tight space (womblike space).*

3. *Sam experiences a feeling of boundaries snuggled next to an adult or in a tight space.*	**Limitation:** *Sam may enjoy the feeling of being snuggled or encased for only a short period of time.* *The issue becomes: How to allow Sam to be in control of his environment*	a. *Read short stories to Sam while he is snuggled until he builds a tolerance for the tactile and proprioceptive sensations this kind of nurturing space provides.* b. c.

After you identify several strategies for overcoming a potential limitation you can consider whether to include one or more of the options in your action plan. Using the "AL-O" Thinking Key helps a therapy guide to consider both sides of an issue in order to avoid being blindsided by a lack of foresight.

"Evaluation Matrix." Use the "Evaluation Matrix" to rate Idea Finding options objectively, using criteria you developed in the Generating Phase of Solution Finding.

Use whatever criteria best suits your need during the evaluation period. In Section 10, for the Nose Blowing Expedition, you used criteria in "TRACS" for the "Evaluation Matrix." Here, for Sam's SI Expedition, we have drawn criteria from the "Will It . . . ?" Thinking Key: Teacher and/or Family Friendly, Practical, Understandable, Effective, and Adaptable.

DIRECTIONS

1. Review the 10 options recorded in the first column.
2. Review the rating scale: Use a smiley face to indicate support for an option; use an unhappy face to indicate lack of support for an option.
3. Evaluate each of the 10 options using the criteria listed. Evaluate all the options against one criterion, drawing in the appropriate faces, before moving on to the criterion in the next column.
4. Count the number of faces that fall into each category and record the totals in the Rating column.

FIELD ORGANIZER

"Evaluation Matrix"

Options	Criteria					Rating
	Teacher and/or Family Friendly	Practical	Understandable	Effective	Adaptable	Scale: ☺ Favorable ☹ Unfavorable
1. Make a laminated picture board of school and home routines.						☺ = _____ ☹ = _____
2. Sam announces changes in the schedule when out with his parents.						☺ = _____ ☹ = _____
3. Sam plays the game "Name That Change" with his parents.						☺ = _____ ☹ = _____
4. Sam's parents and teacher use puppets to talk to Sam about changing from one activity to another.						☺ = _____ ☹ = _____
5. Use a notebook system to communicate between school and home.						☺ = _____ ☹ = _____
6. A student from the middle school helps scribe for Sam in his home/school notebook about something he enjoyed about the school day.						☺ = _____ ☹ = _____

"Evaluation Matrix" (Continued)

Options	Criteria					Rating
	Teacher and/or Family Friendly	Practical	Understandable	Effective	Adaptable	Scale: ☺ Favorable ☹ Unfavorable
7. Sam's parents keep a notebook in which they make an entry on a single page in big letters every time Sam acquires a new skill.						☺ = _____ ☹ = _____
8. Set up a home routine that incorporates main elements of the kindergarten routine in it.						☺ = _____ ☹ = _____
9. Have Sam help make a small board with a pocket to hold a picture of whatever routine activity he is going to begin. As he changes activities, Sam changes the picture that is in the pocket.						☺ = _____ ☹ = _____
10. Have Sam give his mother one-step directions to follow at a designated time in the day.						☺ = _____ ☹ = _____

"PCA." Use the "PCA" (Paired Comparison Analysis) to rate options that are close in value. Unlike the "Evaluation Matrix," the "PCA" does not rely on a criteria-based rating system. Instead it uses a ranking system to prioritize the options.

DIRECTIONS

1. List three options you wish to prioritize in Section I, rows C, D, and E. Begin each option with an action verb that relates to the content of the option. To get you started, options have been listed in rows A and B.
2. Now compare option A to option B.
3. In Section II record your choice of A or B in the Choice box to the right of the Options box in A/B.
4. Continue comparing one option against the next by following the pairs of letters in the Options boxes until you have compared every option to every other option.
5. After you finish rating the options tally the letters by counting the number of times A was recorded, then B, and so on. Record the totals in Section III.
6. Rank order the totals recorded in the boxes and enter them in the designated space in Section III. Rank ordering the options will help you to objectively determine which options you wish to pursue and in what order.

Problem Statement: IWWM a home/school program be develop to help Sam learn how to follow the kindergarten routines?

Section I: Options

A. Have Sam participate in fun activities designed to improve his sensory processing.

B. Sam plays the game "Name That Change" with his parents.

C.

D.

E.

Section II: Option Comparison

Options	Choice	Options	Choice	Options	Choice	Options	Choice
A/B		A/C		A/D		A/E	
		B/C		B/D		B/E	
				C/D		C/E	
						D/E	

Section III: Totals

Total **A**	Total **B**	Total **C**	Total **D**	Total **E**	List Options in Priority Order
					1.
					2.
					3.
					4.
					5.

The "Paired Comparison Analysis" is an effective tool to use when you are making a decision without the help of others or when you are working with a group who share ownership of a problem and need an objective method for considering their options.

Go Forward With an Action Plan: Acceptance Finding

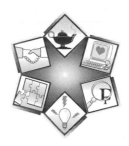

Acceptance Finding: The Generating Phase

"Potential Sources of Support and Resistance." The "Potential Sources of Support and Resistance" Thinking Key will help you to systematically identify the potential sources of support and resistance on the therapy expedition using the 5 Ws & an H question set (who, what, where, when, why, and how).

The "Potential Sources of Support and Resistance" Field Organizer is divided into columns A, B, and C. Each row in column A begins a question from the 5 Ws & a H question set that can be completed by both the phrase in column B and the phrase in column C. Pair up with a partner and practice using the "Potential Sources of Support and Resistance" Field Organizer.

DIRECTIONS

1. Read the proposed idea at the top of the "Potential Sources of Support and Resistance" Field Organizer and the sample questions and answers in row 1.
2. Create the next question by combining the phrase "WHAT things, objects, or activities might be . . . " in column A, row 2, with the word "helpful?" in column B, row 1.
3. Answer the question "What things, objects, or activities might be helpful?" and record in column B those things, objects, or activities that could support the plan.
4. Combine the phrases in column A and column C of row 2 to create the next question. Record those things, objects, or activities that will potentially inhibit the plan from moving forward.
5. Continue creating questions in rows 3 through 6 by combining the phrases in column A with the phrase in column B and column C to trigger thoughts about potential sources of support for and resistance to the proposed plan.
6. Answer the questions in rows 3 through 6 and record the responses in the appropriate rows.

In order to respond to some of the questions using the Sam's SI Expedition you will need to extend your thinking beyond the printed words of the story. All of the sources of support and resistance are not explicitly stated. For this exercise, think "outside of the box" to imagine all sources of support and resistance that you think may possibly impact the therapy expedition.

Proposed idea: *Develop a home/school program to help Sam learn how to follow kindergarten routines.*

A 5 Ws & an H	B Potential Sources of Support	C Potential Sources of Resistance
1. **WHO** might . . .	*contribute time and resources to move the plan forward?* *Sam's parents will support the plan as long as they feel that the time they are investing is producing the desired result.* *Sam's teacher will be supportive if she sees that the plan is practical and easy to implement.*	*limit or restrict the forward movement of the plan?* *If Sam's parents are unclear about the plan they will be unable to put forth their full effort.* *If Sam's teacher feels that the plan for Sam is incompatible with the plan she has for the entire class she will not feel supportive of it.*
2. **WHAT** things, objects, or activities might be . . .	*helpful?*	*an impediment?*
3. **WHERE** are . . .	*locations where the plan can be accomplished?*	*locations that block progress of the plan?*
4. **WHEN** might there be . . .	*an appropriate time to work on the plan (specify hours, day, week, month)?*	*an inappropriate time to work on the plan?*
5. **WHY** might the plan be . . .	*supported?*	*resisted?*
6. **HOW** might I anticipate . . .	*strengths in the plan?*	*weaknesses in the plan?*

"Check the Mindset." The "Check the Mindset" Thinking Key will help you identify mindsets that indicate a person's resistance to, or acceptance of, the action plan. The "Check the Mindset" Field Organizer lists five pairs of mindsets. Each pair represents a continuum from a mindset indicative of resistance to change (on the left side) to a mindset indicative of a readiness for change (on the right). In the "Check the Mindset" Field Organizer each mindset is accompanied by a brief description to trigger your thoughts.

Practice using the "Check the Mindset" Thinking Key by imagining actions that Sam's mother might have taken, knowing what you do about her from the story she wrote. For the following activity, imagine that you are the therapy guide on Sam's SI Expedition.

DIRECTIONS

1. Read the behavior in row 1 that reflects the mindset of Sam's mother as a person who is *willing to take risks* (right side of the continuum).
2. Select one of the mindsets on the continuum in rows 2–5 by filling in the circle next to the mindset. Note: All the mindsets for Sam's mother need not be associated with mindsets indicative of a readiness for change.

3. Imagine a behavior that reflects each of the mindsets you selected for Sam's mother.
4. On the lines below each mindset you chose in rows 2–5, record a behavior you imagined would exemplify the actions of Sam's mother when displaying the mindset selected.

FIELD ORGANIZER

"Check the Mindset"

Resistance to change	Readiness for change
1. ○ **Conforming**	**Willing to take risks** ●
Prefers to act according to the standard or norm.	Willing to expose self to chance; seeks out opportunities that may move the action plan forward.
	Adjusted home routine to include fun sensory integrative activities that encouraged Sam to improve his sensory processing abilities.
2. ○ **Rigid**	**Flexible** ○
Unyielding and consequently unable to change the course of action or switch gears readily.	Able to change the course of action (switch gears) whenever it is necessary to meet the demands of the situation.
3. ○ **Narrow-minded**	**Open-minded** ○
Unreceptive to new ideas or strategies. Prefers to use routine ideas and activities that are familiar.	Acknowledges that there are few absolutes in therapy. Receptive to new ideas or strategies. Open to new possibilities.
4. ○ **Needing to know**	**Tolerant of ambiguity** ○
Needs to have discrete answers.	Feels comfortable waiting for the "better" answer to emerge.
5. ○ **Self-centered**	**Empathetic** ○
Values personal needs and perspectives over the needs of others.	Identifies with the feelings or thoughts of others.

"Generating Potential Actions." Use the Thinking Key "Generating Potential Actions" to generate potential actions that lead to developing an action plan. When you use the "Generating Potential Actions" Thinking Key you answer the following questions:

1. What *possible actions* can be taken to move the action plan forward?
2. What are *possible sources of resistance* to the proposed actions?

Recognizing sources of resistance ahead of time can help a therapy guide plan for ways to deal with them. Practice using the "Generating Potential Actions" Thinking Key with a partner.

DIRECTIONS

1. In column A, rows 11–14, record four more actions that you might take based on information stated or implied in the story.
2. In column B, rows 11–14, record one possible source of resistance to each of the actions recorded in column A. Use the Actions and Sources of Resistance in rows 1–10 to model your responses.

FIELD ORGANIZER

"Generating Potential Actions"

Proposed plan: *Teach the children how to blow their noses through games and relay races.*

A Actions That Move the Plan Forward	B Sources of Resistance That Block the Plan
1. Identify Sam's kindergarten routines.	Kindergarten routines may not be clearly delineated.
2. Set up a home program with activities designed to improve Sam's sensory processing.	Space and equipment, such as a scooter board, mats, and a ramp, are limited. Also limited is knowledge of how to grade the activities with Sam.
3. Set up a school program with activities designed to improve Sam's sensory processing that can be integrated into the existing kindergarten activities.	If Sam's kindergarten teacher is focused on academics as opposed to the developmental needs of the children she may find integrating movement experiences into the classroom a foreign paradigm
4. Obtain baseline data on Sam's level of independence in selected areas of ADL, play, and educational activities by observing him at school and at home.	While Sam is being observed he may perform in a manner unlike his typical behavior because he knows he is being observed.
5. Have Sam's mother gather baseline data on selected subcategories within the ADL performance area.	Sam's mother may consciously or unconsciously record Sam's behavior as better than it is because of her desire to see Sam's ability in a positive light (refer to the Representativeness Bias Mindtrap in Section 10)
6. Provide Sam's parents information about sensory integration problems.	Sam's parents may find it difficult to understand how Sam's behavior is the result of problems with sensory integration.
7. Have an older student assigned to come down in the afternoon to scribe for Sam. The student will ask Sam about what he did that day at school and will write a note to Sam's parents, which Sam dictates.	Unless the student has a high level of empathy and creativity he or she will likely have difficulty being sensitive to Sam's emotional instability.

"Generating Potential Actions" (Continued)

A Actions That Move the Plan Forward	B Sources of Resistance That Block the Plan
8. Have Sam play the "Name That Change" game.	Sam may find the game too difficult or too easy to be a challenge.
9. Use a notebook system to communicate between school and home.	Notebook can be easily misplaced at home and at school.
10. Set up a couple of standard routines for the home.	Sam's parents may have a hectic life with a constantly changing schedule.
11.	
12.	
13.	
14.	

Acceptance Finding: The Focusing Phase

"LIST." The "LIST" Thinking Key helps organize the therapy plan actions into long-term, intermediate, and short-term actions. The "LIST" represents all the actions you foresee at the outset of the therapy expedition. The more thorough the "LIST" the better your ability to plan for successful outcomes and minimize the number of unexpected detours.

Use the "LIST" to organize the actions (previously recorded in the "Generating Potential Actions" Field Organizer) into three categories. After recording and sorting all of the actions from the "Generating Potential Actions" Field Organizer, continue to use the "LIST" to organize and record additional actions as you think of them. Note that in the "LIST" Field Organizer "long-term" refers to actions taken between one and two months, "intermediate" refers to actions to be taken between two weeks and four weeks, and "short-term" refers to actions to be taken within the first two weeks.

DIRECTIONS

1. Turn to the "Generating Potential Actions" Field Organizer and sort the actions you recorded there into long-term, intermediate, and short-term goals. Actions 1 through 10 have already been recorded into one of the three categories in the "LIST."
2. Record the actions you generated into their respective sections.
3. Add to the "LIST" any additional actions that you value to be important but were not included in the original list in the "Generating Action Plans" Field Organizer.

Whenever you think of additional steps along the way be sure to add them to the "LIST."

FIELD ORGANIZER
"LIST"

Long-Term Actions to Take *between the first and second months*

1. Have an older student assigned to come down in the afternoon to scribe for Sam. The student will ask Sam about what he did that day at school and will write a note to Sam's parents, which Sam dictates.
2. Have Sam play the "Name That Change" game.
3. Use a notebook system to communicate between school and home.
4. Set up standard routines for the home that correlate with Sam's kindergarten routines.
5.
6.
7.
8.

Intermediate Actions to Take *between the second and fourth weeks*

1. Set up a home program with activities designed to improve Sam's sensory processing.
2. Set up a school program with activities designed to improve Sam's sensory processing that can be integrated into the existing kindergarten activities.
3.
4.
5.
6.
7.
8.

Short-Term Actions to Take *within the first two weeks*

1. Obtain baseline data on Sam's level of independence in selected areas of ADL, play, and educational activities by observing him at school and at home.
2. Have Sam's mother gather baseline data on selected subcategories within the ADL performance area.
3. Identify Sam's kindergarten routines.
4. Provide Sam's parents with information about sensory integration problems.
5.
6.
7.
8.

Planning for Implementation of the Ideas

"Plan for Action." Use the "Plan for Action" Thinking Key to develop the specific action steps that will be part of the therapy expedition's itinerary. This Thinking Key will focus your thoughts toward the plan's proposed actions. "Plan for Action" uses the 5 Ws & an H question set. Each section of the "Plan for Action" Field Organizer poses a series of questions for each action. The questions are as follows:

> WHAT is the action desired?
>
> WHO will do the action?
>
> WHEN will the action begin and be completed?
>
> WHERE will the action take place?
>
> WHY is the action important?
>
> HOW will you know the action was successful?

The "Plan for Action" Field Organizer is used in conjunction with the "LIST" Field Organizer. Actions are taken from the "LIST" and developed in the Field Organizer "Plan for Action."

DIRECTIONS

1. Read through the six questions and the responses for Long-Term Action #1 (drawn from the "LIST" Field Organizer).
2. Respond to the questions for Long-Term Actions #2 and #3, using #1 as your model.
3. Repeat steps 1 and 2 for Intermediate and Short-Term Actions. (Note that Short-Term Action #1 is a consolidation of the first two actions from the list.)

FIELD ORGANIZER

"Plan for Action"

Long-Term Actions

Long-Term Action #1

1. **WHAT** is the **action** desired? *Identify two older students who will taken turns serving as a buddy to Sam. Sam's buddy will help him write a simple message in his notebook to his parents about something he did each day at school. Sam's buddy needs some brief training as well as intermittent communication with Sam's teacher and therapy guide.*

2. **WHO** will do the **action**? *Therapy guide to speak to principal about buddy program and then to the school counselor or school social worker to identify two qualified students. Teacher and therapy guide interview qualified students and arrange to see how Sam responds to students before they are trained.*

3. **WHEN** will the **action** start? *Fourth week.* finish? *By the eighth week the two students have been selected and trained.*

4. **WHERE** will the **action** take place? *Meetings with principal and counselors in their offices; interview students in classroom before or after school.*

5. **WHY** is the **action** important? *Setting up a buddy system for Sam will offer him some individual help once a day on which he can learn to depend. Buddy could serve as an anchor for Sam since Sam is easily overwhelmed. Sam's buddy could help Sam feel safe and cared for.*

6. **HOW** will you know the **action** was successful? *An appropriate student is identified whom Sam will accept.*

Long-Term Action #2

1. **WHAT** is the **action** desired? _____

2. **WHO** will do the **action**? _____

(continued)

---

3. **WHEN** will the **action** start? _____ finish? _____

4. **WHERE** will the **action** take place? _____

5. **WHY** is the **action** important? _____

6. **HOW** will you know the **action** was successful? _____

Long-Term Action #3

1. **WHAT** is the **action** desired? _____

2. **WHO** will do the **action**? _____

3. **WHEN** will the **action** start? _____ finish? _____

4. **WHERE** will the **action** take place? _____

5. **WHY** is the **action** important? _____

6. **HOW** will you know the **action** was successful? _____

Intermediate Actions

Intermediate Action #1

1. **WHAT** is the **action** desired? *Brainstorm with Sam's parents about activities that could be integrated into their home routine that focus on improving Sam's sensory processing. Set up an initial plan.*

2. **WHO** will do the **action**? *Therapy guide with Sam's parents.*

3. **WHEN** will the **action** start? *Fourth week.* finish? *Fourth week.*

4. **WHERE** will the **action** take place? *At Sam's home.*

5. **WHY** is the **action** important? *Sam's parents are fully invested in helping Sam. They have witnessed the dramatic changes Sam went through after just a brief period of therapy. They want to continue helping him develop his ability to integrate information from the environment.*

6. **HOW** will you know the **action** was successful? *Sam's parents take principles they have learned about sensory processing and start creatively developing activities and ideas of their own.*

Intermediate Action #2

1. **WHAT** is the **action** desired? _____

2. **WHO** will do the **action**? _____

3. **WHEN** will the **action** start? _____ finish? _____

4. **WHERE** will the **action** take place? _____

5. **WHY** is the **action** important? _____

6. **HOW** will you know the **action** was successful? _____

Intermediate Action #3

1. **WHAT** is the **action** desired? _____

2. **WHO** will do the **action**? _____

3. **WHEN** will the **action** start? _____ finish? _____

4. **WHERE** will the **action** take place? _____

5. **WHY** is the **action** important? _____

6. **HOW** will you know the **action** was successful? _____

Short-Term Actions

Short-Term Action #1

1. **WHAT** is the **action** desired? *Therapy guide and Sam's mother gather baseline data on Sam's performance.*

2. **WHO** will do the **action**? *Therapy guide and Sam's mother.*

3. **WHEN** will the **action** start? *First week.* finish? *Second week.*

4. **WHERE** will the **action** take place? *At school and home.*

5. **WHY** is the **action** important? *In order to determine whether Sam's therapy expedition plan is effective it is necessary to measure change in Sam's occupational performance. To measure change accurate baseline data needs to be gathered before the therapy plan is implemented.*

6. **HOW** will you know the **action** was successful? *Baseline date has been gathered on selected performance area subcategories in an easy-to-read table that has designated space to record changes in performance.*

Short-Term Action #2

1. **WHAT** is the **action** desired? _____

2. **WHO** will do the **action**? _____

3. **WHEN** will the **action** start? _____ finish? _____

4. **WHERE** will the **action** take place? _____

5. **WHY** is the **action** important? _____

6. **HOW** will you know the **action** was successful? _____

Short-Term Action #3

1. **WHAT** is the **action** desired? _____

2. **WHO** will do the **action**? _____

3. **WHEN** will the **action** start? _____ finish? _____

(continued)

"Plan for Action" (Continued)

4. **WHERE** will the **action** take place? _____

5. **WHY** is the **action** important? _____

6. **HOW** will you know the **action** was successful? _____

Therapy guides develop the habit of routinely asking the 5 Ws & an H questions about their proposed actions before integrating the actions into the therapy expedition.

After using the 5 Ws & an H questions to uncover the general details related to proposed actions, increase your perspective on the proposed actions by projecting your thoughts further into the future. Envision the proposed actions with as much detail as possible. Ideally, your future vision should include all of the things that you anticipate will "go right" with the action plan as well as those things that may "go wrong."

Each of the following Thinking Keys offers a unique method of systematically projecting your thinking into the future to broaden the perspective of the actions you are about to take. The four Thinking Keys you will revisit here are the "What's Next? Question Series," "If–Then," "What If . . . ? Question Series," and "Think Positive."

"What's Next?" When you ask "What's next?" after each client-directed action, you develop the habit of connecting one action with the next. As the actions become embedded within the therapy expedition's story, they connect sequentially. Asking "What's next?" continually directs your thinking toward issues related to the follow-up actions you will take with a client. The follow-up actions are what makes your initial actions meaningful.

DIRECTIONS

1. In rows 1–4, read the proposed actions recorded in column A, then read the question "What's next?" in column B and the responses in column C.
2. In rows 5–6, read columns A and B and record a logical action in column C that might follow from the proposed action listed in column A.

FIELD ORGANIZER

"What's Next? Question Series"

A Describe *one part* of the therapy plan.	B Ask, "What's next?"	C Respond to the question "What's next?"
1. Identify baseline data in selected subcategories of Sam's occupational performance.	"What's next?"	Identify which occupational performance areas you will focus on at the start of the plan.
2. Provide information to Sam's parents about sensory processing problems.	"What's next?"	Follow up with Sam's parents to help them understand how to relate the information (on sensory processing problems) with Sam's unique behavioral patterns.
3. Use a notebook system to communicate between school and home.	"What's next?"	After a few weeks inquire into the effectiveness of the notebook as a source of communication.

"What's Next? Question Series" (Continued)

A Describe *one part* of the therapy plan.	B Ask, "What's next?"	C Respond to the question "What's next?"
4. *Brainstorm with Sam's parents about activities that could be integrated into their home routine that focus on improving Sam's sensory processing.*	"What's next?"	*Select those activities (for improving Sam's sensory processing) that the parents have the time, willingness, and equipment to carry out.*
5. *Set up a simple method for Sam and his parents to record activities (for improving Sam's sensory processing) in which they engage.*	"What's next?"	
6. *Work with Sam's teacher to integrate into the existing kindergarten routine activities designed to improve Sam's sensory processing.*	"What's next?"	

"If–Then." The "If–Then" Thinking Key helps to structure the hypothesis that provides future direction to the therapy expedition.

DIRECTIONS

1. Read the "If" and "Then" parts of the hypotheses in rows 1–4.
2. Read the "If" parts of the hypotheses in rows 5–6, and complete the "Then" portion of the hypotheses in column B.

FIELD ORGANIZER

"If–Then"

A IF . . .	B THEN . . .
1. **IF** *Sam's parents are provided with pertinant information about sensory processing . . .*	**THEN** *they will better understand Sam's behavior so that they can in turn creatively respond to the challenges Sam's behavior presents.*
2. **IF** *Sam's parents are able to integrate activities into their routine that support enhancing Sam's sensory processing . . .*	**THEN** *Sam will better modulate input in his environment and consequently be better prepared to expand on his skills and abilities.*
3. **IF** *routines at school are reinforced at home . . .*	**THEN** *Sam will come to anticipate what is to occur with certain routines and thus give him a greater sense of control.*
4. **IF** *a notebook system is used to communicate pertinent issues between school and home . . .*	**THEN** *Sam's teacher and parents will have a routine way of maintaining some simple form of communication albeit brief.*
5. **IF** *the therapy guide shares with Sam's parents a few basic principles of sensory processing . . .*	**THEN**
6. **IF** *the therapy guide works closely with Sam's teacher on Sam's issues . . .*	**THEN**

The use of the "If–Then" Thinking Key and "What's Next? Question Series" depends on the situation. These two tools may be used together or independently. The main difference between the two tools is that the "What's Next? Question Series" is designed to sequentially project your thoughts into the future and the "If–Then" Thinking Key helps to develop a hypothesis statement based on the causal relationship between two events.

"What If . . . ?" The "What If . . . ? Question Series" may be used alone or with the "If–Then" Thinking Key and the "What's Next? Question Series." The "What If . . . ? Question Series" also helps you think into the future. The unique function of the "What If . . . ? Question Series" is that it helps you to consider possible outcomes of a certain action. Therapy-related actions can have many possible consequences. Asking "What If . . . ?" stimulates you to think about the worst- and best-case scenarios when planning an action or a series of actions. The more consequences you can anticipate from a proposed action, the better prepared you are when you enter the situation. Practice using the "What If . . . ? Question Series."

DIRECTIONS

1. Read rows 1–2 across columns A and B.
2. Identify a worst-case scenario and a best-case scenario of each of the "What if . . . ?" questions listed in column A, rows 3–4.
3. Record your responses in column B.

FIELD ORGANIZER

"What If . . . ? Question Series"

A "What if . . .	B Worst- and Best-Case Scenario
1. **What if** *Sam got a buddy (older student in his school) to help him once a day?*	**Worst-Case Scenario** *Other children would feel neglected because Sam got a buddy and they did not.* **Best-Case Scenario** *Sam's kindergarten teacher liked the buddy idea and arranged with a seventh or eighth grade classroom to begin a buddy program for all the children in kindergarten. Buddies would come once a week to work with the children as part of a service program for the upper grades.*
2. **What if** *Sam's parents want to incorporate activities to enhance Sam's ability to integrate sensory information from his environment?*	**Worst-Case Scenario** *Sam's parents become frustrated with Sam's progress. They would like to see him making gains at a faster speed.* **Best-Case Scenario** *Sam's parents cherish every small gain Sam makes. They recognize that Sam's sensory processing issues will take time to improve and they are satisfied that he is moving in the right direction.*
3. **What if** *routines at school are reinforced at home?*	**Worst-Case Scenario** **Best-Case Scenario**

"What If . . . ? Question Series" (Continued)

A "What if . . .	B Worst- and Best-Case Scenario
4. **What if** *a notebook system is used to communicate between school and home?*	**Worst-Case Scenario** **Best-Case Scenario**

"Think Positive." The "Think Positive" Thinking Key can be used any time throughout the planning and implementation of the therapy expedition. Use the "Think Positive" Thinking Key whenever you find yourself saying "I can't . . ." to an idea that you would really like to pursue. "Think Positive" helps replace thoughts of "I can't" with thoughts of "How might I?" Practice using the "Think Positive" Thinking Key.

DIRECTIONS

1. Read row 1 to see how an "I can't" statement is transformed into an "In what ways might" statement.
2. Generate an "I can't" statement for rows 2 and 3.
3. Identify and record three statements in column B, rows 2–3, that transform the "I can't" statement in column A into statements beginning with "In what ways might . . ." that create a possibility for accomplishing the desired action.

FIELD ORGANIZER

"Think Positive"

A I can't . . .	B In what ways might . . . ?
1. *get the school district to purchase the necessary equipment to carry out a program in the home.*	a. **IWWM** *Sam's dad construct a ramp for their basement?* b. **IWWM** *I get some equipment on loan?* c. **IWWM** *Sam's parents use outdoor equipment to help facilitate more organized movement?*
2.	a. **IWWM** b. **IWWM** c. **IWWM**

(continued)

"Think Positive" (Continued)

A I can't . . .	B In what ways might . . . ?
3.	a. **IWWM** b. **IWWM** c. **IWWM**

Once a therapy guide has the determination to find a way to reach a goal, she isn't easily deterred. A goal is the vision that fuels the therapy expedition to continue moving forward.

"Action Plan Adoption Checklist." The "Action Plan Adoption Checklist" Thinking Key helps to finalize your plan of action by addressing factors related to advantages, compatibility, complexity, trialability, and visibility. Practice the "Action Plan Adoption Checklist" Field Organizer by asking the two questions under each of the factors to help you examine the effectiveness of the therapy plan.

DIRECTIONS

1. Read the questions in column A.
2. Record your responses in column B. The first question in each of the five sections has been answered.

FIELD ORGANIZER

"Action Plan Adoption Checklist"

A Question	B Response
Advantage: the relative advantage the current plan has over previous actions that were taken to solve the problem. (Consider the "advantage" factor when creating a plan for clients who previously received therapy services.)	
1. What are the benefits to the client and the client's support group for accepting the plan?	*The proposed plan seeks to work on Sam's underlying sensory processing problems while simultaneously creating an environment that supports Sam in learning how to deal with change.*
2. How is this action plan better than previously tried actions?	

"Action Plan Adoption Checklist" *(Continued)*

A Question	B Response
Compatibility: how consistent the plan is with the client's paradigm.	
1. In what ways is the plan consistent with the client's paradigm (values, experiences, needs)?	*The focus of the plan is to create consistency between kindergarten and home routines. The plan is child, family, and teacher friendly. The plan emphasizes helping Sam develop skills and abilities to explore his environment in new and creative ways.*
2. Who among the client's support group will agree with the plan?	
Complexity: the ease with which the plan can (a) be comprehended by others and (b) be implemented.	
1. In what ways can the plan be clearly communicated to others?	*Each month there will be a plan highlighting the activities on which Sam's parents and teacher will focus. The plan will be kept simple and straightforward. Information will be organized in chart form for easy recognition and recall of the activities.*
2. In what ways can the plan be simplified?	
Trialability: the possibility of trying out the plan or having it modified by others and still meet the client's needs.	
1. In what ways can the plan be first implemented on a trial basis?	*Activities which have component parts can be introduced a couple parts at a time e.g., setting up routines at home that parallel routines in kindergarten could be introduced on a trial basis by beginning with two routines.*
2. In what ways can the plan be modified and still accomplish the goal?	
Observability: how visible the outcomes of the plan are to others.	
1. In what ways are the outcomes of the plan visible to all involved with the plan?	*Target behaviors will be identified on the plan so that Sam's parents and teacher know what are the intended outcomes for the period of time under consideration. For example, at the end of the month Sam will transition between three morning routines in kindergarten along with his classmates without an outburst.*
2. In what ways can the outcomes be made easy for others to see and understand?	

"Preparing to Seek Feedback." Use the "Preparing to Seek Feedback" Thinking Key to organize your thoughts as you go about gathering feedback about the effectiveness of the action plan. Seeking feedback from others can help a therapy guide make adjustments in the itinerary in order to ensure that the plan of action is on the right course. The Field Organizer for the "Preparing to Seek Feedback" Thinking Key uses the 5 Ws & an H question series to trigger your thoughts.

DIRECTIONS

1. Read the questions in column A, rows 1–5.
2. Record your responses in column B, rows 3–5. To get you started, possible answers have been provided in rows 1–2.

 FIELD ORGANIZER

"Preparing to Seek Feedback"

A 5 Ws & an H Questions	B Responses to the 5 Ws & an H Questions
1. **Who** might provide feedback?	Sam, Sam's parents, Sam's teacher, the principal at Sam's school.
2. **What** feedback will I seek?	How is Sam handling his kindergarten routines? How is Sam adjusting to changing from one routine to another during the day? What is Sam's tolerance to touch, e.g., materials used for art projects, sand table, dressing, hygiene? How is Sam interacting with children and adults in the classroom?
3. **When and where** are the best times to seek feedback?	
4. **How** might I acquire the feedback?	
5. **Why** do I want to acquire the feedback?	

"Flow Checklist." Use the "Flow Checklist" during your travels to determine whether the experiences planned for the client embrace elements of Flow. Complete the "Flow Checklist" Field Organizer below for Sam's SI Expedition. Since Sam's story was written to provide an overview of life with Sam before and after sensory integration therapy we do not have details of the treatment activities used. Thus, to use the "Flow Checklist" Thinking Key within the context of Sam's SI Expedition, concentrate on Flow experiences Sam's mother described that occurred as a result of treatment.

DIRECTIONS

1. Read the Flow criteria in column A.
2. Record in column B one indication that the criterion for the Flow state was present in the activities during Sam's SI Expedition. To get you started, the first two Flow criteria have been matched with a behavior described in the story.

FIELD ORGANIZER
"Flow Checklist"

A Flow Criterion	B Indication That Flow Criterion Was Present
1. Possesses the *appropriate skills* to perform the activity	*As an outcome of therapy Sam was no longer merely satisfied to jump up and down; instead he started to jump up feet together and land feet apart.*
2. Indicated a sense of the *potential of completion* (goal directed) of the activity.	*Sam climbed across the monkey bars, first one bar to the next, then skipped every other bar.*
3. *Able to concentrate* on activity.	
4. Evidence of *effortless involvement,* while participating in activity.	
5. Experience a *sense of control* while participating in activity.	
6. Indication of *loss of self* (became absorbed) while performing activity.	
7. Indication that the *sense of time was altered* while participating in activity.	

Reflective Journaling: Second Stop

REFLECTIVE JOURNAL ENTRY 13.2

Complete the following thought:

Having completed the therapy expedition as the therapy guide, I feel the primary challenges of Sam's SI Expedition are . . .

Reflective Journaling: Third Stop

REFLECTIVE JOURNAL ENTRY 13.3

Compare your thoughts, feelings, and insights about the challenges you perceived before you applied CPS to your perceptions about the challenges after using CPS.

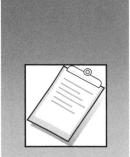

Green dot: I understand the concept and can explain it to a traveling companion.

Red dot: I need to retrace my steps and review the material.

Section 13
SELF-ASSESSMENT

Now that I have completed the thirteenth part of my journey, I can:

○ describe the therapy expedition route of Sam, a child with sensory processing problems.

○ extract relevant information from Sam's story that relates to the occupational therapy process and CPS.

○ use journaling to identify personal thoughts, feelings, and insights about Sam's story.

○ use mind mapping to link information in Sam's story to the therapy expedition itinerary.

○ use Thinking Keys and Field Organizers to creatively solve Sam's therapy-related problems.

Design Your Own Therapy Expedition

Itinerary #14

At the end of the fourteenth part of your journey, you will be able to:

✓ extract relevant information from a story that relates to the occupational therapy process and CPS

✓ use journaling to identify personal thoughts, feelings, and insights about a client's story

✓ use mind mapping to link information in a client's story to the therapy expedition itinerary

✓ use Thinking Keys and Field Organizers to creatively solve therapy-related problems

In this section you will design a therapy expedition for Kaitlyn, a toddler, or Mary, an adolescent. Select one of the two stories that appear in this section and use that story to practice applying CPS to the occupational therapy process. Select the Field Organizers that you feel will help you understand the story and the client's needs. (Blank Field Organizers appear in Appendix B.) This section is set up like Section 13. The only difference is that you are on your own.

We encourage you to use the CPS stages that best help you to make decisions within the context of the story. For example, if you are generating data in the Data Finding stage and all of a sudden you think of another wish statement, feel free to return to Opportunity Finding. Or, if you are in Idea Finding and suddenly think of criteria that might impact the decisions you are about to make, move to the Solution Finding stage.

Keep in mind that the stages are descriptive, not prescriptive; you may use them in any order in the same way therapists use assessment and observations to informally assess a client's status during a therapy session. The initial evaluation is generally the beginning of the occupational therapy process, but the informal assessment goes on throughout the course of treatment. As you develop skill using CPS, you will become more and more proficient. In this final section, try to use the system flexibly; select the CPS stages that most appropriately meet the demands of your specific thinking challenge.

The Thinking Keys: A Review
Before you read the stories and begin to plan your therapy expedition, read through the following for a summary of the Thinking Keys you have used in this field book. They are organized according to the six stages of CPS and the preliminary stage that leads up to CPS.

Preparing to Use CPS Within the Occupational Therapy Process

Thinking Key	*Use this Thinking Key to . . .*
"Watch for Cues and Look for Patterns"	uncover cues from the client's story and look for patterns among the cues that will help you gain insight about the client's problem.
"PACC"	"pack" or frame information from the client's story into an occupational therapy frame of reference.
"Problem Ownership Checklist"	determine a client's level of ownership of a problem.
"Stop, Drop, and Listen"	remind yourself to keep an open mind and listen to what a client is saying by dropping assumptions that may filter and bias the information.
"What Paradigm Is Operating?"	focus in on what paradigms a client might be operating under during the therapy process.
"Consider Other Viewpoints"	actively seek to understand a situation from more than one perspective.
"Well-Structured vs. Ill-Structured Problem Checklist"	determine whether the client's problem can use a ready-made solution or needs a tailor-made solution.

Get Ready to Understand the Problem: Opportunity Finding

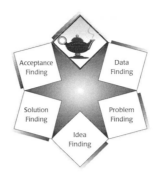

Generating Phase

Thinking Key	*Use this Thinking Key to ...*
"WIBGI . . . ?"	identify the broad challenges, concerns, and opportunities within a client's problem through the use of the invitational stem "Wouldn't it be great if . . . ?" ; generate wish statements that are broad and brief; record *every* wish that crosses your mind.

Focusing Phase

Thinking Key	*Use this Thinking Key to ...*
"Head and Shoulders Test"	determine whether one wish statement stands "head and shoulders" above the rest.
"Highlighting"	identify a wish statement to explore in Data Finding by (1) identifying the Hits among all wish statements, (2) arranging the Hits into Hot Spots (clusters), and (3) relabeling the Hot Spots as new problem statements that reflect the essence of the Hits.

Get Ready to Understand the Problem: Data Finding

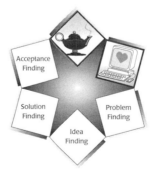

Generating Phase

Thinking Key	*Use this Thinking Key to ...*
"5 Ws & an H"	thoroughly and systematically *gather* and *cluster* data about the wish statement.

| "5 Ws & an H else" | use your imagination to think "off the page," push beyond the information gathered through the "5 Ws & an H" Thinking Key and uncover as much information as possible about the wish. (Keep in mind that the wish statement is like the tip of the iceberg.) |

Focusing Phase

Thinking Key	*Use this Thinking Key to . . .*
"Highlighting" Part 1	identify all the data *you* feel might be relevant to solving the client's problem.
"Storytelling"	connect Hits identified in "Highlighting" so that they tell a story.

Get Ready to Understand the Problem: Problem Finding

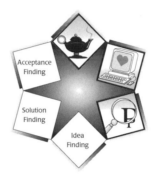

Generating Phase

Thinking Key	*Use this Thinking Key to . . .*
"IWWM . . . Who–Does–What?"	create problem statements by completing the phrase, "In what ways might . . . ?" and answering the question "Who does what?"
"Substitution"	create problem statements by reframing the statements with alternative wording.
"Ladder of Abstraction"	identify a wide range of problem statements by asking "How?" and "Why?" questions. "How?" questions lead to specific details about the client's problem. "Why?" questions lead to general and abstract responses.

Focusing Phase

Thinking Key	*Use this Thinking Key to . . .*
"Head and Shoulders Test"	determine whether one problem statement stands above the rest.
"Highlighting"	begin to identify a wish statement when one wish statement does not stand "head and shoulders" above the rest.

Get Set to Find a Solution: Idea Finding

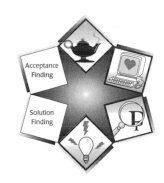

Generating Phase

Thinking Key	*Use this Thinking Key to . . .*
"Brainstorming"	generate a large quantity of ideas.
"CAMPERS"	build flexibility into your thinking by considering the answers to the questions triggered by the words Combine, Adapt, Magnify, Put to other uses, Eliminate, Reverse, Substitute.
"Force Fit"	generate novel ideas by forcing a fit between a random stimulus and the idea under consideration.
"Attribute Listing"	generate ideas by analyzing and altering the parts of the problem statement in an effort to uncover new opportunities.

Focusing Phase

Thinking Key	*Use this Thinking Key to . . .*
"Highlighting" Part 1	identify all ideas that hold promise for solving the client's problem.

Go Forward with an Action Plan: Solution Finding

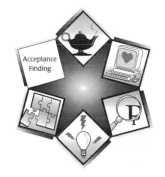

Generating Phase

Thinking Key	*Use this Thinking Key to generate . . .*
"Will It . . . ?"	questions that produce criteria.
"TRACS"	ideas framed by the five broad categories of criteria commonly used in decision making: time, resources, acceptance, costs, space.

| "Making an Idea More Acceptable" | criteria by identifying the essential element in an idea that needs to be improved on. |

Focusing Phase

Thinking Key	*Use this Thinking Key to . . .*
"In-tuit"	use your intuition as criteria for evaluating an idea.
"AL-O"	explore the advantages, limitations, and strategies to overcome the limitations of a limited number of ideas.
"Evaluation Matrix"	systematically evaluate ideas against criteria developed in the Generating Phase of Solution Finding.
"PCA"	rank order a small group of ideas that you perceive to be of equal value.

Go Forward with an Action Plan: Acceptance Finding

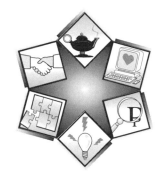

Generating Phase

Thinking Key	*Use This Thinking Key to . . .*
"Potential Sources of Support and Resistance"	systematically identify the potential sources of support and resistance on a therapy expedition.
"Check the Mindset"	identify mindsets that indicate a person's resistance to, or acceptance of, the action plan.
"Generating Potential Actions"	generate actions that might lead to developing an action plan.

Focusing Phase

Thinking Key	*Use This Thinking Key to . . .*
"LIST"	organize the therapy plan actions into long-term, intermediate, and short-term actions.
"Plan for Action"	develop the specific action steps that will be part of the therapy expedition's itinerary.
"What's Next? Question Series"	direct your thinking toward issues related to the follow-up actions you will take with a client. (The follow-up actions are what makes your initial actions meaningful.)

"If–Then"	structure hypothesis statements that provide future direction to the therapy expedition.
"What If . . . ? Question Series"	consider possible outcomes of taking a certain action.
"Think Positive"	replace thoughts of "I can't" with "How might I?"
"Action Plan Adoption Checklist"	finalize your plan of action by addressing factors related to advantages, compatibility, complexity, trialability, and visibility.
"Preparing to Seek Feedback"	organize your thoughts as you go gather feedback about the effectiveness of the action plan.
"Flow Checklist"	examine whether the elements of "Flow" are present during a therapy expedition.

Kaitlyn's Story and Mary's Story

Meet Kaitlyn and Mary. Read their stories and decide whether you want to design a therapy expedition for Kaitlyn or for Mary.

Putting Cosmetic Prostheses to Work

Bruce E. Tapper

1 Working at CareWest La Mariposa, a 99-bed skilled nursing facility in Fairfield, Calif., between San Francisco and Sacramento, Victor Espinoza sought to expand his experience by getting training in hand therapy. He attributes his being able to experiment with such new and different areas to Joice Beatty, his supportive supervisor at IHC Therapy Management, the contractor of occupational therapy services to CareWest; to the rehabilitation director at his facility, Rich Pike, RPT, and to their staff.

2 Espinoza now sees outpatients in part of his nursing facility as well as working after hours in a private clinic with clients having a variety of traumatic hand injuries. This work led Espinoza to achieve success in teaching a former colleague's young daughter to achieve function in a hand that had been transplanted with two toes. The child had a congenital anomaly, missing fingers and having only partial growth of the thumb and index finger. "I was able to teach her how to use her hand functionally in bilateral activities and ADLs using lateral pinch," he said.

3 This work resulted in a referral from Michelle James, MD, in the orthopedic department of Shriner's Hospital for Crippled Children in San Francisco, of a 3-year-old girl with a below-elbow amputation. The child, Kaitlyn, had been fitted with a prosthetic hand device, secured to the shoulder with a harness and operated by elevating the shoulder. Normally, for children of this age such a device is viewed as being mainly of cosmetic significance, Espinoza explained—to enable them and their family to adjust to the notion of wearing a prosthesis.

4 The accepted view was that a child could not learn to use it functionally this early, he said. "But I didn't know that!" he continued. Espinoza said that previously children were fitted with a cosmetic hand from age 1 and ½ but were not instructed in the use of functional terminal devices until they were around 5 or 6. At that point they were encouraged to use a hook, which is far superior for functional tasks.

5 While working with Kaitlyn's cosmetic prosthesis, Espinoza said he felt that it was too difficult to open the hand voluntarily with the glove on. So he removed the long rubber glove worn mainly to protect the hand/cable device. "To my surprise," he said, "within one treatment session she was beginning to pick up large objects such as towels, large square blocks, large dowels, sponges, and beanbags.

6 "Smooth surfaces, such as pens, pencils, or anything made of shiny plastic, would fall out of her prosthetic hand," he observed. So he put thin latex hospital gloves over her hand and experimented with inserting foam padding into the fingers to enable her to pick up smaller objects, such as a penny. The padding took some 15 minutes to wrap—rather long given Kaitlyn's short attention span and the 35–40 minute sessions available.

(continued)

So Espinoza said he got the idea to wrap the fingers with Coban, a substance that sticks to itself. That took only 3 minutes to apply, he said.

7   Kaitlyn used her prosthesis more and more each session, Espinoza said. Now 4 years old, Espinoza said, "She wears the prosthesis all waking hours." And "she's now burning out a glove a month." Espinoza said they had made the gloves a lot looser and shorter in length so as not to inhibit motion.

8   "Shriners Hospital was surprised by the level of function and diversity of Kaitlyn's use of her prosthetic device," Espinoza noted. Kaitlyn was the first child of the age of 3, in the experience of Shriners, who could actually use a cosmetic hand in a functional way.

9   "She improved the most since I've seen hands become available for little kids," said prosthetist James Caywood, CP, who has worked for the past 18 years at Robin-Aids Prosthetics in Vallejo, Calif., the contractor to Shriners for upper extremity devices. "I was really impressed with what he [Espinoza] accomplished," Caywood said. "He was really willing to try a lot of ideas—willing to experiment." Caywood noted that Espinoza was the first to come to the conclusion to take off the original glove and said his techniques have now been incorporated into the work done at Shriners with other children.

10   According to Espinoza, Caywood recommended that he develop a videotape of approximately 20 minutes showing the different activities that can be used for prosthetic device training. Espinoza said the video shows Kaitlyn picking up objects varying in width from 9½ to less than ½ cm. Among the activities shown are picking up a playing card and playing a Mickey Mouse ABC game on a computer using a dowel to hit the keys. Bilateral activities are also stressed, such as holding a bag and getting cookies out with the prosthetic hand, taking a small cup out of a dispenser and filling it with water from a water cooler, and catching and throwing a ball. Espinoza said that Caywood and James are now showing the video throughout northern California to new patients' family members to encourage earlier prosthetic use.

11   As for the effect of pediatric clients coming into a geriatric facility, Espinoza said, "Patients aren't scheduled concurrently but interaction with the patients occurs on a regular basis. The geriatric patients always like to see children of all ages and appear to respond in a positive way to them." The management of the facility, Care Enterprise Northern Division, also has responded in a positive way to activities such as Espinoza's—awarding CareWest La Mariposa the title of "Rehabilitation Facility of the Year." In characteristic expansiveness and generosity, he and the rehabilitation director made sure every member of the staff received a certificate attesting to their share in that achievement.

Reprinted with permission from *OT Week*, January 27, 1994, 14–15.

When Mary Finishes High School

Diana Bal

1   Mary is a 16-year-old girl with multiple disabilities. She is diagnosed with ataxic cerebral palsy. She is non-verbal and non-ambulatory. Mary is wheelchair-dependent but has adequate sitting balance to sit independently in a regular chair. Attendance this year was at a regular middle school, in a self-contained classroom for the orthopedically disabled. Academically, she worked at a kindergarten level. When designing therapeutic pre-vocational tasks that would be beneficial for Mary, it was important to analyze her strengths and upper extremity skills.

2   Occupational therapy was provided to Mary to adapt equipment, to simplify work, and to assess her prevocational skills.[1] During observations and assessment, Mary exhibited a wonderful visual attention to task and was very motivated to finish what she started. As Mary's occupational therapist, I recommended activities to enhance and to accommodate upper extremity coordination and manipulation skills. The ataxia interferes with smooth upper extremity movements of both arms and the increased tone of her right arm impedes further coordination.

3   Mary did much better with a one-pound wrist weight on her left hand. The right hand was secured, given a wrist weight, and stabilized, but it did not improve her skills. The ataxic arm movements of the right upper extremity were needed to stabilize her trunk.

4 The school district's job coach was pleased to see that Mary was motivated and her attention to task was adequate to get a job finished. He stressed the importance of independent toileting. He also suggested analyzing which task she could perform accurately with the fastest speed. Time was spent with Mary's teacher and related staff members training them to enhance toileting and self-care independence. Accommodations, safety bars around the toilet, were made to the bathroom to increase her independence.

5 Stilington[2] stressed the importance of acquainting and giving students the opportunity to try out different work samples. We had received a grant for pre-vocational materials and purchased a kit from Attainment Products. The materials in this kit ranged from easy to more difficult tasks. We found that Mary preferred unilateral sorting tasks. Her long range was a job in an office sorting mail or letters.

6 A sorting box was made with 30 different slots to place envelopes by zip codes. Problems arose because the envelopes were too fragile to hold up under Mary's ataxic movements. Also, she was unable to scan the five number zip code accurately. The task was changed by using popsicle sticks, putting two numbers on each stick. Mary quickly advanced to three and then to five numbers on the stick. Mary's speed increased and she was always accurate. One month later the sticks were changed to 3 × 5 cards with the zip codes written on them. These cards were laminated for durability and stiffness. Mary quickly accommodated to the different material and the change of hand position required to put a card in the slot rather than a popsicle stick. A database was kept to evaluate the speed and accuracy of Mary's skills. In another month, Mary was able to sort eight cards in 15 minutes, all accurately. The cards were then changed to regular envelopes. The envelopes were varied, some of them were typed and some were hand written. Through use the envelopes were bent and mangled, but none ripped or tore.

7 In five months, Mary was sorting 20 envelopes by zip code in 15 minutes, all accurately. This was a major accomplishment for a student who could not sort any envelopes with a five-number zip code at the start of this program.

8 The job coach was thrilled to hear that Mary now went to the bathroom independently with an assistant standing by if help was needed. He was also excited to see how motivated she was to complete her work and that her speed and accuracy had improved greatly. The job coach then recommended that Mary try to sort by name, getting ready to sort mail alphabetically. New envelopes were made and the sorting box was changed from zip codes to names. When first presented with this new activity, Mary was unsure why we had changed everything. However, she quickly generalized her skills and within two weeks she was sorting envelopes and cards by names at the same skill and speed level she had attained with zip codes.

9 With the pre-vocational skills learned this year, Mary is better prepared for high school next year. The sorting skills were not the only tasks that Mary worked on. The prevocational jobs were varied with assembly tasks and bilateral motor skills. Although these were more difficult and not as much fun for Mary, they did help to enhance her manipulation skills and upper extremity stability. The job coach will set up jobs for her in the community and in the school. The occupational therapist will continue to consult and accommodate the jobs for her skill level. We will continue to pursue jobs that require accurate sorting, not speed.

10 Occupational therapy was available at the school twice a month, on a consultative basis. Without the cooperation of the teacher, related staff, and parents, Mary's progress would not have been possible. A table with Mary's job was set up in the classroom. She was given the opportunity to work on her job during the school day. The staff cooperated with the OT to change and update Mary's job. Mary's motivation, willingness to please, and her steady improvement made her a pleasure to work with. A solid pre-vocational program helps her and her family prepare for when Mary finishes high school.

NOTES

1. C. Creighton, "The School Therapist and Vocational Education," *AJOT* 33, no. 6 (1979):373–75.
2. P. Stilington, "Vocational and Special Education in Career Programming for the Mildly Handicapped Adolescent," *Exceptional Child* 47, no. 8 (1981):592–98.

Reprinted with permission from *Occupational Therapy Forum,* June 9, 1995, 14–15.

Reflective Journaling: First Stop
Reread the story you have chosen for your therapy expedition and then complete Reflective Journal Entry 14.1 from the perspective of the therapy guide.

Imagine that you are the therapy guide who will be consulting with Kaityn's therapist or Mary's therapist and complete the following thought.

I feel the primary challenges of _____'s Expedition are . . .

Mind Mapping the Therapy Expedition

Create Layer 1 of your Mind Map for the story you chose. Include information that you consider to be the most pertinent to the expedition. Be the judge and determine what information in the story has relevance to occupational therapy.

Create a Mind Map of the Story

Mind Map Guidelines

1. Place the story's main concept in the center of the space using pictures or words or both.
2. Radiate ideas from the central thought.
   - Headline text—one or two words per line.
   - Print text (for easy reading)
3. Use the following color code for each layer:
   Layer 1 — black
   Layer 2 — green
   Layer 3 — blue
4. Link the main concepts and generate more ideas from the linkages.
5. Have fun!

Remember, the more linkages that you generate between elements, the greater your ability to see how all the elements relate to one another.

Use Thinking Keys to Design a Therapy Expedition

Begin your therapy expedition by reviewing the Thinking Keys in the list "Preparing to Use CPS." When you have selected the Thinking Keys you want to use, locate the corresponding Field Organizers in Appendix B, photocopy them, and complete the work on the photocopies. (Leave the Field Organizers in Appendix B blank so that you can repeatedly photocopy them for your work in the field.)

Continue your expedition by photocopying and completing the Field Organizers you feel are appropriate for Get Ready to Understand the Problem: Opportunity Finding, Data Finding, and Problem Finding.

Reflective Journaling: Second Stop

REFLECTIVE JOURNAL ENTRY 14.2

Complete the following thoughts.

Having completed the therapy expedition as the therapy guide for _____ I now feel that the primary challenges of _____'s Expedition are . . .

Reflective Journaling: Third Stop

REFLECTIVE JOURNAL ENTRY 14.3

Reread your Reflective Journal Entries 14.1 and 14.2. Then complete the following thoughts.

1. Applying CPS to _____'s Therapy Expedition has influenced my perspective of the story as follows . . .

2. My perception of _____'s problems did/did not (circle one) change from the first time I read the story for the following reason: . . .

Green dot: I understand the concept and can explain it to a traveling companion.

Red dot: I need to retrace my steps and review the material.

Section 14
SELF-ASSESSMENT

Now that I have completed the fourteenth section of my journey, I can:

○ extract relevant information from a story that relates to the occupational therapy process and CPS.

○ use journaling to identify personal thoughts, feelings, and insights about a client's story.

○ use mind mapping to link information in a client's story to a therapy expedition itinerary.

○ use Thinking Keys and Field Organizers to creatively solve therapy-related problems.

Appendix A: Answers

Section 2

Nine Dot Exercise
Four-line solution

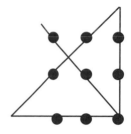

One-line solution
(1) Take a paint brush and swoosh a wide line through all of the dots; (2) cut the paper, line up the dots in a row, and draw one line connecting them. The lesson: Why impose boundaries that are not there?

Section 3

Options for the "What's Next? Question Series" Field Organizer, Column C
3. Consult with Jason's teacher(s) during the trial period to monitor whether the electronic speller has resulted in a reduction in Jason's spelling errors in his class writing assignments and homework assignments. 4. Evaluate through consultation with Jason, Jason's teacher(s), and Jason's parents whether using a water bottle has decreased Jason's habit of sucking on his clothes.

Options for the "If–Then" Field Organizer, Column B
3. THEN he might have fewer spelling errors on his written assignments. 4. THEN he might find less of a need to suck on his clothing

Options for the "What If . . . ? Question Series" Field Organizer, Column B
3. The Energy Corner may draw kids to goof off there and disrupt the classroom. To avoid such a potential disruption, criteria for using the Energy Corner need to be explained to the whole class so they clearly understand the purpose of this space. 4. Other children might want the same "privilege" as Matt. A "special transporting" system may need to be arranged among several teachers that allows other children to transport bags of heavy dictionaries to specified (pre-arranged) classrooms. Most likely, children who do not have a need for this kind of activity would not want to participate in it.

Options for Open-Ended Questions Worksheet, Column B
3. How independent is Shondra in dressing? 4. What day of the week is convenient for you to bring Tasha into therapy? 5. What kinds of toys does Kendall like to play with? 6. What kind of extracur-

ricular activities does Latifah participate in after school? 7. What computer skills has Alexis acquired? 8. How often does Majid complete all of his assignments? 9. What household chores does Marcus perform? 10. How does Jacques express his emotions?

Options for the "Stop, Drop, and Listen" Field Organizer, Columns B and C
2.B. Ms. Cook is narrow-minded and rigid. C. I don't want Bradley to get upset if his toy is lost or broken in school. 3.B. Bradley is a brat. C. I want to hold onto my toy. It makes me feel safe.

Options for the "Watch for Cues and Look for Patterns" Field Organizer, Column C and Part II, 2
5.B. Gregory must be very upset. He has the language development to allow him to express his needs; he seems so upset that he seems unable to use his words to express what he is feeling. II, 2. Gregory is acting peculiar today (not waiting, shouting).

Creative Word Problems
1. Sandbox 2. Man overboard 3. I understand 4. Reading between the lines 5. Long underwear 6. Crossroads 7. Downtown 8. Tricycle 9. Split level 10. 3 degrees below zero 11. Neon light 12. Circles under the eyes 13. High chair 14. Paradise 15. Touchdown 16. Six feet underground 17. Mind over matter 18. He was beside himself 19. Backward glance 20. Life after death

Options for the "Consider Other Viewpoints" Field Organizer, Column B
2. if she uses public transportation, I should also be able to use it. 3. work is my first important priority.

Options for the "Think Positive" Field Organizer, Column B
3. Free up time to perform the evaluation by reworking my schedule to work with three other children within a group session. 4. Ask whether another therapist could work with two students on my caseload for the day in order to free up some time. 5. Ask whether another therapist on the team might have an opening in his or her schedule to perform the evaluation.

Section 4

Crossword Puzzle Solutions

Performance Areas
• Activities of Daily Living

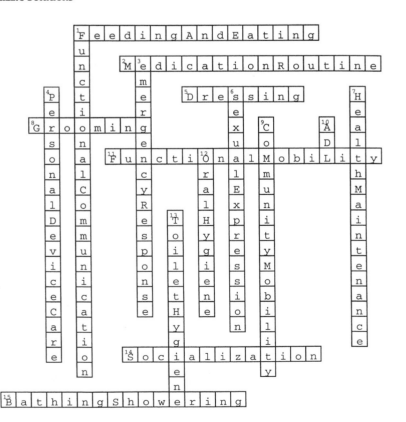

Performance Areas
- **Work and Productive Activities**
- **Play and Leisure**

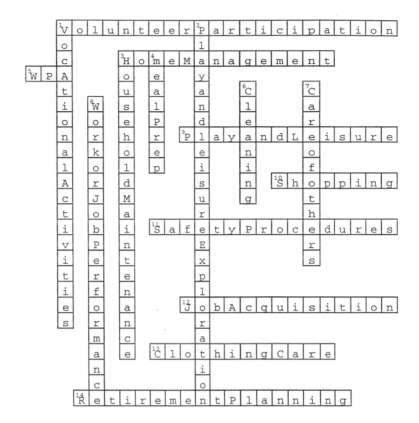

Performance Components
- **Sensorimotor Component**
- **Sensory**
  - **Sensory Awareness**
  - **Sensory Processing**

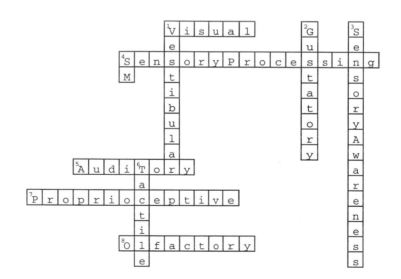

Performance Components
- **Sensorimotor Component**
  - **Sensory**
    - **Perceptual Processing**

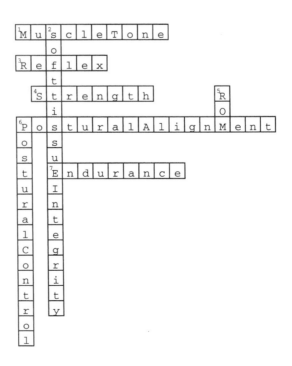

Crossword puzzle (Perceptual Processing):
Across:
2. Depth Perception
6. Kinesthesia
10. Visual Closure
12. Right Left Discrimination
13. Form Constancy

Down:
1. Spatial Relations
3. Topographical Orientation
4. Perceptual Processing
5. Pain Response
7. Stereognosis
8. Figure Ground
9. Position In Space
11. Body Scheme

Performance Components
- **Sensorimotor Component**
  - **Neuromusculoskeletal**

Crossword puzzle (Neuromusculoskeletal):
Across:
1. Muscle Tone
3. Reflex
4. Strength
6. Postural Alignment
7. Endurance

Down:
2. Soft Tissue Integrity
5. ROM
6. Postural Control

Performance Components
- **Sensorimotor Component**
  - **Motor**

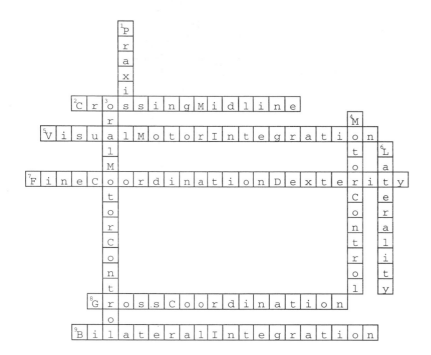

Crossword (Sensorimotor Component):
1. Praxis
2. CrossingMidline
3. MotorControl
4. MotorControl
5. VisualMotorIntegration
6. Laterality
7. FineCoordinationDexterity
8. GrossCoordination
9. BilateralIntegration

Performance Components
- **Cognitive Integration and Cognitive Components**

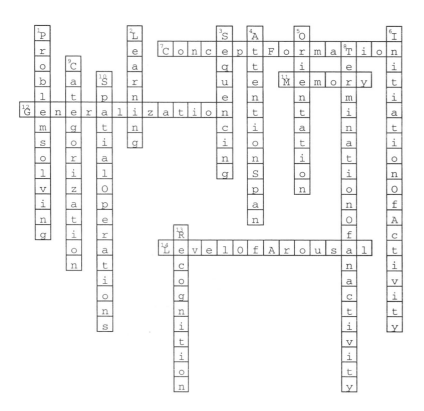

Crossword (Cognitive Integration and Cognitive Components):
1. ProblemSolving
2. Learning
3. SequencingSpan
4. Attention
5. Orientation
6. InitiationOfActivity
7. ConceptFormation
8. TerminationOfActivity
9. Categorization
10. SpatialOperations
11. Memory
12. Generalization
13. Recognition
14. LevelOfArousal

Performance Components
- **Psychosocial Skills**

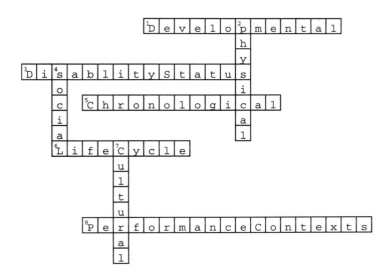

Performance Contexts
- **Temporal Aspects**
- **Environment**

Section 5

Options for the "PACC" Part 2: Performance Components Field Organizer

Sensorimotor Component. 1. Sensory: b. sensory processing (1) tactile: child needs an awareness of the tissue and the skin on his or her nose, including a recognition that the nose may be running. The child also has to sense the inside of the nasal passage in order to clear the nasal passage, since he or she cannot see it; (2) proprioceptive: child needs an awareness of where the arm is in space relative to the nose as he or she blows; also needed is a sense of how hard to squeeze the nose as he or she blows. 2. Neuromusculoskeletal: b. range of motion: necessary for the child to have sufficient range to reach his or her nose and manipulate the tissue; c–f. muscle tone, strength, endurance, postural control: necessary for the child to have a sufficient degree of each of these components to perform the task without having to consciously direct his or her attention toward holding his or her body up in space.

3. Motor: g. fine coordination/motor dexterity: needed to manipulate the tissue inside the nasal passage for waste that is not removed by blowing; f. praxis: necessary to coordinate the actions of blowing with just the right amount of tension and timing to clear the nasal passages, as well as the ability to clean the area around the nose and to dispose of the tissue.

Cognitive Integration and Cognitive Components: Components 1–14 are all involved to a greater or lesser extent. For example, the children need to be oriented in time and space to recognize the need to blow their noses when they are congested. Initiation and termination of an activity comes into play from the point the child retrieves a tissue to the point of proper disposal. Memory and sequencing is called for to remember the steps of how to blow, including closing one nostril and blowing through the opposite side and then reversing that pattern to clear the opposite side. Problem solving is used to manage clearing the nasal passages, which involves blowing and dealing with removal of waste in hard-to-get at places.

Psychosocial Skills. 2. Social: b. social conduct: children need to value learning proper nose blowing etiquette.

3. Self-management: c. self-control: part of having proper nose etiquette is to clear the nasal passage using tissue in place of clothes or other unsanitary means.

Section 7: Options for Field Organizer

FIELD ORGANIZER

"5 Ws & an H" / "5 Ws & an H else" / "Highlighting" Part 1

Wish Statement: *WIBGI the children could learn to blow their noses?*

A *Generate*	B *Hits*	C *Generate*	D *Hits*
Who might be involved in the opportunity?		**Who *else* might be involved in the opportunity?**	
6. principal		6. teacher's family members	
7. speech pathologist		7. aunts and uncles	
8. school nurse		8. other teachers in the school	
9. school social worker		9. preschool parents on the Internet	
10. classroom volunteers		10. preschool teachers on the Internet	

(continued)

"5 Ws & an H"/"5 Ws & an H else"/"Highlighting" Part 1 (Continued)

A *Generate*	B *Hits*	C *Generate*	D *Hits*
What is involved in the opportunity?		**What *else* is involved in the opportunity?**	
6. design a nose blowing program		6. learn to blow through the mouth	
7. medical check for nasal obstruction		7. the children can learn about the concept of germs	
8. blowing nose into tissue on request		8. understand the basic concept of how germs "fly in the air" (are airborne)	
9. blowing through one nostril at a time		9. knowing where a tissue can be located when needed	
10. wiping nose without chafing area below the nose		10. awareness of the sensation of clear nasal passage	
Where might opportunities occur to work on the wish?		**Where *else* might opportunities occur to work on the wish?**	
6. on the rug (during reading time)		6. in the car	
7. at the sand table		7. on public transportation	
8. at the teacher's desk		8. on the way to school	
9. at the water table		9. at the babysitter's	
10. near the wastebasket		10. at the movie theater	
When might there be an opportunity to work on the wish?		**When *else* might there be an opportunity to work on the wish?**	
6. while standing in line for the bathroom		6. while visiting relatives	
7. before lining up to go outside to play		7. in the evening before mealtime	
8. before getting coats on to go home		8. while teaching parents "how to" blow their noses	
9. when nose is running		9. while practicing for a video on nose blowing	
10. before having snack		10. while making an audiotape of funny sounds	
Why is it important to look for opportunities in this area?		**Why *else* is it important to look for opportunities in this area?**	
6. children won't spread their colds to one another in class		6. children will not have to have substitute teachers	
7. teachers won't miss school		7. children will learn to use tissues to blow their noses rather than use their hands to wipe their noses	
8. toys and other objects will stay cleaner		8. teachers will feel good and be healthy	

"5 Ws & an H"/ "5 Ws & an H else"/ "Highlighting" Part 1 (Continued)

A Generate	B Hits	C Generate	D Hits
9. children will be proud of their accomplishments		9. children will have an opportunity to get stronger with a healthy body	
10. children will have their nose blowing skill for life		10. the healthier the children are the more they can ward off infections	
How will you make this wish a reality?		**How *else* will you make this wish a reality?**	
6. buddy system in which children encourage one another to get a tissue to blow their noses		6. children will apply peer pressure to maintain a "proper nose blowing" environment	
7. audiotape the children blowing their noses and see if they can identify themselves on the tape		7. children will carry tissues in a sleeve band for ready use	
8. have the children practice blowing to the beat of a drum		8. capture the funniest pieces of the nose blowing experiences on video and have children view	
9. have the children become a nose/mouth blowing choir where they practice their skill while being videotaped, have children view themselves on tape		9. go to the local museum and walk through a giant size nose model	
10. children accompany the teacher in a song by making sounds created by blowing through their noses		10. provide each child who has a need to use tissue with a small box for discarding the used tissue	

Section 9: Options for Field Organizer

 FIELD ORGANIZER

"Attribute Listing"

Problem Statement: IWWM a program be developed to teach the children how to blow their noses?		
A **Attribute**	B **Elaborate on the Attribute under consideration**	C **Hits**
1. Nose	8. children study how the nose works 9. children make a large paper-mache nose as a class project 10. children make nose sculptures 11. children blow the noses of the stuffed animals in the class 12. children circle noses in magazines	

(continued)

A Attribute	B Elaborate on the Attribute under consideration	C Hits
	13. children make a collage of nose pictures 14. children use their noses to discriminate the smell of scented items (e.g., markers, stickers)	
2. Blow	8. breathing in through the mouth 9. breathing in through one nostril at a time 10. breathing out through one nostril at a time 11. alternate breathing out through one nostril and then the other 12. blowing light objects with the mouth 13. blowing light objects with the nose (e.g., cotton) 14. playing with blow toys (e.g., noisemakers, harmonicas)	
3. Teach	8. teacher's aide teaches the parents 9. teacher's aide teaches the children 10. children teach one another 11. children "teach" the teacher 12. children "teach" the teacher's aide 13. children "teach" the parents 14. children "teach" Louise	
4. Program	8. program is integrated into the movement portion of the curriculum when the children play a series of games that include the nose (e.g., Simon Says, imitating the elephant and other animals) 9. program is integrated into the music and movement portion of the curriculum when the children take turns cueing the rest of the children when to move, using mouth or nose blowing movements 10. program is integrated into the language arts portion of the curriculum when the children make up stories related to nose blowing 11. program includes learning how to put clown make-up on their noses and make funny faces in a mirror using blowing actions of the mouth and nose 12. program includes recording the children's funniest moments on videotape, which children view during the course of the program 13. children receive certificates for successful completion of nose blowing program (certificates are in the shape of a nose) 14. program includes learning a poem about nose blowing, which they recite at the beginning of the school day	

Section 12: Show and Tell Reference Guide

Round 1 (Section 1) Answers
Team A

1. clinical reasoning **2.** During a treatment session, the therapist, like a juggler, manages several issues at once. **3.** Thinking strategies help organize your thoughts and develop your creativity and imagination in order to enhance your problem solving ability within the occupational therapy process. **4.** Thinking Keys **5.** *Clinical* does not fully capture the wide scope of today's practice settings, clinics are only one place among many where therapists see clients. **6.** Creative solutions are tailored to the specific situation in which the problem occurs. Creative solutions are the opposite of ready-made solutions. A ready-made is a prepackaged solution that has been used before to meet a previous challenge under a different set of circumstances at a different time. **7.** fabrication of an assistive device, selection of unusual treatment media and strategies (*other answers are also acceptable*) **8.** "Out of the box" thinking refers to thoughts that are beyond the usual or expected way of looking at something or an event. **9.** "What if" or "How about" **10.** CPS skills allow you the flexibility to respond to change.

Team B

1. Maureen Hayes Fleming, an occupational therapist, and Cheryl Mattingly, an anthropologist **2.** the Three Track Mind **3.** Thinking strategies (the train) help the therapist find a solution (get to the light) to a problem (the tunnel). **4.** Creative Problem Solving **5.** *Reasoning* addresses only the intellectual, rational side of thinking. **6.** Ready-mades are convenient and should be considered first when making a decision because they can save time and money. **7.** fabrication of an assistive device, selection of unusual treatment media and strategies (*other answers, not given by Team A, are acceptable*) **8.** imagination **9.** "What if" or "How about" **10.** A therapist must have the flexibility to respond to change and to the unexpected.

Round 2 (Section 2) Answers
Team A

1. Scott Isaksen, K. B. Dorval, and Donald Treffinger **2.** Alex Osborn **3.** incubation **4.** Get Ready, Get Set, and Go Forward **5.** Get Set: Idea Finding; Go Forward: Solution Finding and Acceptance Finding **6.** Each stage of the process helps you find information that moves you closer to solving a problem. **7.** Referral for therapy services, assessment, goal setting **8.** The Generating Phase is represented by the broadening or expansion of the triangle from its apex; the Focusing Phase is represented by the broad base narrowing or contracting toward the triangle's apex. **9.** The first guideline, striving for quantity, supports the second guideline, stretch your mind. When you strive to generate as many ideas as possible, you stretch your mind to accept any and all options that pop into your head. **10.** (a) Consider all ideas (the possibles, probables, and the impossible ones): value all ideas at first (b) Consider the novelty of an idea: value the originality and the appropriateness of every option (c) Be deliberate and explicit: carefully and clearly evaluate your ideas.

Team B

1. Alex Osborn, an advertising executive created the first CPS model in the late 1930s. Sidney Parnes refined it. **2.** judgment **3.** Get Ready, Get Set, Go Forward **4.** Opportunity Finding, Data Finding, and Problem Finding **5.** No. You may use any of the components (and the stages within them) in any order, depending on the nature of the problem. **6.** The star shape that forms in the middle of the six interconnected diamonds symbolizes the light generated by a bright star. **7.** treatment planning, intervention, discharge planning, and follow-up **8.** Deferred Judgment means that you withhold reviewing your ideas until after you have exhausted generating the list of options. When you use Affirmative Judgment, your thinking shifts into a "critical thinking" evaluative mode. Affirmative Judgment in the Focusing Phase allows you to consider the positives and the negatives. **9.** "Hitchhiking" is attaching one idea on top of the previous one; "free-wheeling," which is "unrestrained behavior," is allowing the ideas—all ideas, even outrageous and silly ones—to flow. **10.** The "doability" scale ranks ideas as possible (has some potential), probable (under certain conditions, the idea might work), and impossible (no chance for the idea to work because of limited resources, inadequate time, or inappropriate place).

Round 3 (Section 3) Answers
Team A

1. The first journey involves moving from section to section, learning the content within each section of the book. The second journey involves moving through the occupational therapy process with a client and his family. **2.** The " 'What's Next?' Question Series" will help to gradually project your thoughts into a future state in which a therapy expedition "lives." (*Accept any response that suggests* *projecting a thought into the future.*) **3.** tolerant of ambiguity, risk taking, flexible, open-minded, empathetic **4.** Asking "What if . . . ?" helps you envision future events by expanding your thoughts about the consequences of an action. (*Accept any response that considers the possible ramifications of a proposed action.*) **5.** *Accept any response that illustrates that the person demonstrated a flexible mindset in response to some changing circumstance.* **6.** When empathy becomes enmeshed with tolerance for ambiguity, flexibility, open-mindedness, and risk-taking, each quality gains in richness, texture, and sensibility. **7.** Occupational therapists learn to reflect on a person's life story, to ponder it, in order to build a therapeutic relationship. **8.** The therapy guide uncovers relevant data, cues, to try to understand the person and the person's life situation that initiated the referral to occupational therapy. The guide assembles the cues into patterns that help him or her visualize the whole picture. **9.** To reframe a problem, you must look at it from a different perspective. To do this, you must shift your paradigm—change the assumptions that underlie a situation—and leave your comfort zone. **10.** *Accept any response that illustrates that the context within which you make a decision has a pervasive influence on your operating paradigms.*

Team B

1. Therapy guides use their heads to retrieve textbook information; they use their hearts to draw on personal beliefs and intuition about the client. **2.** A hypothesis is a forward projection based on some information known about a situation. Sample from text: **If** Jason were seated in the front of the room, **then** his on-task behaviors might improve. (*Accept any example that follows the If . . . Then format provided in the example.*) By continuously generating hypothesis statements in response to the client's performance, the therapy guide is continuously changing and adjusting the therapy process. With these constant changes, the therapy expedition becomes the client's unfolding story. **3.** First, the therapy guide accepts that there are several possible ways to view a problem. Second, he or she welcomes the opportunity to think through each aspect of the problem before deciding on a solution. **4.** The comfort zone is that intangible psychological area that represents the realm of the familiar. It is where you feel safe. When you take a risk and engage in a new, unfamiliar activity and you no longer feel safe. **5.** Thinking positively about a problem sparks the creative energy needed to meet the demands of the challenge by opening up your mind to value all kinds of options. **6.** The therapy guide is on a continuous quest for information in order to get a clear understanding of what the client and the client's family want as a result of the therapy process. **7.** You figuratively drop, or suspend, your point of view so that you can see the problem from the client's point of view. **8.** When we look at the world from a certain point of view, we are using our paradigm as information filters to explain the world as we perceive it. **9.** Using the "Consider Other Viewpoints" Thinking Key helps you distinguish your perception of a situation from the perception of others. With the "Think Positive" Thinking Key you frame your thoughts with positive words that influence your actions toward the possible. With both Thinking Keys you shift your paradigm from an "I can't do it" thought to a "How might I do it?" **10.** Intuition is an internal guidance system that works automatically, like a compass, to point us in a certain direction.

Round 4 (Section 4) Answers
Team A

1. occupation, manifest by one's occupational performance **2.** To capture the total picture of a client, therapy guides assess all three areas of the client's occupational performance. **3.** *Accept any answer that illustrates how a change in the context produced a change in a person's occupational performance.* **4.** Performance Areas broadly define human performance in terms of daily life skills; Performance Components are fundamental human abilities that people demonstrate when they engage in the Performance Areas. **5.** The Uniform Terminology system is organized into Performance Areas, Performance Components, and Performance Contexts. **6.** sensorimotor component, cognitive integration and cognitive components, and psychosocial skills **7.** grooming; oral hygiene; bathing/showering; toilet hygiene; personal device care; dressing; feeding and eating; medication routine; health maintenance; socialization; functional communication; functional mobility; community mobility; emergency response; sexual expression **8.** play and leisure exploration, play and leisure performance **9.** psychological, social, self-management **10.** chronological, developmental, life cycle, disability status

Team B

1. activities of daily living, work and productive activities, play and leisure **2.** Context can powerfully shape the quality of a person's performance and is one of the most significant variables that helps us to remember isolated pieces of information. **3.** The referral is deemed appropriate for occupational therapy services if the client's reason for referral falls within one or more of the three domains of occupational performance. **4.** Uniform Terminology **5.** The chosen category depends on the meaning the activity holds for the client. For one client, socialization might be considered a daily living activity, for another, an activity of play and leisure. **6.** temporal aspects and environment. **7.** home management, care of others, educational activities, vocational activities **8.** sensory, neuromusculoskeletal, motor **9.** level of arousal, orientation, recognition, attention span, initiation of activity, termination of activity, memory, sequencing, categorization, concept formation, spatial operations, problem solving, learning, generalization **10.** physical, social, cultural

Round 5 (Section 5) Answers
Team A
1. "Watch for Cues and Look for Patterns," "Stop, Drop, and Listen," "What Paradigm Is Operating?" "Consider Other Viewpoints," "Problem Ownership Checklist," "Well-Structured vs. Ill-Structured Problem," and the "PACC" **2.** A person who shares ownership of a problem has an internal motivation to close the gap between what is and what should be. **3.** Knowledge of a gap helps an individual close the gap. **4.** Without a need to solve the problem the individual will not make a sincere effort to close the gap between what is and what should be. **5.** *Accept any example that illustrates a therapy guide seeing a problem from the client's perspective.* **6.** Therapy guides work alongside the client as a team to identify the gap between what is and what ought to be. **7.** Well-structured problems have ready-made solutions; ill-structured problems require solutions specially designed to match the unique nature of the situation. **8.** *Accept any response that suggests a unique solution needs to be designed to deal with the situation.* **9.** Louise moved across uncharted territory as she generated a treatment strategy to meet the needs of the children and their teachers. She didn't always know where she was going, but she was willing to take the risk and try new activities, trust her intuition and be willing to take detours along the way. **10.** Performance Areas, Components, and Contexts

Team B
1. Therapy guides must look at the problems in every therapy situation as unique because every client has a unique set of paradigms. **2.** The person must (a) be aware that there is a gap between "what is" and "what should be," (b) be able to measure the gap, (c) have a need to solve the problem, and (d) have access to the resources needed to solve the problem. **3.** Unless a client is able to measure the gap he or she will not perceive when the gap is closed. **4.** Solving problems require resources in the form of time, information, money, and other people. **5.** (a) How does the client define the problem? (b) What are the key issues from the client's point of view? (c) What outcome does the client see as an acceptable solution? **6.** *Accept any problem where at least one answer to the problem is readily available.* **7.** (a) Ill-structured problems lack adequate information, (b) ill-structured problems have unpredictable outcomes, (c) ill-structured problems require custom-made solutions. **8.** Louise had an ill-structured problem because at the beginning, the problem lacked adequate information about what to do. The outcome depended on the cooperation of the children and the follow-through of the teachers and the children's families. Louise had to do research at a day care center and draw on her own creativity to develop a custom-made solution. **9.** In "Highlighting" Part 2, Hits are clustered into groups called Hot Spots and given a label that reflects the focus of the cluster. **10.** Use the "PACC" Thinking Key to organize information about a client's occupational performance as you seek solutions to many of the problems encountered in practice.

Round 6 (Section 6) Answers
Team A
1. The stages in CPS may be used in any order, depending on the needs of the decision maker and the specific situation. **2.** Using the word *opportunity* puts a problem in a positive light and suggests that you are looking for an improved future state for the client. **3.** When the objective of therapy services has been clearly identified by the written referral, you can skip Opportunity Finding and move directly to Data Finding. **4.** "Visionizing" is a combination of "vision" and "actualizing," meaning having thoughts that lead to creating a future state. **5.** You use WIBGI questions to look for potential starting points, not the definitive one. **6.** when you begin repeating opportunity statements **7.** When no one wish statement stands head and shoulders above the rest, use the "Highlighting" Thinking Key. **8.** Hits are promising options that the client is interested in pursuing. **9.** Hits are clustered into groups called Hot Spots and given a label (e.g., dressing, grooming, play). **10.** ½

Team B
1. Opportunity Finding sets the stage for the client to make explicit his wish to close the gap between where he is and where he wants to be. **2.** (a) What do I perceive as the client's opportunities? (b) What is the global objective of the problem? (c) In what ways will the therapy program increase the client's (or the family's or caregiver's) independence? (d) Will I be serving the client directly or indirectly? **3.** Wouldn't it be great if. When you begin your thoughts about a situation with these words, you start to imagine in what ways the situation might be different. **4.** In the Generating Phase of

Opportunity Finding you are looking for possible starting points rather than the definitive one. **5.** Opportunities for success thrive when stated in the affirmative. **6.** Ask the client whether there is one wish that stands head and shoulders above the rest. **7.** Clustering information means putting bits of data into groups or categories to make it easier to relate to. **8.** Hits are identified. **9.** The Restatement of Hot Spots occurs. **10.** a genie's lamp

Round 7 (Section 7) Answers
Team A
1. False. Each of the six stages may be used at any time, in any order, depending on the demands of the situation. **2.** In Data Finding your focus is on finding as much data as you can about the contents of the wish statement in order to help make it a reality. **3.** *Accept any response that names specific kinds of resource people who are defined by the uniqueness of the expedition.* **4.** The data you uncover during Data Finding will serve as a handy reference for the remainder of the CPS process. **5.** The data includes what parts, scope, support systems, objections, difficulties, limitations, or obstacles might be involved in solving the client's problem. **6.** The context is the frame of reference that brings meaning to the situation. **7.** The "5 Ws & an H else" Thinking Key increases your depth of inquiry and further expands your thoughts after using the "5 Ws & an H" Thinking Key. **8.** The aim of "Highlighting" in Data Finding is to identify all the Hits that might help make the Expedition a success, not to find one piece of data to consider. **9.** Use the "Storytelling" Thinking Key to connect selected Hits in such a way as to tell a story. **10.** Information gathered during Data-Finding will serve as a database to expand upon as well as refer back to as you proceed through CPS.
Team B
1. Opportunity Finding, Data Finding, and Problem Finding **2.** Every person who could be involved with making the client's dream come true is potentially a resource on a therapy expedition. **3.** Like the beam cast by the flashlight, a resource person helps you to see the area through which you are traveling more clearly. **4.** The tip of the iceberg hints at what lies below covered by the seawater; the wish statement gives a rough idea of where you are going on a therapy expedition. **5.** "How" questions identify the steps, activities, or actions involved in the situation. **6.** The more minds, the more perspectives. **7.** In the Focusing Phase of Opportunity Finding, you try to select one wish statement; in the Focusing Phase of Data Finding you try to understand how the pieces of data relate to each other. **8.** to look for relationships among Hits identified in Part 1 of the "Highlighting" process **9.** Extracting themes helps you deal with a large amount of information by categorizing each item. **10.** The computer symbolizes the process of collecting data to understand the wish statement. The heart on the icon's computer monitor is a reminder that in addition to facts, data includes feelings, impressions, observations, and questions.

Round 8 (Section 8) Answers
Team A
1. Problem Finding identifies the specific gap between "what is" and "what should be"; Opportunity Finding seeks to describe the broad challenges within a situation. **2.** When you begin therapy with an end in mind the process has a clear direction in which it is headed. **3.** To reframe a problem, you must shift your paradigm in order to look at a situation from a different perspective. (Reframing a problem statement in a positive form elicits a flow of ideas.) **4.** To complete a thought that you begin with "IWWM . . . " answer the question "Who does what?" **5.** to create alternative wording for your problem statement when you need to see a problem with a fresh perspective **6.** the specific action to be taken **7.** offers the opportunity to state a problem in many different ways in order to see a problem in a new light. **8.** allows you to look for specific answers and methods **9.** to identify all the problem statements that show the most promise of shining a light on the path to the solution **10.** The more inclusive (without becoming unwieldy) the problem statement, the more comprehensive the solution will be.
Team B
1. Once you have a clear vision of the journey ahead, the development of appropriate and realistic therapy goals become a natural part of the therapy expedition. **2.** When a client has a clear vision of therapy outcomes, a detour need only deter the client temporarily from arriving at his destination. **3.** Framing a problem statement in a positive manner will help elicit a flow of ideas. **4.** helps keep a positive mindset toward the client and his therapy-related challenge. **5.** identifies who will carry out the action addressed in the problem statement **6.** the issue you want to address **7.** Asking "Why" questions broadens the problem statement and suggests new problem statements. **8.** "Head and Shoulders Test" and "Highlighting" **9.** Part 2 **10.** The magnifying glass symbolizes the process of focusing in on the problem area that will be used to solve the client's problem.

Round 9 (Section 9) Answers
Team A
1. One stage, Idea Finding **2.** (a) personal experiences, (b) ability to combine, adapt, and rearrange information from personal experiences, (c) imagination **3.** to increase your options for finding solutions based on novel, creative ideas **4.** fluency **5.** restricts the free flow of ideas **6.** As ideas recorded on self-sticking notes are evaluated, they can easily be moved into clusters. **7.** flexibility **8.** originality **9.** an object, a word from a dictionary, a geographical location, for example **10.** You elaborate on your thinking about a problem by analyzing the parts (the attributes) of the problem.
Team B
1. the Generating Phase **2.** the more ideas you generate, the higher the quality of your ideas **3.** fluency, flexibility, originality, elaboration **4.** For brainstorming to be successful, everyone must feel free to express whatever ideas come to mind; judging ideas inhibits the free flow of ideas. **5.** facilitator **6.** Eliciting the help of others has a way of moving you out of your comfort zone in order to see a problem from another perspective. **7.** Combine, Adapt, Modify, Put to other uses, Eliminate, Rearrange, Substitute **8.** A new stimulus gets the mind working in a new direction. **9.** elaboration **10.** to examine whether a solution should involve novel strategies ("reach for the sky") or be conservative because of limited resources and the need for gradual change ("stick to the basics")

Round 10 (Section 10) Answers
Team A
1. Solution Finding and Acceptance Finding **2.** Evaluating criteria will help you make objective decisions. **3.** Time, Resources, Acceptability, Cost, Space **4.** Once the essential criteria of an idea is identified, the extraneous parts can be removed and the essential element(s) reworked in order to arrive at an acceptable idea. **5.** Sensing what you feel can carry a deep kind of certainty about it, feelings can be indispensable when making rational decisions. **6.** Advantages, Limitations, Overcome (as in, overcome the limitations) **7.** to objectively compare and rate Idea Finding options against criteria you generated in the Generating Phase of Solution Finding **8.** Rating each option against each criterion encourages objectivity. **9.** When rules of thumb are relied on to an extreme they become mindtraps. **10.** "First time" presented information is perceived to have a greater value even though it is not of greater importance.
Team B
1. the Focusing Phase **2.** Completing the statement "Will it . . . ?" leads to the random and spontaneous development of criteria. **3.** The "TRACS" Thinking Key keeps you on track during the therapy expedition by helping you evaluate your proposed actions using the five most common categories of criteria within the decision making process. **4.** internal physiological factors that manifest psychologically **5.** Therapy guides build their confidence using intuition to make decisions by reflecting on the outcomes of their intuitive decisions. **6.** In using the "AL-O" a therapy guide can anticipate possible negative consequences and plan ahead by preparing strategies to overcome the limitations. **7.** a rating scale based on a series of numbers or on a series of symbols to represent a level of choice. **8.** The "Evaluation Matrix" relies on a criteria-based rating system; the "PCA" uses a ranking system to prioritize the options. **9.** ease of recall, retrievability, and presumed associations **10.** *Accept any response that illustrates an insensitivity to baseline information or sample size.*

Round 11 (Section 11) Answers
Team A
1. In Solution Finding you use criteria to transform ideas into solutions, in Acceptance Finding you lead the client from the present to a desired future state by creating a therapy expedition plan of action. **2.** *Accept any answer that illustrates a person being supportive of one part of a plan but resistant or uncooperative about another part.* **3.** One kind of change involves creating a new paradigm for the client. The second kind of change relates to improving the client's performance within a familiar, recognized paradigm. **4.** time, continuity of people, and stability of resources **5.** A therapy guide develops the long-term actions (the end point) first so that all the members of the therapy expedition have a clear vision of the destination point. Establishing long-term actions at the start of an expedition helps to avoid unnecessary detours that may take up time and delay progress. **6.** (a) WHAT is the action desired? (b) WHO will do the action? (c) WHEN will the action start, finish? (d) WHERE will the action take place? (e) WHY is the action important? (f) HOW will you know the action is successful? **7.** (a) "What's Next? Question Series" (b) "If–Then" (c) "What If . . . ?" (d) "Think Positive" **8.** The therapy guide must collect feedback from everyone involved in the therapy expedition in order to determine if the client is making progress toward reaching the goals set forth in the action plan. **9.** Activities that are not challenging may lead to boredom; activities that are too much of a challenge may raise the client's state of arousal and lead to undue anxiety. **10.** Clients who are empowered to

make choices (have a sense of control) during therapy gain confidence to solve their own problems creatively outside of the therapy setting.

Team B

1. Sources of support are the persons, places, times, or things that support an environment or "climate" conducive to moving the plan forward; resisters are persons, places, times, or things that block or inhibit the therapy process. **2.** (a) type of change, (b) mindset of the individuals impacted by the change, (c) context in which the change will occur **3.** (a) conforming–willing to take risks (b) rigid–flexible, (c) narrow-minded–open-minded, (d) needing to know–tolerant of ambiguity, (e) self-centered–empathic **4.** When you use the Thinking Key "Generating Potential Actions" you answer the following two questions: (a) What possible actions can be taken to move the action plan forward? (b) What are possible sources of resistance to the proposed actions? **5.** The "LIST" Thinking Key helps you organize the therapy plan actions into long-term, intermediate, and short-term actions. **6.** the "LIST" Field Organizer **7.** (a) advantages, (b) compatibility, (c) complexity, (d) trialability, (e) visibility **8.** Flow **9.** When a client is engaged in an activity that holds meaning for him, he is more likely to focus his attention, thus establishing the conditions for effortless involvement. **10.** The more elements of Flow you are able to promote, the more likely you will increase the client's productivity within the treatment process.

Section 13: Options for Field Organizers

FIELD ORGANIZER

"Watch for Cues and Look for Patterns"

Part I: Cues

Story Paragraph #	A Cue	B What might this cue mean?
6	Emotionally fragile	Sam must be a handful to the family because they avoid taking him out in public and limit the visitors into their home. What does the mother do when she takes Sam out? What are her coping mechanisms when he begins to cry?
7	Medical diagnosis	Sam's medical diagnosis may be cerebral palsy (CP), but this diagnosis does not explain his behavior toward his mother. CP is a nonprogressive lesion to the motor cortex. How does that relate to the behaviors that Sam exhibits when he is touched or when he is around strangers?
8	Two cues: a. Atypical motor development	Sam went from crawling to running. I wonder whether he had difficulty with modulating slow movements. How did he manage movement situations in which balance was threatened? Did he fall often? What was his muscle tone like? His mother described his body as "very floppy"; Sam leaned against nearby objects or persons for support. If he's floppy, I wonder what else is going on if he always runs.
	b. Arousal level	Sam "never slept well" at night yet he "never stopped running"? "He tired easily" according to his mother. The paradoxical observations of Sam's activity level reported by his mother raises questions about Sam's ability to modulate incoming sensory information. Typically, children who are active during the day generally sleep well at night. But the observation that Sam displays periods of spacing out, followed by periods of rapid head-shaking or frenzied running may be an indication that intuitively Sam is trying to influence his arousal level through self-directed sensorimotor activities.

(continued)

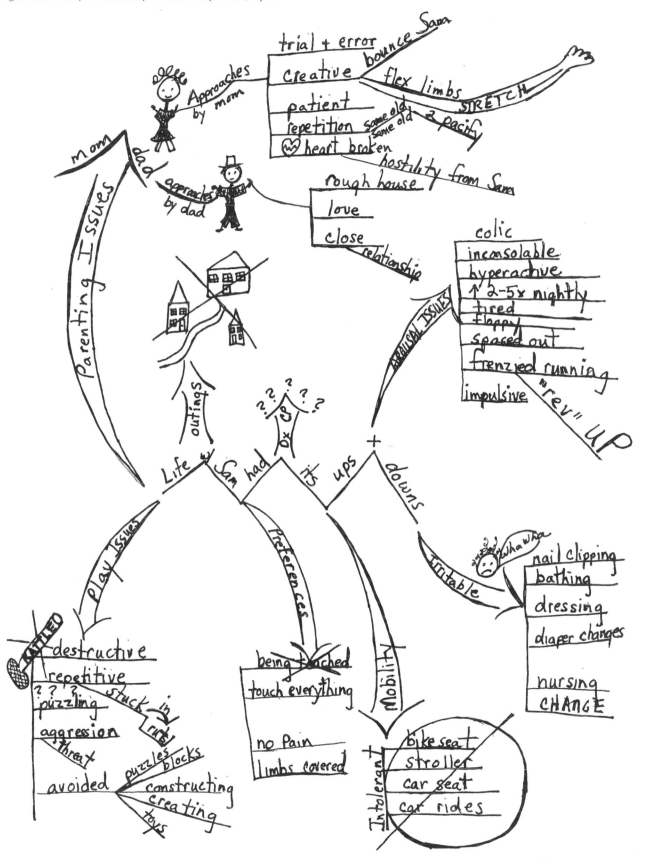

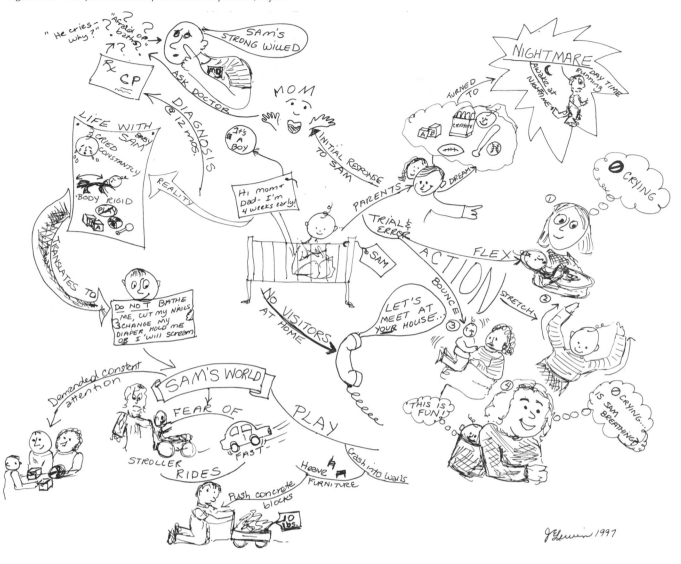

J.E. Lewin 1997

FIELD ORGANIZER

"Watch for Cues and Look for Patterns" (Continued)

Part I: Cues		
Story Paragraph #	**A Cue**	**B What might this cue mean?**
9	Low tolerance for being passively moved through space	Sam cannot tolerate a bike seat, stroller, car seat, or car rides for longer than five minutes without screaming nonstop. I wonder about the integrity of his vestibular system. His mother describes him as floppy (paragraph 8); there is a neurophysiological connection between the vestibular system and the integrity of the muscles. Sam's intolerance for passive movement and his apparently low muscle tone may imply poor modulation of sensory information being interpreted by the vestibular system. He also may have an altered sense of proprioception when he is moved through space by others.

Part I: Cues

Story Paragraph #	A Cue	B What might this cue mean?
10	No interest in constructive play activities	Sam avoids puzzles, blocks, drawing with crayons on paper, and other activities that demand constructional praxis skills. Requests to make representational objects with play dough (e.g., animals, monsters, pretend food) are met with anger and frustration. I wonder about Sam's body scheme awareness and motor planning abilities. With a diagnosis of cerebral palsy, he must have atypical muscle tone; abnormal muscle tone most likely influences his proprioceptive and kinesthetic sensory perception. Some of the difficulties he exhibits with motor planning may be tied in with the status of his muscle tone and the way he is processing incoming sensory information within his central nervous system.
11	Three cues: a. Never plays with toys	Perhaps Sam doesn't play with toys because he doesn't know what to do with them. He demands his mother's constant attention because, unlike toys, which are static objects, she can adapt her responses to his needs. Playing with toys is not intrinsically rewarding for Sam because he doesn't experience the same sense of control over them as he does when he vies for his mother's attention.
	b. No interest in TV, radio, or noise of any sort	I wonder whether the sounds emitted from the TV or radio are too fast for Sam to decode the content. His lack of interest in auditory stimuli may be another indication of Sam's difficulty with processing sensory information from his environment.
	c. Tolerates self-initiated sounds	The voices of others seem to upset Sam, although he tolerates the sounds he makes himself, even though they get increasingly loud as he makes them. Perhaps because Sam is in control of the pitch and the volume of the sounds he makes himself, he doesn't become defensive to his own sounds. From the parents' viewpoint, Sam had difficulty modulating the volume of his sounds. I wonder whether Sam can whisper or carry a melody when singing.
12	Two cues: a. Enjoys repeatedly engaging in previously learned, familiar activities	Repeating familiar activities has a calming influence on the central nervous system. Perhaps Sam felt overly aroused much of the time. Repeating activities that he felt he could do well was one way to boost his self-esteem and calm himself.
	b. Pushing a heavy cartload of concrete blocks	Pushing a heavy load stimulates the proprioceptive system. Proprioceptive stimulation can have a calming or an alerting influence on the nervous system. Perhaps Sam enjoys the activity because it helps calm him. I also wonder whether Sam enjoys pushing the heavy cart because the activity empowers him with a definition of where he is in space and contributes to the development of his body scheme.
13	Two cues: a. Enjoys roughhousing	Sam's apparent enjoyment of being tossed in the air and spun as well as being bounced on the bed and wrestled on the floor suggests that vestibular and proprioceptive input are satiating to Sam's nervous system.
	b. Hostility toward mother	I wonder how Sam's mother responds when she feels Sam is hostile toward her. Family teaching will need to be a priority of the treatment program to help Sam's parents understand that the underlying causes for his behavior are manifestations of his inability to accurately perceive and process information from the environment.

(continued)

Part I: Cues

Story Paragraph #	A Cue	B What might this cue mean?
14	Two cues: a. Insists on keeping arms and legs covered by clothing	Being touched by others must cause Sam great pain if he insists on wearing long-sleeved shirts and slacks all of the time, including the summer. I wonder whether he is able to discriminate where he is touched. Perhaps some of his difficulties interacting with peers is related to his resistance to being touched.
	b. Irritated by passive touch yet actively touches everything	Just as Sam will self-initiate sounds, he will touch but responds aversively to being touched by others. When he is in control and can stop and start the activity on his own he seems better able to engage in it.
15	Impervious to pain	Pain is a very primitive sensation and an important survival mechanism. The issue that Sam seems, to his mother, to be "impervious to pain" raises questions about the severity of his ability to process sensory information. Since pain, temperature, and touch are mediated physiologically through the same tracts, I wonder whether Sam can distinguish between hot and cold temperatures. How does he respond when he picks up an ice cube? How long can he hold it? Does he have a history of unknowingly getting burned on the stove, for example?
16	Two cues: a. Aggressive with peers	Physical aggression is a form of proprioceptive input. Sam seems to crave proprioceptive input; therefore, why would he understand that physical aggression is a threat to other children? I wonder whether he ever engages in adult-supervised play on playground equipment. If he does, I wonder what types of equipment he enjoys most (e.g., monkey bars, swings, teeter-totter).
	b. Unable to direct his own activities constructively	Sam seems to have problems with planning nonhabitual activities that involve the sensorimotor system. He may be unable to conceptualize what he needs to do in order to develop a plan, before acting. Based on previous cues, he lacks adequate intersensory communication within his central nervous system. This communication from within would allow Sam to develop the appropriate neuronal models necessary to develop a motor plan to act.
17	Traditional behavior management techniques unsuccessful	Sam may not have responded positively to time-outs, rewards, and removal of privileges if he was unaware that he was doing anything wrong. Perhaps he perceived the spankings as another form of proprioceptive stimulation, which he enjoyed. Sam's apparently high threshold for pain may explain why spanking him was not perceived as punishment.

Part II: Patterns

Story Paragraph #	Patterns that emerged from cues found in the story
1, 4, 5	Developmental delays in prereadiness skills for academic preparation
2–4, 8–17	Difficulty interpreting sensory information
4, 9	Atypical balance and/or movement patterns
3–5, 8–11, 12–17	Sam's mother is an astute observer of her son's behaviors and seems willing to explore creative ways to meet his atypical needs

"PACC"

Part 2: Performance Components

Performance Component	Story Paragraph #	Story Element
Sensory awareness	2, 12	Cuddling did not console; enjoyed repetition of familiar activities; change was upsetting
Tactile	3, 14	Any skin exposure sent him into hysterics; kept arms and legs covered
Proprioceptive	12, 5, 9	Deliberately crashed into walls; joint traction was calming; heaved heavy objects; pushed cartload of concrete blocks; enjoyed walks while scrunched up in a knapsack
Vestibular	5	Bouncing calmed him
Auditory	11	Avoided anything to do with noise (e.g., TV; radio)
Pain response	15	Seemed impervious to pain
Visual-closure	10	No interest in puzzles, blocks, or any play with put-together parts
Strength	8	Body seemed floppy
Endurance	8	Sam tired easily
Postural control	8	Sam leaned against nearby objects for support
Motor control	8	Went from crawling to running
Praxis	12	Same activity, same path; difficulty initiating new tasks
Fine coordination/dexterity	10	Avoided puzzles or any play that involved putting parts together
Level of arousal	8	Hyperactive; awakened several times during the night; "spaced out" at times
Initiation of activity	12, 16	Aversion to engaging in any new activities; no idea how to enter play with other children
Termination of activity	12	Repeats same activity over and over
Problem solving	10	No interest in blocks, puzzles, forming objects with play dough
Learning	17	Cried if he didn't get his own way
Generalization	6	Cried for hours following the briefest change in his environment
Psychological	13	Hostility toward mother; wanted her total attention
Interests	12	Limited repertoire of activities
Self-concept	17	Became hysterical if he didn't get his own way
Social conduct	6, 16	Cried hysterically when taken out in public; aggressive with other children
Interpersonal skills	17	Like a wild animal, out of control

(continued)

Part 2: Performance Components

Performance Component	Story Paragraph #	Story Element
Self-expression	6	Cried a lot
Coping skills	6	Cried at briefest change in his environment
Self-control	6, 14	Emotionally fragile; impulsive

Part 3: Performance Contexts

Performance Context	Story Paragraph #	Story Element
Developmental	9	Atypical play behaviors for age 2 ½ years (e.g., no interest in puzzles, crayons, table-top activities; low tolerance for stroller rides; heaving heavy objects)
Life cycle	8, 2	Early childhood
Disability status	7	Medical diagnosis: mild cerebral palsy
Physical		Sam seemed to have greatest difficulties in nonstructured environments. He seemed most at peace when experiencing vestibular or proprioceptive input.
Social		Parents expected Sam to engage in table-top activities, manipulative play, and enjoy stroller rides
Cultural		Sam lived at home with both parents; he was an only child

FIELD ORGANIZER

"Problem Ownership Checklist"

2. Is the person **able to measure the gap**?   Yes ✔   No ☐

   Parent compared Sam's behavior to the behavior of children in the Sunday School.

3. Does the person **need to solve the problem**?   Yes ✔   No ☐

   Implicit in the story, the parent realized the devastating social and learning implications for Sam if his atypical behaviors were to continue.

4. Does the person **have access to the resources** needed to solve the problem?   Yes ✔   No ☐

   Sam's mother has demonstrated that she is very resourceful. Sam's parents also had insurance coverage that permitted him to have his surgery at the rehabilitation center.

FIELD ORGANIZER

"Stop, Drop, and Listen"

Story Paragraph #	A WHO said WHAT?	B Assumption to Be Dropped	C Behind these words or actions the person is saying . . .
3	Mother said, "Any skin exposure at all sent him into hysterics."	Mother overreacts.	I'm very frustrated with Sam's behaviors because he doesn't enjoy the activities that typically bring joy to parents.
4	Mother said that Sam never played with baby toys, yet he wasn't satisfied being a passive observer.	Mother didn't spend enough time playing with Sam.	I've observed what Sam does. Help me understand why he acts the way he does.
8	Mother said, "Sam never slept well at night, awakening between 2 and 5 times a night."	Mother put Sam to bed too early so that she wouldn't have to deal with his behaviors.	When Sam awakens at night, I am also awake. Sam is wearing me down.

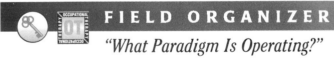

FIELD ORGANIZER

"What Paradigm Is Operating?"

Story Paragraph #	A Record a behavior to be analyzed.	B Identify the operating paradigm that could explain the behavior described in column A.
3	"Sam obviously felt terrorized" by routine skin exposure, including having his nails clipped and hair washed.	I am Sam's mother. I don't want to hurt Sam, I just want to take care of him. So why does Sam act as if he is being tortured when I dress and bathe him, change his diaper, or cut his nails?
5	"By trial and error, I eventually discovered two remedies to stop the crying. One was to bounce him vigorously on my knees. The other was to flex and stretch his arms and legs."	Because I am Sam's mother, I am responsible for finding some way to help Sam and myself. I am a fighter like Sam and I will not be defeated.
6	"Because of his emotional fragility, we avoided taking him out in public and seldom had visitors."	Helping Sam cope is more important than having a social life and going places.
12	"I was continually and unsuccessfully trying to draw him into new activities.	Sam should enjoy learning about new things. I will find a way for Sam to learn.

FIELD ORGANIZER

"Consider Other Viewpoints"

Story Paragraph #	It was **Anne's** perspective that . . .	On the other hand, **you** perceive that perhaps . . .
14	Sam insisted on having his arms and legs covered at all times.	Sam was overly sensitive to being touched by others and therefore protected himself from discomfort by insisting on wearing long sleeves and pants at all times.
15	Sam was almost impervious to pain.	Sam's high threshold for pain was a manifestation of a problem Sam had with registering sensory input.
16	Sam was extremely aggressive with other children.	Sam's physical aggressiveness toward his peers was a sign of his inability to modulate his strength because of lack of awareness of how to move his body while interacting with people and things in his environment.

FIELD ORGANIZER

"Well-Structured vs. Ill-Structured Problem Checklist"

Well-Structured Problem	Ill-Structured Problem
2. ☐ Predictable outcome(s)	✔ Unpredictable outcome(s) Sam's behaviors are unique and complex; he's young and therefore his future is undetermined.
3. ☐ Ready-made solution(s)	✔ Custom-made solution(s). The treatment program for Sam must be individualized to his unique sensorimotor needs. The treatment program will be tailor-made to meet the ever-evolving needs of Sam and his parents.

FIELD ORGANIZER

"WIBGI... ?"/"Highlighting"

Generate			Focus		
			Part 2: Clustering Hits into Hot Spots		
Wouldn't it be great if ...		**Part 1: Hits**	**A Performance Area**	**B Performance Area Subcategory**	**C Location**
11.	Sam was able to take a walk without tripping on every sidewalk crack?	●	ADL	Community mobility	Home and school
12.	Sam slept through the night?				
13.	Sam gave his mother hugs?				
14.	Sam liked being hugged and cuddled?				
15.	Sam responded to typical behavior management strategies?	●	ADL	Socialization	Home and school
16.	Sam went on errands with his mother?				
17.	Sam controlled his need to throw objects at others?	●	ADL	Socialization	Home and school
18.	Sam had favorite activities that were calming to him?	●	ADL	Health maintenance	Home and school
19.	Sam played simple games on the computer?	●	Play and leisure	Play and leisure performance	Home and school
20.	Sam could dress himself?	●	ADL	Dressing	Home and school

FIELD ORGANIZER

"Head and Shoulders Test"

Ask the client:

"Do any wish statements in the group stand **head and shoulders** above the rest?"

WIBGI Sam enjoyed kindergarten?

Proceed to Data Finding using this wish statement.

FIELD ORGANIZER
"Highlighting" Part 3

Hot Spots from Column A: **Using Performance Areas *to Cluster Hits***
Area I: Clusters **Cluster One Labeled:** *Play and leisure*
WIBGI . . .
19. Sam played simple games on the computer?
Cluster Two Labeled: *ADL*
WIBGI . . .
11. Sam was able to take a walk without tripping on every sidewalk crack?
15. Sam responded to typical behavior management strategies?
17. Sam controlled his need to throw objects at others?
18. Sam had favorite activities that were calming to him?
20. Sam could dress himself?
Area II: Restatements
Hot Spot Two: WIBGI Sam could eagerly participate in a wide range of activities of daily living?
Hot Spot Three: WIBGI Sam could demonstrate the readiness skills for school?

FIELD ORGANIZER
"Highlighting" Part 3

Hot Spots from Column B: **Using Performance Areas Categories *to Cluster Hits***
Area I: Clusters **Cluster One Labeled:** *Play and leisure performance*
WIBGI . . .
19. Sam played simple games on the computer?
Cluster Two Labeled: *Community mobility*
WIBGI . . .
11. Sam was able to take a walk without tripping on every sidewalk crack?
Cluster Four Labeled: *Socialization*
WIBGI . . .
15. Sam responded to typical behavior management strategies?

Hot Spots from Column B: *Using* **Performance Areas Categories** *to Cluster Hits*
17. Sam controlled his need to throw objects at others?
Cluster Six Labeled: *Health Maintenance*
WIBGI . . .
18. Sam had favorite activities that were calming to him?
Cluster Seven Labeled: *Dressing*
WIBGI . . .
20. Sam could dress himself?
Area II: Restatements
Hot Spot Two: WIBGI Sam enjoyed moving in and about the community?
Hot Spot Three (Clusters 3, 7): WIBGI Sam could cooperate during daily dressing and eating routines?
Hot Spot Four (Clusters 4, 5, 6): WIBGI Sam could develop the self-control necessary to focus his attention on activities and interactions with others?

FIELD ORGANIZER

"Highlighting" Part 3

Hot Spots from Column C: *Using* **Location** *to Cluster Hits*
Area I: Clusters **Cluster One Labeled:** *Wishes that can be worked on at home and school*
WIBGI . . .
15. Sam responded to typical behavior management strategies?
17. Sam controlled his need to throw objects at others?
18. Sam had favorite activities that were calming to him?
19. Sam played simple games on the computer?
Cluster Three Labeled: *Wishes best worked on at home*
WIBGI . . .
11. Sam was able to take a walk without tripping on every sidewalk crack?
20. Sam could dress himself?
Area II: Restatements
Hot Spot Three: WIBGI skills and abilities Sam learned at home could transfer to school?

FIELD ORGANIZER

"5 W's & an H"/ "5 W's & an H else"/ "Highlighting" Part 1

Wish Statement: WIBGI Sam enjoyed kindergarten?

A Generate	B Hits	C Generate	D Hits
Who might be involved in the opportunity?		**Who *else* might be involved in the opportunity?**	
9. occupational therapist from the rehabilitation center	●	9. Internet support group for parents with children with special needs	
10. school principal		10. coordinator of local toy lending library	
11. school counselor		11. parent advocacy groups	
12. parent support group for children with cerebral palsy		12. babysitter	
13. respite care worker		13. high school student "buddy program"	
14. special education director, local school		14. Park District program directors (art program, movement program)	
15. classroom aide	●	15. school custodian	
What is involved in the opportunity?		**What *else* is involved in the opportunity?**	
9. Explore details related to the kindergarten curriculum.	●	9. Establish a schedule for regular meetings with Sam's teacher.	●
10. Set up a simple communication system that can go back and forth between school and home.	●	10. Investigate the availability of a high school student who might be interested in working with Sam during school or at home.	●
11. Explore with parents how they might incorporate therapy experiences into their daily routine (home program).	●	11. Observe Sam at various times during his day at school (observe transitions between activities and on-task behavior).	●
12. Work with educational team to plan Sam's school program.	●	12. Investigate the potential of using the local toy-lending library.	●
13. Explore whether music helps Sam cope with change.		13. Obtain an Internet address for a parent support group for parents with children with special needs.	
14. Explore whether Sam responds positively to massage as a form of tactile and proprioceptive input.		14. Meet with the school principal.	
15. Gather information about all the activities that Sam enjoys doing.		15. Seek a contact with a parent advocacy group.	

"5 W's & an H"/ "5 W's & an H else"/ "Highlighting" Part 1 (Continued)

Wish Statement: *WIBGI Sam enjoyed kindergarten?*

A Generate	B Hits	C Generate	D Hits
Where might opportunities occur to work on the wish?		**Where *else* might opportunities occur to work on the wish?**	
9. neighborhood playground	●	9. Children's Museum	
10. Sunday School		10. community swimming pool	
11. shopping for clothes		11. neighborhood block	
12. barbershop		12. homes of extended family	
13. Sam's playroom		13. in front of the television when it's turned on	
14. bathroom at home		14. on family outings	
15. Sam's bedroom	●	15. on location during field trips	
When might there be an opportunity to work on the wish?		**When *else* might there be an opportunity to work on the wish?**	
9. entering the classroom at the beginning of the day	●	9. dressing for the day	●
10. circle time in the classroom	●	10. undressing at bath- and bedtime	●
11. group activities at school	●	11. during mealtimes at home	●
12. following directions	●	12. drying hair with towel or blow-dryer	●
13. when play wrestling		13. during haircuts	●
14. playing simple musical instruments		14. sharing toys	
15. standing in line at school	●	15. when getting in and out of the car	
Why is it important to look for opportunities in this area?		**Why *else* is it important to look for opportunities in this area?**	
9. so that Sam will tolerate being physically close to other children in the classroom	●	9. so that Sam demonstrates self-sufficiency in managing his coat when he comes to and leaves school	●
10. successes from learning to read and write will help him develop his self-concept and self-esteem	●	10. so that Sam can work on little projects he can display to his family	

(continued)

"5 W's & an H"/ "5 W's & an H else"/ "Highlighting" Part 1 (Continued)

Wish Statement: WIBGI Sam enjoyed kindergarten?

A Generate	B Hits	C Generate	D Hits
Why is it important to look for opportunities in this wish?		**Why *else* is it important to look for opportunities in this wish?**	
11. so that Sam can learn from the stories that are read to him	●	11. so that Sam can begin to develop his personality	
12. so that Sam can start to make up his own stories one day		12. so that Sam enjoys being with his classmates	
13. so that Sam can become interested in learning		13. Sam may physically hurt other children if his needs are not addressed	●
14. so that Sam can learn to develop his impulse control		14. Sam may be hurt by other children who defend themselves against Sam's aggressive behaviors	●
15. so that Sam's teacher will enjoy working with Sam		15. so that Sam can learn the rudiments of cutting with scissors	
How will you make this wish a reality?		**How *else* will you make this wish a reality?**	
9. Videotape Sam during a calm period and show Sam the video.		9. See if Sam responds positively to playing regularly in a pool.	
10. Take a picture of Sam performing at his best and post this picture in a visible space in the house.		10. Experiment with Sam's interest in playing with mud, sand, clay, and water (outside) to create a fun mess (while addressing some of his intense sensory needs).	
11. Play wrestle with Sam to provide an outlet for his need to roughhouse.		11. Experiment with Sam's interest in sliding down a kiddy slide into a kiddy pool in the backyard.	
12. Experiment whether a punching bag would help Sam channel some of his need to roughhouse.		12. Experiment with Sam's interest in moving to different styles of music.	
13. Suspend a hook in Sam's basement to hang a bolster that Sam could use under supervision with his parents.		13. Explore Sam's ability to use a drum to beat out music for other people to move to.	
14. Set up a ramp in Sam's basement that would permit fun movement experiences that could be graded to Sam's ability.		14. Explore Sam's interest in going to an indoor play center where Sam could crawl and jump around in a safe, protected environment.	
15. Experiment with having Sam chew bubble gum as a heavy work pattern that can tap off some of his excess energy.		15. Try rolling Sam up in a blanket and slowly rock him (to produce calming).	

FIELD ORGANIZER

"IWWM . . . Who–Does–What?"/"Highlighting" Part 1

Opportunity Finding Statement: WIBGI Sam enjoyed kindergarten?				
Generate				**Focus**
IWWM . . .				
	Who?	**Does?**	**What**	**Hits**
11.	principal	help	Sam transition from home into his new kindergarten classroom?	●
12.	Sam's mother	help	Sam to keep a journal about school?	
13.	Sam	"write"	a daily journal with the help of an audiocassette to record his day at school?	
14.	children's television	help	Sam look forward to going to kindergarten through modeling Big Bird and Mr. Rogers?	
15.	Sam	follow	the daily routines in his classroom?	●
16.	teacher	direct	Sam throughout his day?	
17.	teacher's aide	work	with Sam during the day at school?	
18.	high school student	help	Sam during his day in school?	●
19.	social worker	help	Sam during his day in school?	
20.	Sam's mother	design	an "art gallery" at home to display Sam's school drawings and art projects?	●

 FIELD ORGANIZER

"Substitution"/"Highlighting" Part 1

Problem Statement: IWWM Sam learn to follow the daily classroom routine?			
IWWM . . .			
	Who?	**Does?**	**What?**
5.	Sam's teacher	engage	Sam learn to follow the daily classroom routines?
6.	Sam's teacher	demonstrate	Sam learn to follow the daily classroom routines?
7.	Sam's teacher	redirect	Sam learn to follow the daily classroom routines?
8.	Sam's teacher	encourage	Sam learn to follow the daily classroom routines?

(continued)

"Substitution"/ "Highlighting" Part 1 (Continued)

Problem Statement: IWWM Sam learn to follow the daily classroom routine?	

Part B		**Hits**
5.	IWWM Sam's teacher engage Sam to direct other students in the class to follow the classroom routines?	
6.	IWWM Sam's teacher demonstrate to Sam how he might participate in classroom routines?	
7.	IWWM Sam's teacher redirect Sam to participate in the "activity of the moment"?	●
8.	IWWM Sam's teacher build on Sam's successes to encourage him to participate in the classroom routines?	●

FIELD ORGANIZER

"Ladder of Abstraction"/"Highlighting" Part 1

	7 New Problem Statement IWWM Sam develop coping strategies that will transfer to other situations?	8 ● New Problem Statement IWWM Sam learn to "switch gears" from one activity to another when playing with friends?	9 ● New Problem Statement IWWM Sam learn to plan for change when change is about to occur?
L E V E L C	Why Else? so Sam can develop strategies that will transfer to other situations	Why? so that Sam will be able to "switch gears" from one activity to another when playing with friends	Why Else? so Sam can learn to plan for change when change is about to occur
	4 ● New Problem Statement IWWM Sam learn to anticipate change in his routine during the day?	5 ● New Problem Statement IWWM Sam learn to accept change in his routine?	6 New Problem Statement IWWM Sam learn that school is a continuous cycle of beginning and ending tasks?
L E V E L B	Why Else? so that he learns to anticipate change in routine during the day.	Why? so that he can accept change in the routine	Why Else? so he learns that school is a continuous series of beginning and ending tasks

"Ladder of Abstraction"/"Highlighting" Part 1 (Continued)

	1 New Problem Statement IWWM Sam learn to cooperate with his peers and teachers in structured and unstructured activities?	2 ● New Problem Statement IWWM Sam learn to transition from one task to the next?	3 New Problem Statement IWWM Sam learn from the daily classroom activities?
LEVEL A	Why Else? so Sam can learn to cooperate with his peers and teachers in structured and unstructured activities	Why? so Sam can learn to transition from one task to the next.	Why Else? so Sam can learn from the daily classroom activities

Start Here → ***Initial Problem Statement:*** *IWWM Sam learn to follow the daily kindergarten routine?*

LEVEL A	How Else? by Sam's mother posting Sam's daily home routine schedule at home	How? by Sam's mother setting up a home schedule that includes a snack and bathroom, painting, and reading time	How Else? by developing a home schedule of "special" responsibilities, like those at school
	1 New Problem Statement IWWM Sam visit the classroom in the fall?	2 ● New Problem Statement IWWM Sam's mother simulate kindergarten routines at home, such as snack, bathroom, and reading time?	3 New Problem Statement IWWM Sam meet his teacher before school starts?
LEVEL B	How Else? by Sam's visting the classroom before school starts in the fall	How? by Sam's mother simulating kindergarten routines at home, such as snack, bathroom, and reading time	How Else? by Sam meeting his teacher before school starts in the fall
	4 ● New Problem Statement IWWM Sam's mother post Sam's daily home routine schedule?	5 ● New Problem Statement IWWM Sam's mother set up a home schedule that includes a snack and painting and reading time?	6 ● New Problem Statement IWWM Sam's mother develop a home schedule of "special" responsibilities like those at school?

(continued)

"Ladder of Abstraction"/"Highlighting" Part 1 (Continued)

L E V E L C	How Else? by eliciting Sam's help in planning the home schedule	How? by creating a picture-board schedule from which Sam removes the picture after completing the activity	How Else? by eliciting Sam's teacher's help in planning the home schedule
	7 New Problem Statement IWWM Sam's mother elicit Sam's help in planning the home schedule?	8 New Problem Statement IWWM Sam's mother develop a picture board that Sam can use to help him sequence his daily activities at home?	9 New Problem Statement IWWM Sam's mother elicit Sam's teacher's ideas for what to include in the home schedule?

FIELD ORGANIZER

"Highlighting" Part 2

Wish Statement: *WIBGI Sam enjoyed kindergarten?*

Area I: Hits	Central Theme
IWWM . . .	
16. Principal help Sam transition from home into his new kindergarten classroom?	change
17. Sam follow the daily routines in his classroom?	school routine
18. High school student help Sam during his day in school?	school routine
19. Sam's mother design an "art gallery" at home to display Sam's school drawings and art projects?	play school at home
20. Sam's teacher redirect Sam to participate in the "activity of the moment?"	change
21. Sam's teacher build on Sam's successes to encourage him to participate in the classroom routines?	school routine
22. Sam learn to anticipate change in his routine during the day?	change
23. Sam learn to plan for change when change is about to occur?	change
24. Sam's mother post Sam's daily home routine schedule?	school routine
25. Sam's mother develop a home schedule of "special" responsibilities, like those at school?	school routine
26. Sam's mother elicit Sam's help in planning the home schedule?	school routine
27. Sam's mother elicit Sam's teacher's ideas for what to include in the home schedule?	play school at home
Area II: Hot Spots Labels	
4. School routine	
5. Play school at home	
6. Change	

FIELD ORGANIZER

"Highlighting" Part 3

Area I: Hot Spots **Hot Spot I Labeled: *Handling change***
IWWM . . .
16. Principal help Sam transition from home into his new kindergarten classroom?
20. Sam's teacher redirect to participate in the "activity of the moment"?
22. Sam learn to anticipate change in his routine during the day?
23. Sam learn to plan for change when change is about to occur?
Labeled: *Play school at home*
IWWM . . .
19. Sam's mother design an "art gallery" at home to display Sam's school drawings and art projects?
27. Sam's mother elicit Sam's teacher's ideas for what to include in the home schedule?
Hot Spot III Labeled: *School routine*
IWWM . . .
17. Sam follow the daily routines in his classroom?
18. High school student help Sam during his day in school?
21. Sam's teacher build on Sam's successes to encourage him to participate in the classroom routines?
24. Sam's mother post Sam's daily home routine schedule?
25. Sam's mother develop a home schedule of "special" responsibilities, like those at school?
26. Sam's mother elicit Sam's help in planning the home schedule?
Area II: Restatements
Hot Spot II: IWWM kindergarten routines be used at home in a fun way to prepare Sam for school?
Hot Spot III: IWWM the adults in Sam's life help Sam adjust to his school and home routines?

FIELD ORGANIZER

"What If . . . ? Question Series"

A "What if . . .	B Worst- and Best-Case Scenario
3. **What if** routines at school are reinforced at home?	*Worst-Case Scenario* Sam becomes frustrated at school with routines that are now imposed on him at home. *Best-Case Scenario* Sam gains comfort from the constancy provided in his environment. The sameness of the routines at home and school help Sam cope with the school environment.
4. **What if** a notebook system is used to communicate between school and home?	*Worst-Case Scenario* Sam's parents or his teacher find communicating in the notebook a chore. *Best-Case Scenario* Sam's parents and teacher appreciate the insight they derive from the brief, daily two-way communication. A simple charting system could be devised with a couple of items that the teacher and parents could check off (or direct Sam's buddy to check off) as an alternate to writing.

Appendix B: Blank Field Organizers

"Watch for Cues and Look for Patterns"
"PACC" Part 1: Performance Areas
"PACC" Part 2: Performance Components
"PACC" Part 3: Performance Contexts
"Problem Ownership Checklist"
"Stop, Drop, and Listen"
"What Paradigm Is Operating?"
"Consider Other Viewpoints"
"Well-Structured vs. Ill-Structured Problem Checklist"
"Head and Shoulders Test" (for Wish Statement)
"WIBGI . . . ?"/"Highlighting"
"Highlighting" Part 3
"5 Ws & and H"/"5 Ws and an H else"/"Highlighting" Part 1
"Storytelling"
"IWWM . . . Who–Does–What?"/"Highlighting" Part 1
"Substitution"/"Highlighting" Part 1
"Ladder of Abstraction"/"Highlighting" Part 1
"Head and Shoulders Test" (for Problem Statement)
"Highlighting" Part 2
"Highlighting" Part 3
"Brainstorming"
"CAMPERS"

"Force Fit"
"Attribute Listing"
"Highlighting" Part 1
"Will It . . . ?"
"TRACS"
"Making an Idea More Acceptable"
"In-tuit"
"AL-O"
"Evaluation Matrix"
"Paired Comparison Analysis"
"Potential Sources of Support and Resistance"
"Check the Mindset"
"Generating Potential Actions"
"LIST"
"Plan for Action"
"What's Next? Question Series"
"If–Then"
"What If . . . ? Question Series"
"Think Positive"
"Action Plan Adoption Checklist"
"Preparing to Seek Feedback"
"Flow Checklist"

Part I: Cues

Story Paragraph #	A Cue	B What might this cue mean?
1		
2		
3		
4		
5		
6		
7		
8		

Part II: Patterns

Story Paragraph #	Patterns that emerged from cues found in the story

Performance Area	Story Paragraph #	Story Element
A. Activities of daily living		
1. Grooming		
2. Oral hygiene		
3. Bathing/showering		
4. Toilet hygiene		
5. Personal device care		
6. Dressing		
7. Feeding and eating		
8. Medication routine		
9. Health maintenance		
10. Socialization		
11. Functional communication		
12. Functional mobility		
13. Community mobility		
14. Emergency response		
15. Sexual expression		
B. Work and productive activities		
1. Home management		
a. Clothing care		
b. Cleaning		
c. Meal preparation and cleanup		
d. Shopping		
e. Money management		
f. Household maintenance		
g. Safety procedures		
2. Care of others		
3. Educational activities		
4. Vocational activities		
a. Vocational exploration		
b. Job acquisition		
c. Work or job performance		

(continued)

"PACC" Part 1: Performance Areas (Continued)

Performance Area	Story Paragraph #	Story Element

d. Retirement planning
    e. Volunteer participation
 	
C. Play and leisure
   1. Play and leisure exploration
   2. Play and leisure performance		

"PACC" Part 2: Performance Components

Performance Component	Story Paragraph #	Story Element
A. Sensorimotor component		
1. Sensory		
a. Sensory awareness		
b. Sensory processing		
(1) Tactile		
(2) Proprioceptive		
(3) Vestibular		
(4) Visual		
(5) Auditory		
(6) Gustatory		
(7) Olfactory		
c. Perceptual processing		
(1) Stereognosis		
(2) Kinesthesia		
(3) Pain response		
(4) Body scheme		
(5 Right-left discrimination		
(6) Form constancy		
(7) Position in space		
(8) Visual closure		
(9) Figure ground		
(10) Depth perception		
(11) Spatial relations		
(12) Topographical orientation		
2. Neuromusculoskeletal		
a. Reflex		
b. Range of motion		
c. Muscle tone		
d. Strength		
e. Endurance		

(continued)

"PACC" Part 2: Performance Components (Continued)

Performance Component	Story Paragraph #	Story Element
f. Postural control		
g. Postural alignment		
h. Soft tissue integrity		
3. Motor		
a. Gross coordination		
b. Crossing midline		
c. Laterality		
d. Bilateral integration		
e Motor control		
f. Praxis		
g. Fine coordination/ dexterity		
h. Visual-motor integration		
i. Oral-motor control		
B. Cognitive integration and cognitive components		
1. Level of arousal		
2. Orientation		
3. Recognition		
4. Attention span		
5. Initiation of activity		
6. Termination of activity		
7. Memory		
8. Sequencing		
9. Categorization		
10. Concept formation		
11. Spatial operations		
12. Problem solving		
13. Learning		
14. Generalization		
C. Psychosocial skills		
1. Psychological		
a. Values		
b. Interests		
c. Self-concept		

"PACC" Part 2: Performance Components (Continued)

Performance Component	Story Paragraph #	Story Element
2. Social		
a. Role performance		
b. Social conduct		
c. Interpersonal skills		
d. Self-expression		
3. Self-management		
a. Coping skills		
b Time management		
c. Self-control		

Performance Context	Story Paragraph #	Story Element

A. Temporal aspects
   1. Chronological
   2. Developmental
   3. Life cycle
   4. Disability status
B. Environment
   1. Physical
   2. Social
   3. Cultural		

1. Is the person **aware that there is a gap** between what is and what should be?
Yes ☐   No ☐

2. Is the person **able to measure the gap?**   Yes ☐   No ☐

3. Does the person **need to solve the problem?**   Yes ☐   No ☐

4. Does the person **have access to the resources** needed to solve the problem?
Yes ☐   No ☐

"Stop, Drop, and Listen"

Story Paragraph #	A WHO said WHAT?	B Assumption to Be Dropped	C Behind these words or actions the person is saying ...

FIELD ORGANIZER

"What Paradigm Is Operating?"

Story Paragraph #	A Record a behavior to be analyzed.	B Identify the operating paradigm that could explain the behavior described in column A.

"Consider Other Viewpoints"

	A It is (was) _____'s (record name of person) perspective that . . .	**B** On the other hand _____ (record name of person) perceives that perhaps . . .
Source	(Record target view.)	(Record other person's perspective.)

FIELD ORGANIZER

"Well-Structured vs. Ill-Structured Problem Checklist"

Well-Structured Problem	Ill-Structured Problem
1. ☐ sufficient information	☐ insufficient information
2. ☐ predictable outcome(s)	☐ unpredictable outcome(s)
3. ☐ ready-made solution(s)	☐ custom-made solution(s)

FIELD ORGANIZER

"Head and Shoulders Test"

Ask the client:

"Does one wish statement in the group stand **head and shoulders** above the rest?"

If the client is very interested in pursuing one of the statements or a combination of statements at this point, confirm the wish statement with the client and write it on the line below.

WIBGI _____ ?

Proceed to Data Finding using this wish statement.

"WIBGI . . . ?"/"Highlighting"

Generate		Focus		
	Part 1:	**Part 2: Clustering Hits into Hot Spots**		
Wouldn't it be great if . . .	**Hits**	**A**	**B**	**C**
1.				
2.				
3.				
4.				
5.				
6.				
7.				
8.				
9.				
10.				
11.				
12.				
13.				
14.				
15.				

Area I: Wish Statements

Hot Spots from Using _____ *to Cluster Hits*

Cluster One Labeled:

WIBGI . . .

Cluster Two Labeled:

WIBGI . . .

Cluster Three Labeled:

WIBGI . . .

Area II: Restatements

Hot Spot One: WIBGI

Hot Spot Two: WIBGI

Hot Spot Three: WIBGI

Wish Statement: *WIBGI* _____?

A Generate	B Hits	C Generate	D Hits
Who might be involved in the opportunity?		**Who *else* might be involved in the opportunity?**	
1.		1.	
2.		2.	
3.		3.	
4.		4.	
5.		5.	
6.		6.	
7.		7.	
8.		8.	
9.		9.	
10.		10.	
What is involved in the opportunity?		**What *else* is involved in the opportunity?**	
1.		1.	
2.		2.	
3.		3.	
4.		4.	
5.		5.	
6.		6.	
7.		7.	
8.		8.	
9.		9.	
10.		10.	
Where might opportunities occur to work on the wish?		**Where *else* might opportunities occur to work on the wish?**	
1.		1.	
2.		2.	
3.		3.	

(continued)

A *Generate*	B *Hits*	C *Generate*	D *Hits*
Where might opportunities occur to work on the wish?		**Where *else* might opportunities occur to work on the wish?**	
4.		4.	
5.		5.	
6.		6.	
7.		7.	
8.		8.	
9.		9.	
10.		10.	
When might there be an opportunity to work on the wish?		**When *else* might there be an opportunity to work on the wish?**	
1.		1.	
2.		2.	
3.		3.	
4.		4.	
5.		5.	
6.		6.	
7.		7.	
8.		8.	
9.		9.	
10.		10.	
Why is it important to look for opportunities in this area?		**Why *else* is it important to look for opportunities in this area?**	
1.		1.	
2.		2.	
3.		3.	
4.		4.	
5.		5.	
6.		6.	
7.		7.	
8.		8.	

"5 Ws & an H"/ "5 Ws & an H else"/ "Highlighting" Part 1 (Continued)

A *Generate*	B *Hits*	C *Generate*	D *Hits*
Why is it important to look for opportunities in this area?		**Why *else* is it important to look for opportunities in this area?**	
9.		9.	
10.		10.	
How will you make this wish a reality?		**How *else* will you make this wish a reality?**	
1.		1.	
2.		2.	
3.		3.	
4.		4.	
5.		5.	
6.		6.	
7.		7.	
8.		8.	
9.		9.	
10.		10.	

FIELD ORGANIZER

"Storytelling"

Part A

Wish Statement: _____ . . .

1. _____
   _____
   _____

   ↓

2. _____
   _____
   _____

   ↓

3. _____
   _____
   _____

   ↓

4. _____
   _____
   _____

   ↓

5. _____
   _____
   _____

   ↓

6. _____
   _____
   _____

Part B: Themes from the Story

1. _____

2. _____

3. _____

4. _____

5. _____

6.

Opportunity Finding Statement: *WIBGI* _____ . . .

Generate				Focus
IWWM . . . ?				
Who?	**Does?**	**What?**		**Hits**
Ex.: Teacher	decrease	the absenteeism in the class during the "cold season"?		
1.				
2.				
3.				
4.				
5.				
6.				
7.				
8.				
9.				
10.				
11.				
12.				
13.				
14.				

Part A

Circle those parts of the sentence for which you wish to find substitutions.

Problem Statement: IWWM _____?

IWWM . . .

	Who?	Does?	What?
1.			
2.			
3.			
4.			
5.			
6.			
7.			
8.			
9.			
10.			

Part B

		Hits
1.	IWWM	
2.	IWWM	
3.	WWM	
4	IWWM	
5.	IWWM	
6.	IWWM	
7.	IWWM	
8.	IWWM	
9.	IWWM	
10.	IWWM	

FIELD ORGANIZER

"Ladder of Abstraction"/ "Highlighting" Part 1

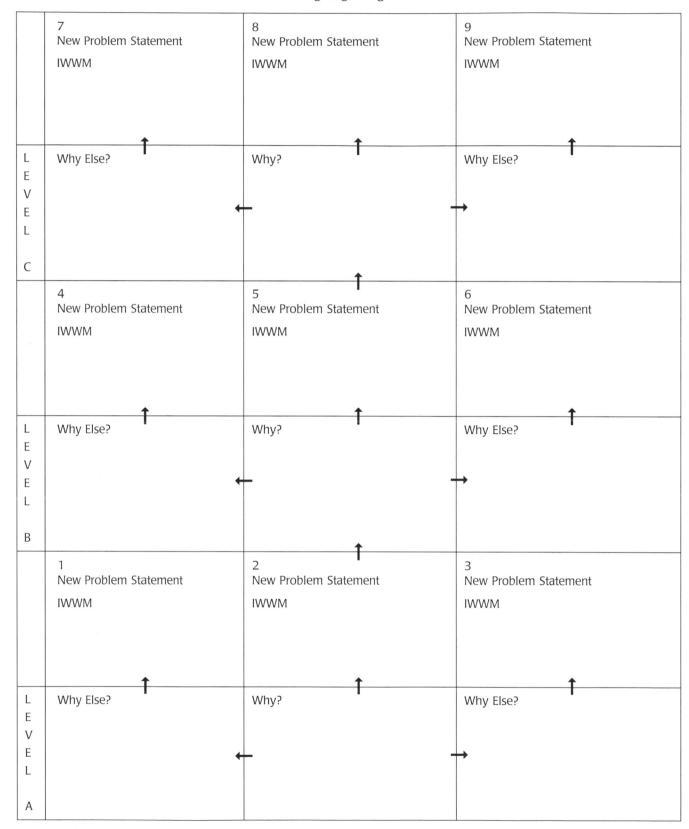

	7 New Problem Statement IWWM	**8** New Problem Statement IWWM	**9** New Problem Statement IWWM
L E V E L C	Why Else?	Why?	Why Else?
	4 New Problem Statement IWWM	**5** New Problem Statement IWWM	**6** New Problem Statement IWWM
L E V E L B	Why Else?	Why?	Why Else?
	1 New Problem Statement IWWM	**2** New Problem Statement IWWM	**3** New Problem Statement IWWM
L E V E L A	Why Else?	Why?	Why Else?

"Ladder of Abstraction"/ "Highlighting" Part 1 (Continued)

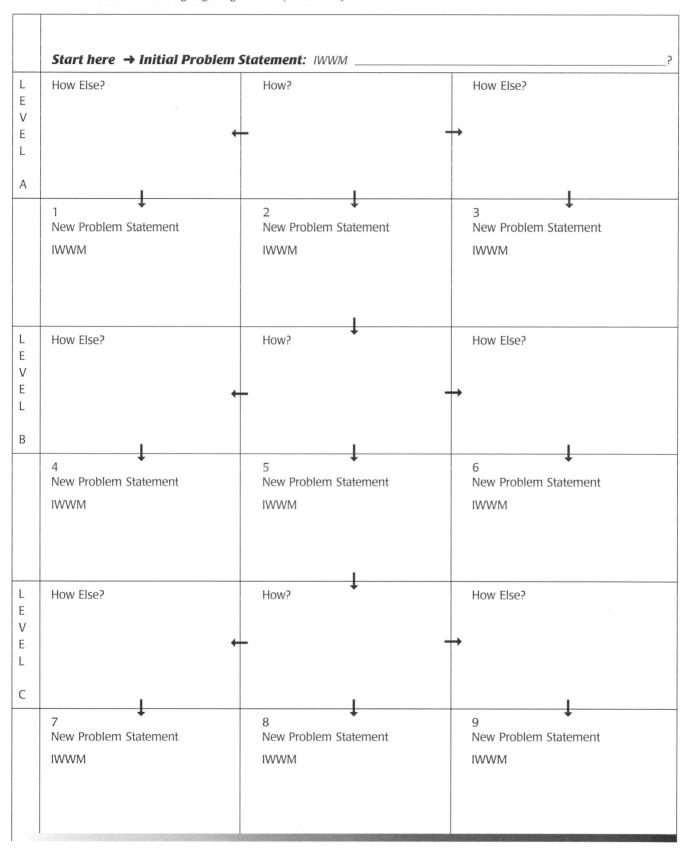

FIELD ORGANIZER

"Head and Shoulders Test"

Ask the client:

"Does one problem statement in the group stand **head and shoulders** over the rest?"

If the client is very interested in pursuing one of the statements or a combination of statements at this point, confirm the problem statement with the client and write it on the line below.

IWWM _____?

Proceed to Idea Finding using this problem statement.

Opportunity Finding Statement: *WIBGI* _____ ?

Part A

"Hits"	Central Theme
IWWM . . .	
1.	
2.	
3.	
4.	
5.	
6.	
7.	
8.	
9.	
10.	
11.	
12.	
13.	
14.	
15.	
16.	
17.	
18.	
19.	
20.	

Part B

Hot Spots Labels

1. _____   4. _____
2. _____   5. _____
3. _____   6. _____

Opportunity Finding Statement: WIBGI ————————————————————————?

Area I: Hot Spots

Hot Spot I Labeled:

IWWM . . .

_____
_____
_____
_____
_____
_____
_____

Hot Spot II Labeled:

IWWM . . .

_____
_____
_____
_____
_____
_____
_____

Hot Spot III Labeled:

IWWM . . .

_____
_____
_____
_____
_____
_____
_____

Part B Restatements

Hot Spot I IWWM
_____
Hot Spot II IWWM
_____
Hot Spot III IWWM
_____

FIELD ORGANIZER

"Brainstorming"

Problem Statement: IWWM _____ ?

A Idea	B Hits	C Idea	D Hits	E Idea	F Hits
1.		2.		3.	
4.		5.		6.	
7.		8.		9.	
10.		11.		12.	
13.		14.		15.	
16.		17.		18.	
19.		20.		21.	

Problem Statement: IWWM _____ ?

A Sample questions to develop flexibility in your thinking	B Responses to questions in column A	C Hits
What can I Combine?		
Can I combine units, purposes, ideas, steps, or different types of people, disciplines, or groups?		
How about a blend, or an assortment?		
What can I Adapt?		
Can I use existing materials, processes, or personnel to solve the problem?		
What can I use from a past experience?		
What can I Modify?		
How can a new twist be added to an obvious situation?		
How can I duplicate, exaggerate, condense, streamline?		
What can I Put to other uses?		
In what other contexts might what I choose work?		
What are some "out of the box" ways to use it?		
What can I Eliminate?		
Could fewer steps, materials, or people be involved?		
How can I make less be more?		
What can I Rearrange?		
What part of the process can be reversed?		
Can I interchange things or people?		
What can I Substitute?		
Who else might be recruited?		
What other ingredients, materials, processes, places, or approaches could be used?		

FIELD ORGANIZER
"Force Fit"

Problem Statement: IWWM _____ ?		
A **Random Input**	**B** **Force a Fit Between the Random Input and the Current Problem**	**C** **Hits**
1.	1. 2. 3. 4. 5. 6. 7. 8. 9. 10.	
2.	1. 2. 3. 4.	

(continued)

A **Random Input**	B **Force a Fit Between the Random Input and the Current Problem**	C **Hits**
	5.	
	6.	
	7.	
	8.	
	9.	
	10.	
3.	1.	
	2.	
	3.	
	4.	
	5.	
	6.	
	7.	
	8.	
	9.	
	10.	

"Attribute Listing"

Problem Statement: *IWWM* ———?

A Attribute	B Elaborate on the Attribute under consideration	C Hits
1.	1. 2. 3. 4. 5. 6. 7. 8. 9. 10.	
2.	1. 2. 3.	

(continued)

"Attribute Listing" (Continued)

A Attribute	B Elaborate on the Attribute under consideration	C Hits
	4. 5. 6. 7. 8. 9. 10.	
3.	1. 2. 3. 4. 5. 6. 7. 8. 9. 10.	

FIELD ORGANIZER

"Highlighting" Part 1

Problem Statement: *IWWM* —— ?

"Hits" Transfer

1.

2.

3.

4.

5.

6.

7.

8.

9.

10.

11.

12.

13.

14.

(continued)

"Highlighting" Part 1 (Continued)

"Hits" Transfer

15. _____

16. _____

17. _____

18. _____

19. _____

20. _____

21. _____

22. _____

23. _____

24. _____

25. _____

26. _____

27. _____

28. _____

29. _____

"Hits" Transfer

30.

31.

32.

FIELD ORGANIZER
"Will It . . . ?"

Idea: _____

_____

A Will it . . . ?	B Criteria
1.	
2.	
3.	
4.	
5.	
6.	
7.	
8.	
9.	
10.	

FIELD ORGANIZER

"TRACS"

A Option	B Criterion	C Consideration
1.	what _____ would be involved?	1. 2. 3.
2.	what _____ would be involved?	1. 2. 3.
3.	what _____ would be involved?	1. 2. 3.
4.	what _____ would be involved?	1. 2. 3.
5.	what _____ would be involved?	1. 2. 3.

A Idea to Be Improved	B Essential Criterion to Consider	C Possible Improvements
1.		a. b. c.
2.		a. b. c.
3.		a. b. c.
4.		a. b. c.

FIELD ORGANIZER

"In-tuit"

A Do I sense that this idea will help solve the problem?	B Yes	C No	D Rework
1.			
2.			
3.			
4.			
5.			
6.			
7.			
8.			
9.			
10.			

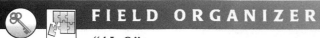

Idea: _____

_____

A Advantages	B Limitations	C How to Overcome a Limitation
1.	**Limitation:** *The issue becomes:* **How to**	a. b. c.

Idea: _____

_____

	Limitation: *The issue becomes:* **How to**	a. b. c.
2.		

Idea: _____

_____

	Limitation: *The issue becomes:* **How to**	a. b. c.
3.		

Options	Criteria					Rating Scale ☺ Favorable ☹ Unfavorable
1.						☺ = _____ ☹ = _____
2.						☺ = _____ ☹ = _____
3.						☺ = _____ ☹ = _____
4.						☺ = _____ ☹ = _____
5.						☺ = _____ ☹ = _____
6.						☺ = _____ ☹ = _____
7.						☺ = _____ ☹ = _____
8.						☺ = _____ ☹ = _____
9.						☺ = _____ ☹ = _____
10.						☺ = _____ ☹ = _____

FIELD ORGANIZER
"Paired Comparison Analysis"

Problem Statement: *IWWM* _____ ?

Section I: Options

A.

B.

C.

D.

E.

Section II: Option Comparison

Options	Choice	Options	Choice	Options	Choice	Options	Choice
A/B		A/C		A/D		A/E	
		B/C		B/D		B/E	
				C/D		C/E	
						D/E	

Section III: Totals

Total **A**	Total **B**	Total **C**	Total **D**	Total **E**	List Options in Priority Order
					1. 2. 3. 4. 5.

FIELD ORGANIZER

"Potential Sources of Support and Resistance"

Proposed idea: _____

_____

A 5 Ws & an H	B Potential Sources of Support	C Potential Sources of Resistance
1. **WHO** might . . .	*contribute time and resources to move the plan forward?*	*limit or restrict the forward movement of the plan?*
2. **WHAT** things, objects, or activities might be . . .	*helpful?*	*an impediment?*
3. **WHERE** are . . .	*locations where the plan can be accomplished?*	*locations that block progress of the plan?*
4. **WHEN** might there be . . .	*an appropriate time to work on the plan (specify hours, day, week, month)?*	*inappropriate time to work on the plan?*
5. **WHY** might the plan be . . .	*supported?*	*resisted?*
6. **HOW** might I anticipate . . .	*strengths in the plan?*	*weaknesses in the plan?*

Resistance to change	Readiness for change
1. ○ **Conforming**	**Willing to take risks** ○
Prefers to act according to the standard or norm.	*Willing to expose self to chance; seeks out opportunities that may move the action plan forward.*
2. ○ **Rigid**	**Flexible** ○
Unyielding and consequently unable to change the course of action or switch gears readily.	*Unable to change the course of action (switch gears) whenever it is necessary to meet the demands of the situation.*
3. ○ **Narrow-minded**	**Open-minded** ○
Unreceptive to new ideas or strategies. Prefers to use routine ideas and activities that are familiar.	*Acknowledges that there are few absolutes in therapy. Receptive to new ideas or strategies. Open to new possibilities.*
4. ○ **Needing to know**	**Tolerant of ambiguity** ○
Needs to have discrete answers.	*Feels comfortable waiting for the "better" answer to emerge.*
5. ○ **Self-centered**	**Empathetic** ○
Values personal needs and perspectives over the needs of others.	*Identifies with the feelings or thoughts of others.*

"Generating Potential Actions"

Proposed plan: _____

A **Potential Actions That Could Move the Plan Forward**	B **Potential Sources of Resistance to the Action**
1.	
2.	
3.	
4.	
5.	
6.	
7.	
8.	
9.	
10.	
11.	
12.	
13.	

(continued)

"Generating Potential Actions" (Continued)

A **Potential Actions That Could Move the Plan Forward**	B **Potential Sources of Resistance to the Action**
14.	
15.	
16.	
17.	
18.	

FIELD ORGANIZER
"LIST"

Long-Term Actions to Take Between _____

1. _____

2. _____

3. _____

4. _____

5. _____

6. _____

7. _____

8. _____

9. _____

Intermediate Actions to Take Between _____

1. _____

2. _____

3. _____

4. _____

5. _____

6. _____

7. _____

(continued)

Intermediate Actions to Take Between _____

8. _____

9. _____

Short-Term Actions to Take Within _____

1. _____

2. _____

3. _____

4. _____

5. _____

6. _____

7. _____

8. _____

9. _____

Long-Term Actions

Long-Term Action #1

1. **WHAT** is the **action** desired? _____

   _____

2. **WHO** will do the **action**? _____

   _____

3. **WHEN** will the **action** start? _____ finish? _____

4. **WHERE** will the **action** take place? _____

   _____

5. **WHY** is the **action** important? _____

   _____

6. **HOW** will you know the **action** was successful? _____

   _____

Long-Term Action #2

1. **WHAT** is the **action** desired? _____

   _____

2. **WHO** will do the **action**? _____

   _____

3. **WHEN** will the **action** start? _____ finish? _____

4. **WHERE** will the **action** take place? _____

   _____

5. **WHY** is the **action** important? _____

   _____

6. **HOW** will you know the **action** was successful? _____

   _____

(continued)

Long-Term Action #3

1. **WHAT** is the **action** desired? _____

   _____

2. **WHO** will do the **action**? _____

   _____

3. **WHEN** will the **action** start? _____ finish? _____

4. **WHERE** will the **action** take place? _____

   _____

5. **WHY** is the **action** important? _____

   _____

6. **HOW** will you know the **action** was successful? _____

   _____

Intermediate Actions

Intermediate Action #1

1. **WHAT** is the **action** desired? _____

   _____

2. **WHO** will do the **action**? _____

   _____

3. **WHEN** will the **action** start? _____ finish? _____

4. **WHERE** will the **action** take place? _____

   _____

5. **WHY** is the **action** important? _____

   _____

6. **HOW** will you know the **action** was successful? _____

   _____

Intermediate Action #2

1. **WHAT** is the **action** desired? _____

   _____

2. **WHO** will do the **action**? _____

   _____

3. **WHEN** will the **action** start? _____ finish? _____

4. **WHERE** will the **action** take place? _____

   _____

5. **WHY** is the **action** important? _____

   _____

6. **HOW** will you know the **action** was successful? _____

   _____

Intermediate Action #3

1. **WHAT** is the **action** desired? _____

   _____

2. **WHO** will do the **action**? _____

   _____

3. **WHEN** will the **action** start? _____ finish? _____

4. **WHERE** will the **action** take place? _____

   _____

5. **WHY** is the **action** important? _____

   _____

6. **HOW** will you know the **action** was successful? _____

   _____

(continued)

Short-Term Actions

Short-Term Action #1

1. **WHAT** is the **action** desired? _____

_____

2. **WHO** will do the **action**? _____

_____

3. **WHEN** will the **action** start? _____ finish? _____

4. **WHERE** will the **action** take place? _____

_____

5. **WHY** is the **action** important? _____

_____

6. **HOW** will you know the **action** was successful? _____

_____

Short-Term Action #2

1. **WHAT** is the **action** desired? _____

_____

2. **WHO** will do the **action**? _____

_____

3. **WHEN** will the **action** start? _____ finish? _____

4. **WHERE** will the **action** take place? _____

_____

5. **WHY** is the **action** important? _____

_____

6. **HOW** will you know the **action** was successful? _____

_____

"Plan for Action" *(Continued)*

Short-Term Action #3

1. **WHAT** is the **action** desired? _____

   _____

2. **WHO** will do the **action**? _____

   _____

3. **WHEN** will the **action** start? _____ finish? _____

4. **WHERE** will the **action** take place? _____

   _____

5. **WHY** is the **action** important? _____

   _____

6. **HOW** will you know the **action** was successful? _____

   _____

A *Describe <u>one part</u> of the therapy plan.*	B *Ask, "What's next?"*	C *Respond to the question "What's next?"*
1.	"What's next?"	
2.	"What's next?"	
3.	"What's next?"	
4.	"What's next?"	
5.	"What's next?"	
6.	"What's next?"	

FIELD ORGANIZER
"If–Then"

A If . . .	B Then . . .
1. **IF**	**THEN**
2. **IF**	**THEN**
3. **IF**	**THEN**
4. **IF**	**THEN**
5. **IF**	**THEN**
6. **IF**	**THEN**

FIELD ORGANIZER

"What If . . . ? Question Series"

A What if . . .	B Worst- and Best-Case Scenario
1. **What if**	*Worst-Case Scenario* *Best-Case Scenario*
2. **What if**	*Worst-Case Scenario* *Best-Case Scenario*
3. **What if**	*Worst-Case Scenario* *Best-Case Scenario*

FIELD ORGANIZER

"Think Positive"

A I can't . . .	B In what ways might . . . ?
1.	a. **IWWM** b. **IWWM**
2.	a. **IWWM** b. **IWWM**

FIELD ORGANIZER

"Action Plan Adoption Checklist"

A Questions	B Responses
Advantage	
1. What are the benefits to the client and the client's support group for accepting the plan?	
2. How is this action plan better than previously tried actions?	
Compatibility	
1. In what ways is the plan consistent with the client's paradigm (values, experiences, needs)?	
2. Who among the client's support group will agree with the plan?	
Complexity	
1. In what ways can the plan be clearly communicated to others?	
2. In what ways can the plan be simplified?	
Trialability	
1. In what ways can the plan be first implemented on a trial basis?	
2. In what ways can the plan be modified and still accomplish the goal?	
Observability	
1. In what ways are the outcomes of the plan visible to all involved with the plan?	
2. In what ways can the outcomes be made easy for others to see and understand?	

A 5 Ws & an H Question	B Responses to the 5 Ws & an H Question
1. **Who** might provide feedback?	
2. **What** feedback will I seek?	
3. **When and where** are the best times to seek feedback?	
4. **How** might I acquire the feedback?	
5. **Why** do I want to acquire the feedback?	

FIELD ORGANIZER

"Flow Checklist"

A **Flow Criteria**	B **Indication That Flow Criteria Was Present**
1. Possessed the *appropriate skills* to perform the activity	
2. Indicated a sense of the *potential of completion* (goal directed) of the activity.	
3. Was *able to concentrate* on activity.	
4. Evidence of *effortless involvement* while participating in activity.	
5. Experienced a *sense of control* while participating in activity.	
6. Indication of *loss of self* (became absorbed) while performing activity.	
7. Indication that the *sense of time was altered* while participating in activity.	

Glossary

Acceptance Finding. The CPS stage in which the plan of action for the therapy expedition is defined.

Affirmative Judgment. The constructive analysis applied to all alternatives before a decision is made; a principle of the critical, evaluative, or Focusing Phase of each stage of CPS.

"a-ha!" experience. The sudden emergence of a great idea that seems to jump into one's head after a period of relative mental inactivity, referred to as incubation.

AOTA. American Occupational Therapists Association.

attributes. The characteristics of a situation; knowledge of these characteristics may lead to possibilities for recombining them to create a different perception of the situation.

brainstorming. A group technique developed by Alex Osborn for generating options; among the guidelines for the Generating Phase of each stage of CPS. This technique requires that the participants defer judgment, strive for quantity, free wheel, and hitchhike one idea on another.

CAMPERS. Acronym for the following idea-generating concepts introduced by Alex Osborn in *Applied Imagination* (1963): combine, adapt, modify, put to other uses, eliminate, reverse, substitute.

client. The person or persons to whom the therapy guide relates during the therapy expedition. In this field book, "client" is the person who was referred for therapy services and that person's adult family member or primary caregiver with whom the therapy guide discusses the person's therapy schedule, program, goals, and progress and discharge. In many cases the client is the child and the child's parent or parents.

clustering. The act of grouping similar statements, thoughts, or ideas that have attributes in common.

comfort zone. A psychological area that represents the realm of the familiar, where one feels at ease to think and act freely without threat of failure or rejection; the "mental space" in which one feels a sense of comfort, positive energy, and a low level (if any) of psychological turbulence or fear. Therapy guides are risk-takers who venture out of their comfort zones when making decisions.

CPS component. An aspect of the problem solving model that includes one or more stages of the six-stage CPS model. The three major CPS components are Get Ready to understand the problem, Get Set to find a solution, and Go Forward with an action plan. (These are adapted from Isaksen, Treffinger, and Dorval, who identified the components as Understanding the Problem, Generating Ideas, and Planning for Action.)

CPS stage. Any of the six elements of the CPS model (Opportunity Finding, Data Finding, Problem Finding, Idea Finding, Solution Finding, and Acceptance Finding) that are embedded in each CPS component.

Creative Problem Solving model (CPS). A nonsequential, contextual organizing framework for solving ill-structured problems. The model consists of three components and six stages; each stage contains a generative (Generating) and an evaluative (Focusing) phase. The stages are descriptive and may be used in any order. The order depends on the context in which the elements of the problem emerge.

cues. A hint or intimation of information that is a piece of a greater whole of a story or "picture."

Data Finding. The stage of CPS in which the problem solvers gather all information to be considered to help understand and define the problem; data includes need-to-know, want-to-know, and nice-to-know information, feelings, impressions, and observations.

Deferred Judgment. A principle of CPS used in the Generating Phase of each stage, an adaptation of the Divergent Phase described by Isaksen, Treffinger, and Dorval; focuses on refraining from evaluating with criticism or praise while generating as many options as possible.

field book. A workbook with ideas to apply in the field of occupational therapy practice; the thinking strategies in this field book are presented in Field Organizers designed to be used in the field of occupational therapy wherever the practitioner needs to solve ill-structured problems.

Field Organizer. A form designed for use in the field of occupational therapy that serves as an explicit prompt to strategically monitor specific thinking processes. There is one Field Organizer for every Thinking Key.

Focusing Phase. The evaluative phase of each stage of CPS, an adaptation of the Convergent Phase described by Isaksen, Treffinger, and Dorval. Using Affirmative Judgment is a principle of this phase.

free wheel. To allow an unrestrained flow of ideas, including those that initially appear to be silly or wild; an important part of the Generating Phase of each stage of CPS.

Generating Phase. The expansive phase of each stage of CPS, an adaptation of the Divergent Phase described by Isaksen, Treffinger, and Dorval. Using divergent thinking, the problem solver concentrates on producing a quantity of options in response to open-ended questions such as "Wouldn't it be great if . . . ?" (Opportunity Finding) and "In what ways might . . . ?" (Idea Finding). Using Deferred Judgment is a principle of this phase.

highlighting. An evaluative thinking technique; used during the Focusing Phase of each stage of CPS to compress the options under consideration. After the "Hits" are identified, relationships are identified; clusters of Hits then are highlighted.

hitchhike ideas. To allow one idea to trigger another, similar thought.

Hits. Options selected by the client and the therapy guide as having the most potential for consideration in the development of a solution to the problem both are trying to solve for the client.

Idea Finding. The stage of CPS in which the client and the therapy guide generate many ideas related to a specific problem statement; the ideas that hold the most promise are refined and developed and may become part of the final action plan.

ill-structured problem. A problem that lacks adequate information, has an undetermined outcome, and requires a custom-made solution.

incubation. The phenomenon that occurs when one continues to percolate ideas subconsciously after the conscious thinking about the challenge or concern has passed for the moment.

itinerary. The detailed plan for a journey or expedition; in this field book, the plan for a therapy expedition.

Mind Map. A graphic representation of one's thoughts that taps into the whole brain; contains a focus in the center of the page from which ideas flow freely without judgment, with key words representing ideas. The ideas are connected or "webbed" to the central idea through lines. Mindmapping is a registered trademark belonging to Tony Buzan.

occupational therapy process. A seven-stage process including referral, assessment, goal setting, treatment planning, treatment implementation, discharge planning, and follow-up.

Opportunity Finding. The stage of CPS in which the general goals or "wish" statements are developed in the Generating Phase and created for further consideration in the Focusing Phase, a modification of Mess-Finding, described by Isaksen, Treffinger, and Dorval. The opportunity statement that begins with the phrase "Wouldn't it be great if" is a broad area of concern related to an ill-structured problem.

OT practitioner. An occupational therapist or occupational therapy assistant who delivers occupational therapy services; referred to in this field book as the therapy guide, who facilitates the therapy expedition.

out-of-the-box thinking. Off-the-wall, free-wheeling thinking associated with unique, creative thoughts that are not bound by conventional rules and regulations.

paradigm. An information filter through which one sees and defines what is real to one; one's "world view" or rules by which one plays the "game of life." What may be obvious to one person may be invisible to someone with a different paradigm. Creative thinking challenges the rules of the paradigm.

paradigm shift. A change to a new game or set or rules; one of the keys to innovative behaviors, frequently instigated by trends.

pattern. A definitive cluster of behaviors that characterize the performance of an individual or a group of individuals within a specific context.

Performance Areas. Broadly defined human activities that are part of daily life. As defined by the AOTA Uniform Terminology, the Performance Areas are activities of daily living, work and productive activities, and play and leisure.

Performance Components. Fundamental human abilities that all individuals demonstrate when they successfully engage in the Performance Areas. As defined by the AOTA Uniform Terminology, the Performance Components are sensorimotor, cognitive integration, and cognitive and psychosocial skills.

Performance Contexts. The situations in which an individual performs, which profoundly influence the quality of one's performance. As defined by the AOTA Uniform Terminology, the Performance Contexts are divided into two categories: temporal aspects and environment.

Problem Finding. The stage of CPS in which the problem solver generates a variety of ways to state the problem and defines the problem statement.

ready-made solution. A predetermined solution to a well-structured problem

Reflective Journal Entry. An opportunity for the learner to anchor new concepts by explicitly pondering, reflecting, and writing about personal life experiences and perceptions that correspond to content in this field book.

reframing the problem. Reorganizing one's thinking about a situation in such a way that one creates a different perspective of the situation; shifting one's paradigm.

Solution Finding. The stage of CPS in which ideas are selected after being evaluated against set criteria.

therapeutic process and therapy-related process. All activities related to the occupational therapy process; the systematic series of therapist-client relationships or actions basic to all therapy interactions.

therapy expedition. In this field book, the client's "journey" facilitated by the occupational therapy practitioners, the therapy guide.

therapy guide. The occupational therapy practitioner who directs the client's therapy expedition.

Thinking Key. A thinking strategy.

thinking strategy. A mental system that directs the way one thinks by using a systematic framework to conceptualize thought patterns; referred to in this field book as a Thinking Key.

TRACS. Acronym for time, resources, acceptance of options, costs, and space; an adaptation of CARTS, categories of criteria described by Isaksen, Treffinger, and Dorval. TRACS keeps a therapy guide on track when generating criteria during the Solution Finding stage.

Uniform Terminology. Developed by AOTA to provide a generic outline of the domains of concern in occupational therapy.

visionizing. A term coined by Sidney Parnes, from "vision" and "actualizing" to describe the visual transformation that occurs when one proactively looks for opportunities, relationships, and implications in a challenging situation to find the necessary steps that translate the dream into a reality.

well-structured problem. A problem that can be solved with routine procedures because it has sufficient information and a predetermined outcome with ready-made solutions.

Bibliography

Adizes, I. *Corporate Lifecycles: How and Why Corporations Grow and Die and What to Do About It*. New York: Prentice Hall, 1988.

Amabile, T. M. *Growing Up Creative: Nurturing a Lifetime of Creativity*. Buffalo, N.Y.: The Creative Educational Foundation, 1989.

Anderson-Inman, L., and L. Zeitz. "Computer-Based Concept Mapping: Active Studying for Active Learners." *The Computing Teacher*, August–September 1993, 6–10.

AOTA. "Uniform Terminology for Occupational Therapy—Third Edition." *American Journal of Occupational Therapy* 48, no. 11 (1994): 1047–54.

Armstrong, T. *Seven Kinds of Smart: Identifying and Developing Your Many Intelligences*. New York: Plume, 1993.

Ayres, A. J. *Sensory Integration and the Child*. Los Angeles: Western Psychological Services, 1979.

Barker, J. *Paradigms: The Business of Discovering the Future*. New York: Harper Business, 1993.

Barrell, J. "Like an Incredibly Hard Algebra Problem: Teaching for Metacognition." In A. Costa, J. Bellanca, and R. Fogarty, eds., *If Minds Matter: A Foreword to the Future*, 1:257–66. Palatine, Ill.: Skylight, 1992.

Bazerman, M. *Judgment in Managerial Decision Making*. 3d ed. New York: John Wiley & Sons, 1994.

Black, R. A. *Broken Crayons: Break Your Crayons and Draw Outside the Lines*. Dubuque, Iowa: Kendall/Hunt, 1995.

Bobath, K. *A Neurophysiological Basis for the Treatment of Cerebral Palsy*. Suffolk, England: The Laverham Press, 1980.

Brenner, P. *From Novice to Expert: Excellence and Power in Clinical Nursing Practice*. Reading, Mass.: Addison-Wesley, 1984.

Burke, K. *How to Assess Thoughtful Outcomes*. Palatine, Ill.: IRI/Skylight, 1993.

Buzan, T. *Use Both Sides of Your Brain*. 3d ed. New York: Penguin Books, 1989.

Caine, G., R. Caine, and S. Crowell. *Mindshifts: A Brain-Based Process for Restructuring Schools and Renewing Education*. Tucson, Ariz.: Zephyr Press, 1994.

Caine, R. N., and G. Caine. *Making Connections: Teaching and the Human Brain*. New York: Addison-Wesley, 1994.

Cameron, J., and M. Bryan. *The Artist's Way: A Spiritual Path to Higher Creativity*. New York: G. P. Putnam's Sons, 1992.

Carnegie, D. *How to Win Friends and Influence People*. New York: Pocket Books, 1936.

Chapman, L. J., and J. G. Chapman. "Genesis of Popular but Erroneous Diagnostic Observations." *Journal of Abnormal Psychology* 72 (1967): 193–204.

Childre, D. L. *Freeze Frame*. Boulder Creek, Colo.: Planetary Publications, 1994.

Chopra, D. *Ageless Body, Timeless Mind*. New York: Harmony Books, 1993.

Clark, J. Edward. "The Search for a New Educational Paradigm." In A. Costa, J. Bellanca, and R. Fogarty, eds., *If Minds Matter: A Foreword to the Future*, 1:25–40. Palatine, Ill.: Skylight, 1992.

Cooper, R. K. *The Performance Edge*. Boston: Houghton Mifflin Company, 1991.

Costa, A., J. Bellanca, and R. Fogarty, eds. *If Minds Matter: A Foreword to the Future*. Palatine, Ill.: Skylight, 1992.

Covey, S. *The Seven Habits of Highly Effective People*. New York: Simon & Schuster, 1989.

———. *First Things First*. New York: Simon & Schuster, 1994.

Creighton, C., M. Dikers, N. Bennett, and K. Brown. "Reasoning and the Art of Therapy for Spinal Cord Injury." *American Journal of Occupational Therapy* 49, no. 4 (1995): 311–17.

Creton, M., and O. Davies. *The American Renaissance*. New York: St. Martin's Press, 1989.

Csikszentmihalyi, M. *Creativity: Flow and the Psychology of Discovery and Invention*. New York: HarperCollins, 1996.

———. *Flow: The Psychology of Optimal Experience*. New York: HarperCollins, 1991.

Dawes, R. M. *Rational Choice in an Uncertain World*. New York: Harcourt Brace Jovanovich, 1988.

de Bono, E. *Lateral Thinking: Creativity Step by Step*. New York: Harper & Row, 1970.

———. *Six Thinking Hats*. New York: Penguin Books, 1985.

———. *CoRT Thinking: Teacher's Notes*. Des Moines, Iowa: Advanced Practical Thinking Training, Inc., 1986.

———. *I Am Right, You Are Wrong*. New York: Penguin Books, 1990.

———. *Handbook for the Positive Revolution*. New York: Penguin Books, 1991.

DePorter, B., and M. Hernacki. *Quantum Learning: Unleashing the Genius in You*. New York: Dell, 1992.

Dey, J. "Intelligence in Down's Syndrome." *Australian Journal of Mental Retardation* 1 (1971): 154.

Draze, D. *Creative Problem Solving for Kids*. San Luis Obispo, Calif.: Dandy Lion, 1994.

Dreyfus, H. L., and S. E. Dreyfus. *Mind over Machine: The Power of Human Intuition and Expertise in the War of the Computer*. New York: Free Press, 1986.

Dunn, W., ed. *Pediatric Occupational Therapy: Facilitating Effective Service Provision*. Thorafare, N.J.: Slack, 1991.

Dutton, R. *Clinical Reasoning in the Physical Disabilities*. Baltimore, Md.: Williams & Wilkins, 1995.

Eberle, B. *SCAMPER*. New York: D.O.K, 1971.

Ferguson, M. *The Aquarian Conspiracy*. Los Angeles: Jeremy P. Tarcher, 1980.

Firestein, R. L., and D. Treffinger. "Ownership and Converging: Essential Ingredients of Creative Problem Solving." *Journal of Creative Behavior* 17, no. 1 (1983): 32–38.

Fleming, M. H. "Clinical Reasoning in Medicine Compared with Clinical Reasoning in Occupational Therapy." *American Journal of Occupational Therapy* 45 (1991): 988–96.

———. "The Therapist with the Three-Track Mind." *American Journal of Occupational Therapy* 45 (1991): 1007–14.

Fobes, R. *The Creative Problem Solver's Toolbox*. Corvallis, Ore.: Solutions through Innovation, 1993.

Fogarty, R., and J. Bellanca. *Patterns for Thinking—Patterns for Transfer*. Palatine, Ill.: IRI/Skylight, 1993.

Fogarty, R., D. Perkins, and J. Barell. *How to Teach for Transfer*. Palatine, Ill.: Skylight, 1992.

Frankl, Victor. *Man's Search for Meaning*. 3d ed. New York: Simon & Schuster, 1984.

Fusco, E., and G. Fountain. "Reflective Teacher, Reflective Learner." In A. Costa, J. Bellanca, and R. Fogarty, eds., *If Minds Matter: A Foreword to the Future*, 1:239–55. Palatine, Ill.: Skylight, 1992.

Gardner, H. *Frames of Mind*. New York: HarperCollins, Basic Books, 1983.

Goldberg, N. *Writing Down the Bones: Feeling the Writer Within*. Boston: Shambhala, 1986.

Goldberg, P. *The Intuitive Edge*. New York: Jeremy P. Tarcher, 1983.

Goleman, D. *Emotional Intelligence*. New York: Bantam Books, 1995.

Goleman, D., P. Kaufman, and M. Ray. *The Creative Spirit*. New York: Penguin Books, 1992.

Grandin, T. *Thinking in Pictures and Other Reports from My Life with Autism*. New York: Random House, Vintage Books, 1995.

Grinder, M. *Righting the Educational Conveyor Belt*. Portland, Ore.: Metamorphous Press, 1991.

Gryskiewicz, S. S. "Predictable Creativity." In S. G. Isaksen, ed., *Frontiers in Creativity Research: Beyond the Basics*. Buffalo, N.Y.: Bearly, 1987.

Guilford, J. P. *Way Beyond the IQ*. Buffalo, N.Y.: The Creative Education Foundation, 1997.

Guilford J. P., and Sidney Parnes, eds. *Source Book for Creative Problem Solving*. Buffalo, N.Y.: Creative Education Foundation Press, 1992.

Helfgott, D., M. Helfgott, and B. Hoof. *Inspiration*. Portland, Ore.: Inspiration Software, 1993.

Helmstetter, S. *You Can Excel in Times of Change*. New York: Pocket Books, 1991.

Higgs, J. "Developing Clinical Reasoning Competencies." *Physiotherapy* 78, no. 8 (1992): 575–81.

Himes, G. K. "Stimulating Creativity: Encouraging Creative Ideas." In A. D. Timpe, ed., *Creativity*. New York: Kend Publishing, 1987.

Hoff, B. *The Tao of Pooh*. New York: Penguin Books, 1982.

Hopkins, H. L. "Problem Solving." In H. L. Hopkins and H. D. Smith, eds., *Willard and Spackman's Occupational Therapy*. 8th ed. Philadelphia, Pa.: Lippincott, 1993.

Hopkins, H. L., and H. D. Smith, eds. *Willard and Spackman's Occupational Therapy*. 8th ed. Philadelphia, Pa.: Lippincott, 1993.

Horgan, J. "Profile: Reluctant Revolutionary: Thomas S. Kuhn Unleashed Paradigm on the World." *Scientific American*, May 1991, 40.

Hyams, J. *Zen in the Martial Arts*. New York: Bantam Books, 1992.

Isaksen, S., K. B. Dorval, and D. Treffinger. *Creative Approaches to Problem Solving*. Dubuque, Iowa: Kendall/Hunt, 1994.

Isaksen, S., and D. Treffinger. *Creative Problem Solving: The Basic Course*. Buffalo, N.Y.: Bearly, 1985.

Jensen, E. *Superteaching: Master Strategies for Building Student Success*. Delmar, Calif.: Turning Point for Teachers, 1988.

Jeroski, S., F. Brownlie, and L. Kaser. *Reading and Responding: Evaluation Resources for Your Classroom*. Scarborough, Ontario: Nelson Canada, 1990.

Johnson, S. *"Yes" or "No": The Guide to Better Decisions*. New York: HarperCollins, 1992.

Kanter, R. M. "Change Master Skills: What It Takes to Be Creative." In R. Kuhn, ed., *Handbook for Creative and Innovative Managers*. New York: McGraw-Hill, 1988.

———. *The Change Masters*. New York: Simon & Schuster, 1983.

Kirton, M. J. "Adapters, Innovators, and Paradigm Consistency." *Psychological Reports* 57, no. 7 (1985): 487–90.

———. "Adapters and Innovators: Why New Initiatives Get Blocked." In J. Henry, ed., *Creative Management*, 209–21. London: Sage, 1991.

Kline, P. *The Everyday Genius: Restoring Children's Natural Joy of Learning—and Yours, Too*. Arlington, Va.: Great Ocean Publishers, 1988.

Kuhn, R., ed. *Handbook for Creative and Innovative Managers*. New York: McGraw-Hill, 1988.

Kuhn, T. *The Structure of Scientific Revolutions*. Chicago: University of Chicago Press, 1962.

Langer, E. *Mindfulness*. New York: Addison-Wesley, 1989.

Lister, M., ed. *A Contemporary Management of Motor Control Problems: Proceedings of the 11 Step Conference*. Alexandria, Va.: Foundation for Physical Therapy, 1991.

Loye, D. *The Sphinx and the Rainbow*. Boulder, Colo.: Shambhala, 1983.

Marcia, E. *Intuition Workbook*. Englewood Cliffs, N.J.: Prentice Hall, 1994.

Margulies, N. *Mapping Inner Space*. Tucson, Ariz.: Zephyr Press, 1991.

———. *Maps, Mindscapes, and More*. Tucson, Ariz.: Zephyr Press, 1993.

Markova, D. *The Art of the Possible: A Compassionate Approach to Understanding the Way People Think, Learn, and Communicate*. Berkeley, Calif.: Conari Press, 1991.

Mattingly, C. "The Narrative Nature of Clinical Reasoning." *American Journal of Occupational Therapy* 45 (1991): 998–1005.

———. "What Is Clinical Reasoning?" *American Occupational Therapy Association* 45 (1991): 979–86.

Mattingly, C., and M. H. Fleming. *Clinical Reasoning: Forms of Inquiry in a Therapeutic Practice*. Philadelphia, Pa.: F. A. Davis, 1993.

May, B., and J. Newman. "Developing Competence in Problem Solving." *Physical Therapy* 60, no. 9 (1980): 1140–45.

McCarthy, M. J. *Mastering the Information Age*. Los Angeles: Jeremy P. Tarcher, 1991.

McVey, V. *The Sierra Club Wayfinding Book*. San Francisco: Sierra Club Books, 1989.

Michalko, M. *Thinkertoys*. Berkeley, Calif.: Ten Speed Press, 1991.

Miller, W. C. *The Creative Edge*. Reading, Mass.: Addison-Wesley, 1986.

Moore, J. C. *Concepts from the Neurobehavioral Sciences*. Dubuque, Iowa: Kendall/Hunt, 1973.

Moore, L. P. *You're Smarter Than You Think*. New York: Holt, Rinehart and Winston, 1985.

Myers, I. B., and M. H. McCaulley. *Manual: A Guide to the Development and Use of the Myers-Briggs Type Indicator*. Palo Alto, Calif.: Consulting Psychologists Press, 1985.

Naisbitt, J., and P. Aburdene. *Megatrends 2000*. New York: William Morrow, 1990.

Neustadt, R., and E. May. *Thinking in Time: The Uses of History for Decision-Makers*. New York: Free Press, 1986.

Osborn, Alex. *Applied Imagination*. 3d ed. rev. New York: Charles Scribner's Sons, 1963.

Parham, D. "Nationally Speaking—Toward Professionalism: The Reflective Therapist." *American Journal of Occupational Therapy* 41 (1987): 555–61.

Parker, T. *Rules of Thumb*. Boston: Houghton Mifflin, 1983.

Parnes, S. *Visionizing*. Buffalo, N.Y.: Creative Education Foundation Press, 1992.

———, ed. *Source Book for Creative Problem Solving*. Buffalo, N.Y.: Creative Education Foundation Press, 1992.

Pearson, J. *Drawing on the Inventive Mind*. Los Angeles: Jon Pearson, 1992.

Perkins, D. *Schools of Thought: The Necessary Shape of Education*. New York: Basic Books, 1992.

Perkins, D., and G. Salomon. "The Science and Art of Transfer." In A. Costa, J. Bellanca, and R. Fogarty, eds., *If Minds Matter: A Foreword to the Future*, 1:201–9. Palatine, Ill.: Skylight, 1992.

Peters, T. *The Pursuit of WOW: Every Person's Guide to Topsy-Turvy Times*. New York: Vintage Books, 1994.

Pike, B. "Time to Take Our Own Advice and 'Break out of the Box.' " *Creative Training Techniques*, July 1995, 1–2.

Plattelli-Palmarini, M. *Inevitable Illusions: How Mistakes of Reason Rule Our Minds*. New York: John Wiley & Sons, 1994.

Prince, F. *C & the Box: A Paradigm Parable*. San Diego, Calif.: Pfeiffer, 1993.

Prince, G. "The Mindspring Theory: A New Development from Synectics Research, 177–93." In J. P. Guilford and S. Parnes, eds., *Source Book for Creative Problem Solving*. Buffalo, N.Y.: Creative Education Foundation Press, 1992.

Pritchett, L. *Stop Paddling and Start Rocking the Boat: Business Lessons from the School of Hard Knocks*. New York: Harper Business, a division of HarperCollins, 1995.

Rainer, T. *The New Diary*. New York: J. P. Tarcher, 1978.

Reed, K. "The Beginnings of Occupational Therapy." In Helen L. Hopkins and Helen D. Smith, eds., *Willard and Spackman's Occupational Therapy*. Philadelphia, Pa.: Lippincott, 1993.

Resnick, L. B. *Education and Learning to Think*. Washington, D.C.: National Academy Press, 1987.

Rico, G. *Writing the Natural Way*. Los Angeles: Jeremy P. Tarcher, 1983.

Rogers, E. M. *Diffusion of Innovations*. New York: Free Press, 1983.

Rogers, J. C. Eleanor Clarke Slagle Lectureship, 1983, "Clinical Reasoning: The Ethics, Science, and Art." *American Journal of Occupational Therapy* 37 (1983): 601–16.

Rogers, J. C., and M. B. Holm. "Occupational Therapy Diagnostic Reasoning: A Component of Clinical Reasoning." *American Journal of Occupational Therapy* 45 (1991): 1045–53.

Rosanoff, N. *Intuition Workout: A Practical Guide to Discovering and Developing Your Inner Knowing*. Santa Rosa, Calif.: Aslan Publishing, 1988.

Royeen, C. B. (1995). "A Problem-Based Learning Curriculum for Occupational Therapy Education." *American Journal of Occupational Therapy*, 49 (12), 338–46.

Ruben, B. "For Maine OT, Community-Based Care Is Key to Recovery." *OT Week*, March 8, 1990.

Rubenfeld, M. G., and B. K. Scheffer. *Critical Thinking in Nursing: An Interactive Approach*. Philadelphia, Pa.: Lippincott, 1995.

Russell, P. *The Brain Book*. New York: E. P. Dutton, 1979.

Samples, B. *Open Mind/Whole Mind*. Rolling Hills Estates, Calif.: Jalmar Press, 1987.

Schöen, D. A. (1983). *The Reflective Practitioner: How Professionals Think in Action*. New York: Basic Books, 1983.

Schwartz, R., and S. Parks. *Infusing the Teaching of Critical and Creative Thinking into Elementary Instruction*. Pacific Grove, Calif.: Critical Thinking Press & Software, 1994.

Senge, P. *The Fifth Discipline: The Art and Practice of the Learning Organization*. New York: Currency, Doubleday, 1990.

Senge, P. M., C. Roberts, R. B. Ross, B. J. Smith, and A. Kleiner. *The Fifth Discipline Fieldbook: Strategies and Tools for Building a Learning Organization*. New York: Currency, Doubleday, 1994.

Shallcross, D. J., and D. A. Sisk. *Intuition: An Inner Way of Knowing*. Buffalo, N.Y.: Bearly, 1989.

Simon, H. A. *The New Science of Management Decisions*. Rev. Ed. Englewood Cliffs, N.J.: Prentice Hall, 1977.

Slater, D. Y., and E. S. Cohn. "Staff Development Through Analysis of Practice." *American Journal of Occupational Therapy* 45 (1991): 1038–44.

Smith, F. *To Think*. New York: Teachers College Press, 1990.

Swartz, R., and S. Parks. *Infusing the Teaching of Critical and Creative Thinking into Elementary Instruction: A Lesson Design Handbook*. Pacific Grove, Calif.: Critical Thinking Press & Software, 1994.

Timpe, A. D., ed. *Creativity*. New York: Kend Publishing, 1987.

Torrance, E. P. *Creativity: Just Wanting to Know*. Pretoria, South Africa: Benedic Books, 1994.

Treffinger, Donald. *Assessing CPS Performance*. Sarosota, Fla.: Center for Creative Learning, 1992.

———. *The Real Problem Solving Handbook*. Sarasota, Fla.: Center for Creative Learning, 1994.

———. *Creative Problem Solving and School Improvement*. Idea Capsules. Sarasota, Fla.: Center for Creative Learning, 1996.

Treffinger, D., S. Isaksen, and K. B. Dorval. *Creative Problem Solving, Introduction*. Rev. ed. Sarasota, Fla.: Center for Creative Learning, 1994.

Treffinger, D., and P. McEwen. *Fostering Independent Creative Learning: Applying Creative Problem Solving to Independent Learning*. East Aurora, Ill.: D.O.K., 1989.

Tversky, A., and D. Kahnemann. "The Belief in the 'Law of Numbers.' " *Psychological Bulletin* 76 (1971): 105–10.

———. "Extensional Versus Intuitive Reasoning: The Conjunction Fallacy in Probability Judgment." *Psychological Review* 90 (1983): 293–315.

———. "Judgment under Uncertainty: Heuristics and Biases." *Science* 185 (1974): 1124–31.

———. "Rational Choice and the Framing of Decisions." *Journal of Business* 59 (1986): 251–94.

———. "The Framing of Decisions and the Psychology of Choice." *Science* 211 (1981): 453–64.

Uretsky, A. *Teacher's Helper Plus Crossword Companion*. Eugene, Ore.: Visions Technology in Education, 1995.

Uretsky, A., and M. Albert. *Teacher's Helper Plus*. Springfield, Ore.: Visions Technology in Education, 1996.

VanGundy, A. *Techniques of Structured Problem Solving*. 2d ed. New York: Van Nostrand, 1988.

———. *Idea Power: Techniques and Resources to Unleash the Creativity in Your Organization*. New York: American Management Association, 1992.

VanLeit, B. "Using the Case Method to Develop Clinical Reasoning Skills in Problem-Based Learning." *American Journal of Occupational Therapy* 49 (1995): 349–53.

Vitale, B. M. *Unicorns Are Real: A Right-Brained Approach to Learning*. Rolling Hills Estates, Calif.: Jalmar Press, 1982.

———. *Free Flight: Celebrating Your Right Brain*. Rolling Hills Estates, Calif.: Jalmar Press, 1986.

von Oech, R. *A Kick in the Seat of the Pants*. New York: Harper & Row, 1986.

———. *A Whack on the Side of the Head*. New York: Warner Books, 1990.

Williams, D. *Nobody Nowhere*. New York: Avon Books, 1992.

———. *Somebody Somewhere: Breaking Free from the World of Autism*. New York: Random House, 1994.

Wujec, T. *Five Star Mind: Games and Puzzles to Stimulate Your Creativity and Imagination*. New York: Doubleday, 1995.

Wycoff, J. *Mindmapping*. New York: The Berkley Publishing Group, 1991.

Yong, L. "Managing Creative People." *Journal of Creative Behavior* 28 no. 1 (1994): 16–20.

Zigler, Z. *Top Performance: How to Develop Excellence in Yourself and Others*. New York: Berkley Books, 1986.

Index

Page numbers followed by *f* indicate figures.

Motor component skills
  concept map, 107f
  definitions of, 115–16
Motor control skills, definition of, 116
Muscle tone skills, definition of, 115

Narrow-mindedness and resistance to change.
    See "Check the Mindset" Thinking Key
Neuromusculoskeletal component skills
  concept map, 106f
  definitions of, 115
New practice areas, developing skills in, 5
Nine Dot exercise, 26f, 26–27
"The Nose Blowing Expedition" (Betteridge),
    162–63
Novice level of practice, definition of, 5

Objective finding stage, 174
Occupation, definition of, 76
Occupational performance. See Performance
Occupational therapy (OT)
  as expedition, 36–38
  fitting to client's paradigms, 59–60
  flexibility of, 23–24
  integrating CPS into, 23–24
  language of, 79–151
  practice of, 5
  as reflective practice, 54
Olfactory skills, definition of, 114
Open-ended questions, 52–53
Openmindedness
  in people on an expedition. See "Check
      the Mindset" Thinking Key
  in therapy guide, 43
Opportunity Finding stage, 21
  Focusing Phase of, 179–87, 373–80
    summary of Thinking Keys for, 445
  Generating Phase of, 175–79, 371–73
    summary of Thinking Keys for, 445
  origin of name, 174–75
  and referral process, 174–75
  symbol for, 187
Opportunity statements, clustering of, 180–81
Oral hygiene tasks, definition of, 89
Oral-motor control skills, definition of, 116
Orientation skills, definition of, 116
Originality of ideas, Thinking Keys associated
    with, 234, 240–43, 403
Osborn, Alex
  and brainstorming, 20
  and creation of CPS model, 20
  on generating ideas, 28–29, 232, 234
  on note-taking, 259
Osborn-Parnes CPS model, 20
OT. See Occupational therapy
"The Other Side of the Mirror" (Gidewell),
    44–47
Outcome(s), predictability of, in problem
    solving, 159–60
Out-of-the-box thinking, 8–13, 27

Ownership of a problem. See Problem
    ownership

"PACC" Thinking Key, 154, 164–70, 362–66
  uses of, 359, 444
Pain response skills, definition of, 114
Paired Comparison Analysis. See "PCA"
    Thinking Key
Paradigm(s). See also "What Paradigm Is
    Operating?" Thinking Key
  characteristics of, 62
  context as factor in, 67–69
  definition of, 59–62
  paralysis of, 62
  shifts in, 60–61
    generating for clients, 296–97
    to reframe a problem, 63–69, 211
Parent(s)
  amount of contact with children, 13
  with children with disabilities, challenges
      faced by, 45–47
Parnes, Sidney, 20, 176
Patterns, watching for. See "Watch for Cues
    and Look for Patterns" Thinking Key
"PCA" (Paired Comparison Analysis) Think-
    ing Key, 272–73, 423–24
  uses of, 419, 448
People, importance of continuity of, 300
Perceptual frame(s), as mindtraps, 274–86
Perceptual processing skills
  concept map, 105f
  definition of, 114
Performance
  and client assessment, 76
  context and, 76–78
Performance areas, 76, 79, 81f–88f
  categories of, 81f
  definitions of specific, 89–91
  field evaluation of. See "PACC" Thinking
      Key
  subcategories of, 82f
"Performance Areas, Components, and Con-
    texts" Thinking Key. See "PACC" Think-
    ing Key
Performance components, 103–109
  categories of, 81f
    subcategories, 103f
  definition of, 79
  field evaluation of. See "PACC" Thinking
      Key
Performance contexts, 143f–144f
  categories of, 81f
    subcategories of, 143f
  concept map, 144
  definition of, 79
  field evaluation of. See "PACC" Thinking
      Key
Personal device care tasks, definition of, 89
Personal inner knowledge, vs. technical
    knowledge, 4
Perspectives, shifting of, 233
Physical aspects of environment, definition
    of, 146

"Plan for Action" Thinking Key, 307–10,
    431–34
  uses of, 448
Plan of action. See Action plan
Play and leisure activities
  assessment of, 76
  concept map, 83f
  definitions of, 91
  field evaluation of. See "PACC" Thinking
      Key
  subcategories of, 82f
Point of view, altering. See Paradigm(s),
    shifts in
Position in space skills, definition of, 114
Postural alignment skills, definition of, 115
Postural control skills, definition of, 115
"Potential Sources of Support and Resis-
    tance" Thinking Key, 294–96, 425–26
  uses of, 448
Praxis skills, definition of, 116
"Preparing to Seek Feedback" Thinking Key,
    316–17, 440
  uses of, 449
Presumed Associations mindtrap, 278–79, 284
Problem(s)
  vs. challenge, in problem solving, 6, 43
  defining from client's point of view, 159
  developing understanding of, 174–75
  expanding statement of, with "Ladder of
      Abstraction" Thinking Key, 217–22,
      395–97
  reframing of, by shifting paradigms, 63–69
  rephrasing of, to gain new insight, 211,
      214–16
  well-structured vs. ill-structured. See Well-
      structured vs. ill-structured
      problem(s)
Problem Finding stage, 21, 210–11
  Focusing Phase of, 222–27, 397–402
    summary of Thinking Keys for, 446
  Generating Phase of, 211–22, 392–93
    summary of Thinking Keys for, 446
  symbol for, 227
Problem ownership, establishing, 155–58
"Problem Ownership Checklist" Thinking
    Key, 154–55, 157–58, 367
  uses of, 444
Problem solving. See also Creative problem
    solving model (CPS)
  definition of, 117
  and imagination, 8–9
  and mindset, 9, 12
  and uniqueness of every client, 154–55
Procedural reasoning, definition of, 4
Proficient level of practice, definition of, 5
Proprioceptive skills, definition of, 114
Psychological boundaries. See Paradigm(s)
Psychological skills
  concept map, 109f
  definition of, 117
  field evaluation of. See "PACC" Thinking
      Key
"Putting Cosmetic Prostheses to Work"
    (Tapper), 449–50
Putting things to other uses, and flexibility,
    236, 239